AF775217

PHYSICAL THERAPY EFFECTIVENESS

Edited by **Mario Bernardo-Filho, Danúbia da Cunha de Sá-Caputo** and **Redha Taiar**

Physical Therapy Effectiveness
http://dx.doi.org/10.5772/intechopen.76735
Edited by Mario Bernardo-Filho, Danúbia da Cunha de Sá-Caputo and Redha Taiar

Contributors

Tsung-Hsien Wang, Mario Bernardo-Filho, Danúbia Sá-Caputo, Redha Taiar, Dani Zoorob, Sara Anderson, Joseph Balogun, Yoshibumi Bunno, Luciana Auxiliadora De Paula Vasconcelos, Sandro Dos Santos Ferreira, Simona Maria Carmignano, Henry Puff, Vincent Grote, Elke Böttcher, Alexandra Unger, Hilde D. G. Nielsen, Jirakrit Leelarungrayub, Yothin Pothasak, Jynwara Kaju, Rungtiwa Kanthain, Andre Nyberg, Erik Frykholm, Andrea Foglia, Paolo Bizzarri, Terry Ellapen, Yvonne Paul, Marco Barnard, Mariette Swanepoel

© The Editor(s) and the Author(s) 2020
The rights of the editor(s) and the author(s) have been asserted in accordance with the Copyright, Designs and Patents Act 1988. All rights to the book as a whole are reserved by INTECHOPEN LIMITED. The book as a whole (compilation) cannot be reproduced, distributed or used for commercial or non-commercial purposes without INTECHOPEN LIMITED's written permission. Enquiries concerning the use of the book should be directed to INTECHOPEN LIMITED rights and permissions department (permissions@intechopen.com).
Violations are liable to prosecution under the governing Copyright Law.

(cc) BY

Individual chapters of this publication are distributed under the terms of the Creative Commons Attribution 3.0 Unported License which permits commercial use, distribution and reproduction of the individual chapters, provided the original author(s) and source publication are appropriately acknowledged. If so indicated, certain images may not be included under the Creative Commons license. In such cases users will need to obtain permission from the license holder to reproduce the material. More details and guidelines concerning content reuse and adaptation can be found at http://www.intechopen.com/copyright-policy.html.

Notice

Statements and opinions expressed in the chapters are these of the individual contributors and not necessarily those of the editors or publisher. No responsibility is accepted for the accuracy of information contained in the published chapters. The publisher assumes no responsibility for any damage or injury to persons or property arising out of the use of any materials, instructions, methods or ideas contained in the book.

First published in London, United Kingdom, 2020 by IntechOpen
IntechOpen is the global imprint of INTECHOPEN LIMITED, registered in England and Wales, registration number: 11086078, 7th floor, 10 Lower Thames Street, London,
EC3R 6AF, United Kingdom
Printed in Croatia

British Library Cataloguing-in-Publication Data
A catalogue record for this book is available from the British Library

Additional hard and PDF copies can be obtained from orders@intechopen.com

Physical Therapy Effectiveness, Edited by Mario Bernardo-Filho, Danúbia da Cunha de Sá-Caputo and Redha Taiar
p. cm.
Print ISBN 978-1-83880-075-8
Online ISBN 978-1-83880-076-5
eBook (PDF) ISBN 978-1-78985-145-8

We are IntechOpen, the world's leading publisher of Open Access books

Built by scientists, for scientists

4,700+
Open access books available

121,000+
International authors and editors

135M+
Downloads

151
Countries delivered to

Our authors are among the
Top 1%
most cited scientists

12.2%
Contributors from top 500 universities

BOOK CITATION INDEX
CLARIVATE ANALYTICS
INDEXED

WEB OF SCIENCE™

Selection of our books indexed in the Book Citation Index in Web of Science™ Core Collection (BKCI)

Interested in publishing with us?
Contact book.department@intechopen.com

Numbers displayed above are based on latest data collected.
For more information visit www.intechopen.com

For EU product safety concerns:
IN TECH d.o.o., Prolaz Marije Krucifikse Kozulić 3, 51000 Rijeka, Croatia,
info@intechopen.com or visit our website at intechopen.com.

Meet the editors

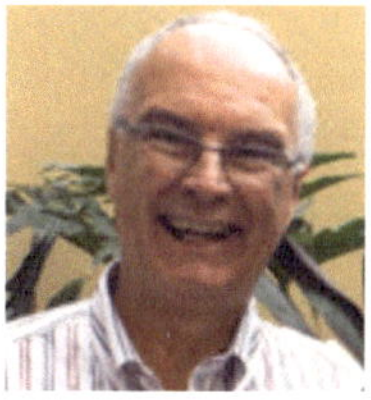

Mario Bernardo-Filho is the Head of the *Laboratório de Vibrações Mecânicas e Práticas Integrativas-LAVIMPI, Instituto de Biologia Roberto Alcantara Gomes, Departamento de Biofísica e Biometria, Policlínica Piquet Carneiro, UERJ.* He has completed the academic courses of biomedicine and physiotherapy, and obtained his PhD (1988). In 1999, he became a Full Professor (UERJ). He has started and supervised research (2010) involving integrative and complementary medicine (auriculotherapy and acupuncture) and mechanical vibrations generated from a vibrating platform that produces whole body vibration exercises (WBVE) when a subject is in contact with a platform. Studies to evaluate the consequences of WBVE and extracts of medicinal plants in rats are ongoing. Investigations on the effects of the WBVE in individuals with different diseases and healthy people are ongoing too. He is the supervisor of Master of Sciences and PhD theses and has participated and lectured in various national and international congresses. He is Editor-in-Chief of the Brazilian Journal of Health and Biomedical Sciences, and guest editor of some scientific journals. He is the reviewer of several scientific journal indexed in the PubMed and Scopus.

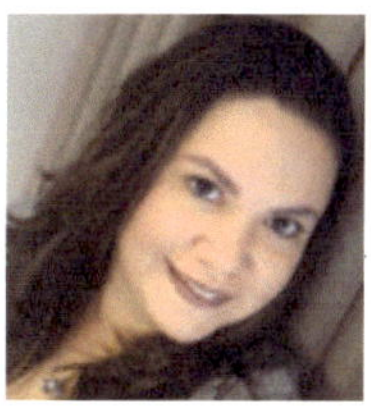

She has been a postdoctoral fellow of the Laboratory of Mechanical Vibration and Integrative Practices, Universidade do Estado do Rio de Janeiro, Brazil since 2016. She has been a professor and researcher in the Faculdade Bezerra de Araújo since 2017. She completed her academic course of Physiotherapy in 2004. She obtained her Master's degree in 2015 and her PhD degree in 2016 with studies involving whole-body vibration exercises in chronic diseases. She performed her first postdoctorate in Université de Reims in 2018 and a second in Universidade do Estado do Rio de Janeiro in 2019. Nowadays, she researches the biological, biophysical, and biomechanical effects in individuals with different clinical conditions and healthy individuals that are exposed to mechanical vibration from a vibrating platform.

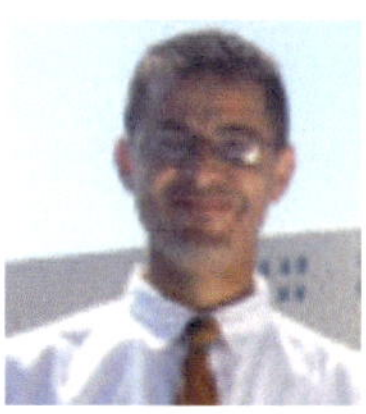

He is a biomechanic and a Professor at the University of Reims Champaign France. He is Head of the RTBE (Redha Taiar Biomechanical Engineering) Society developed for sport and medical advice for the industry. His research focuses on the industry engineering for medicine and high-level sport. He is an engineer for different industries such as high-level sport and Sidas, Medicapteur for the medical development. In the industry, his last work was for the Notrax Society on conception and validation of anti-fatigue mats. For sport, his last work focused on the development of a swimsuit for triathlons and swimming for the Brazil Olympic Games (2016) and suit fabrics for skiing in the Olympic Games at Sotchi in 2014. He is responsible for different patents such as the development of a new kind of knee rehabilitation tool for high-level athletes and pathological subjects, and the conception of a new shoe for high-level athletes and pathological subjects.

Contents

Preface

Physical therapy involves non-pharmacological interventions in various clinical conditions. Therefore, it is important to highlight the procedures that are suitable, effective and, in general, do not have side effects or complications when properly performed. Physical therapy can be valuable in different situations along various steps of an individual's life and in various clinical disorders. Indeed, the editors wanted to select chapters that could be useful for readers and could contribute to improving their professional performance. In this book, there are six sections and the topics and chapters are highly engaging.

The sections are (i) *physical therapy interventions for the pelvic floor* will bring new findings about the interventions in women's health and in the management of reproductive disorders; (ii) *musculoskeletal rehabilitation with physical therapy approaches* will explore the relevance of the whole-body vibration exercise as an intervention to improve musculoskeletal performance and the medical quality outcomes and achievements of a multi-disciplinary inpatient musculoskeletal system rehabilitation; (iii) *neurophysiological aspects and physical therapy interventions* will discuss neuroscience and the effectiveness of motor imagery on physical therapy and its neurophysiological aspects and interventions in Parkinson´s disease rehabilitation indicating the effectiveness of the approaches and new perspectives; (iv) *physical therapy interventions related to pulmonary conditions* with the application of a single case study or case research design to present the rehabilitation effectiveness in a clinic, in the targeting of limb muscle dysfunction in chronic obstructive pulmonary disease and the early mobilization in patients with mechanical ventilation; (v) *physical therapy interventions associated with chronic clinical conditions* will demonstrate the relevance of actions in clinical chronic conditions of physical activity in non-communicable diseases and of the extracorporeal shock wave therapy in chronic wound care, and finally; (vi) *conceptual approaches of physical therapy interventions* discusses the effect and exercise, the conceptual framework for the inclusion of recreational therapy within South African healthcare paradigms and the question of "Is manual therapy art or science?".

The readers will have the opportunity to read about the latest findings related to various approaches of interventions in several fields related to health sciences. It is expected that this book might contribute to health promotion, wellbeing, and human development.

At the end, the editors would like to thank the publisher IntechOpen and all the authors of the chapters for their contributions.

Mario Bernardo-Filho
Laboratory of Mechanical Vibration and Integrative Practices
Rio de Janeiro State University, Brazil

Danúbia da Cunha de Sá-Caputo
Laboratory of Mechanical Vibration and Integrative Practices
Rio de Janeiro State University, Brazil
Faculty Bezerra de Araújo, Physiotherapy Course, Brazil

Redha Taiar
University of Reims Champagne-Ardenne, France

Section 1

Physical Therapy Interventions in Pelvic Floor

Chapter 1

Pelvic Floor Physical Therapy and Women's Health

Dani Zoorob and Sara Anderson

Additional information is available at the end of the chapter

http://dx.doi.org/10.5772/intechopen.88740

Abstract

Personalized approaches for the management and maintenance of women's pelvic health are increasingly in demand. As pelvic floor dysfunction is multifactorial and origins vary, it is essential as a clinician, to be familiar with available interventions to address each of these dysfunctions and their causes. This chapter will discuss the role of physical therapy in the management of female patients presenting with pelvic floor dysfunction related to bowel, bladder and sexual health with focus on variations associated with age. Each section addresses a specific type of pelvic floor dysfunction, discusses the methodology for management, as well as the efficacy of the physical therapy intervention related to treatment of each diagnosis.

Keywords: pelvic floor physical therapy, sexual dysfunction, urinary incontinence, pelvic organ prolapse, constipation

1. Introduction

Addressing the muscular strength, coordination and mobility required for healthy pelvic floor function, in addition to providing education regarding healthy bowel and bladder habits and establishing diet and lifestyle modifications, physical therapists are poised to provide care that directly impacts women's overall well-being and quality of life. Physical therapists who treat pelvic floor dysfunction have completed post-graduate training in the specific anatomy, physiology, functions and treatment of impairments of the pelvis. Pelvic floor physical therapists complete internal vaginal as well as external vulvar, abdominal, hip and spine screenings to establish differential diagnosis [1]. Interventions employed by physical therapists are varied and dependent upon diagnosis as well as patient and clinician preference but can include internal and external manual therapy, therapeutic exercise and neuromuscular reeducation, and utilization of modalities such as biofeedback, rectal balloon manometry,

IntechOpen

© 2019 The Author(s). Licensee IntechOpen. This chapter is distributed under the terms of the Creative Commons Attribution License (http://creativecommons.org/licenses/by/3.0), which permits unrestricted use, distribution, and reproduction in any medium, provided the original work is properly cited.

electrical stimulation and transcutaneous electrical nerve stimulation (TENS) [2]. Pelvic floor physical therapists establish plans of care based on physician's referral orders, patient goals and baseline functional measurements. These plans of care utilize home exercise programs to supplement in-clinic treatment and maximize efficacy of physical therapy intervention [1].

Pelvic floor physical therapy is an important tool in the conservative management of sexual dysfunction, urinary incontinence, pelvic organ prolapse and constipation [2]. Understanding of the role and efficacy of physical therapy intervention in the treatment of these impairments is important in providing patients with thorough and optimal care.

2. Management of types of sexual dysfunction through pelvic floor physical therapy

Sexual function from a physical perspective involves the integrity and synchronization of neurologic, hormonal, vascular and muscular systems [3]. The adaptations these systems undertake throughout a woman's lifespan to accommodate gestation, delivery, post-partum healing and menopause can result in physiologic disruption resulting in sexual dysfunction. Common presentations of sexual dysfunction in women include chronic pelvic pain syndromes, musculoskeletal conditions and sexual pain disorders [4].

Chronic pelvic pain is multifactorial and greatly affects sexual function. Pelvic pain may develop following somatic dysfunction, after pelvic or psychological trauma, childbirth or surgical intervention, and it may be idiopathic or pathologic [5–7]. Of the multitude of factors contributing to chronic pelvic pain, perhaps the most responsive to physical therapy intervention is the condition of overactivity of pelvic floor musculature—also known as high tone pelvic floor dysfunction. Prolonged overactivity of pelvic floor muscles (PFM) can lead to hypertonicity and functional tissue shortening [6]. In addition to decreased length of contractile tissue, mobility restrictions can affect neural and fascial function, resulting directly in pelvic pain or worsening of the condition. Physical therapy intervention aimed at improving tissue length, mobility, and decreasing trigger points has been shown to positively impact sexual function. In a 2012 study by Fitzgerald, 60% of women who underwent treatment for interstitial cystitis/painful bladder syndrome with myofascial physical therapy (PT) reported moderate to marked improvement in symptoms, compared to 26% in the control group treated with non-pelvic/global massage only [8]. Interventions for the treatment group consisted of internal and external techniques aimed at connective tissue manipulation for tissue lengthening and proprioceptive awareness.

Musculoskeletal conditions can impact the actual structure and anatomy of the pelvic floor and create mechanical impairments leading to sexual dysfunction [4]. Coccygeal fractures from falls, perineal tears and episiotomy scars and pelvic surgeries change the mobility and angle of pull of pelvic floor musculature. Kinematic changes to pelvic floor soft tissue increase likelihood of dysfunction including hypertonicity, weakness, and loss of coordination. For example, increased tone of the obturator internus or piriformis may result in impingement of the pudendal nerve causing pain with sitting, numbness, and tingling along the ipsilateral thigh as well as pain with intercourse [7]. In many cases, manual internal soft tissue mobilization of these muscles—along with neural mobilization and core stability training—has been shown to help relieve even severe pudendal nerve pain. Musculoskeletal conditions can also present in conjunction with other diagnoses. A study by Mieritz et al. showed lumbosacral mobility impairments and positive pain provocation tests for sacroiliac joint dysfunction in 51% of study participants with chronic pelvic pain and suspected endometriosis [9]. Musculoskeletal restriction in thoracolumbar spine can impair ilioinguinal, iliohypogastric and genitofemoral nerve function, while sacral disruption can affect pudendal and posterior femoral cutaneous nerves, adding to pelvic floor dysfunction [7]. An important population to consider with musculoskeletal conditions affecting sexual function is that of postpartum women. These patients develop loss of pelvic floor muscle strength and function following vaginal delivery, and this state negatively impacts the stimulation and arousal required for orgasm [10].

Sexual pain disorders are classified as dyspareunia and vaginismus by the DSM-5. Dyspareunia includes provoked, localized vulvodynia and vestibulodynia, with suggested etiologies ranging from hormonal and neurologic changes to inflammatory response and high tone pelvic floor disorder [11]. Each of these proposed etiologies can be impacted by physical therapy interventions as part of a multidisciplinary approach. Use of manual techniques to improve fascial, visceral, neural and muscular mobility has been shown to improve sexual outcome scores in women with levator-related pelvic pain. In a 2014 study by Zoorob et al., two groups of women reporting dyspareunia were treated with either pelvic floor PT or levator-directed trigger-point injections. Results from this study demonstrated improvement in both groups, however the group receiving PT demonstrated a greater overall improvement in sexual function based on sexual function scores [12]. In addition to decreasing pain with intercourse, some studies have shown that pelvic floor physical therapy intervention can actually help increase sexual pleasure [13, 14]. Improvements in sexual pleasure may include better orgasmic and arousal potential, desire, excitement and lubrication [13]. While PT intervention alone has been shown to be effective in a patient's functional recovery, it is important to consider a multimodal approach to sexual dysfunction to address physical, psychological and social barriers to optimize function on all levels.

3. The role of physical therapy in treatment of urinary incontinence

Urinary incontinence is a significant concern for women globally, with proposed incidence of 41% in women over the age of 40 [15]. Incidence of urinary incontinence has been observed to increase with age, parity, and obesity [7, 16] Hormonal changes with age, including decreasing estrogen and testosterone levels have an effect on urethral patency and pelvic floor muscle strength. Aging is also associated with a decrease in overall activity level, which contributes to disuse atrophy of the supportive pelvic floor musculature. It also results in a higher incidence of weight gain due to hormonal changes, increasing abdominal girth and intra-abdominal pressure (IAP). As parity increases, so do the effects of labor, including tissue laxity and neuropathy.

Physical therapy intervention is appropriate for management of all these physiologic changes and has been shown to be effective as first-line treatment for urinary incontinence. In a Cochrane review by Dumoulin et al. in 2014, pelvic floor physical therapy (PFPT) was shown to be more effective than no treatment or placebo drug in women with stress urinary incontinence (SUI) or a combination of urinary incontinence types. Subjects treated with PFPT alone reported better quality of life, fewer episodes of urinary incontinence and improved sexual functioning [17]. Improving pelvic floor muscle coordination and strength allows for improved bladder and urethral support, decreasing visceral translation during periods of increased IAP such as coughing, sneezing and laughing, and also increases urethral pressure, preventing urine leakage [18]. A 2013 study by McLain et al. demonstrated reduced bladder neck mobility during coughing and increased cross-sectional area of the urethra musculature in patients who underwent 12 sessions of weekly pelvic floor physical therapy [19]. The observed hypertrophy of the urethra sphincter is important in demonstrating the role of pelvic floor physical therapy in treatment of urinary incontinence in women who do not have intact pelvic floor muscles or who have strong pelvic floor muscles but have impaired urethral sphincters. In addition to hypertrophy of the urethral sphincter, increased strength of levator ani in the pelvis and increased clamping of the compressor urethrae while increasing urethral pressure markedly help in preventing incontinence [20]. Pelvic Floor physical therapy interventions are not isolated to training of intrapelvic musculature and benefit may be extended when paired with strength training of accessory muscles, such as the gluteal muscles, hip adductors and anterior abdominal wall musculature. Strengthening of the transverse abdominis (TrA)—in addition to intrapelvic musculature–has been shown to decrease effects of SUI and improve quality of life (QOL) in multiparous women [21]. Although pelvic floor physical therapy is available as an option for treating urge urinary incontinence, this is rarely considered in isolation to address and counteract the detrusor contractions [17, 22]. Physical therapy intervention for urinary incontinence also includes behavioral training related to urge suppression and voiding mechanics, dietary changes to avoid bladder irritants and neuromuscular retraining to address tonal abnormalities affecting muscle function [7].

Weight management, as demonstrated by the PRIDE study, is an important factor in the restoration of urinary continence. The study showed a 50% reduction in frequency and severity of SUI when subjects lost 10% of their bodyweight [16]. Despite the benefits of weight loss, many patients are hesitant to begin a weight loss program due to fear of injury or re-injury, lack of information or guidance on initiating a diet or exercise regimen, or even lack of resources, such as access to a gym. Physical therapists are uniquely positioned to establish safe and effective exercise programs and give nutritional guidance to patients attempting to reach a healthier weight to improve their incontinence. Many women also report decreasing or ceasing participation in regular exercise due to urinary incontinence experienced with physical activity. Participation in pelvic floor physical therapy to improve pelvic floor muscle strength and coordination prior to and during initiation of an exercise program will allow a woman to enjoy bladder control while engaging in physical activity. Evaluation of dysfunctional movement patterns and treatment of chronic pains and recurrent injuries are well within a physical therapist's scope of practice and will allow patients to feel confident increasing their activity level.

Gestation and delivery are both major factors in development of urinary incontinence [23]. Loss of anterior abdominal wall muscular strength with the progressing gestation results in limiting of the body's ability to recruit accessory musculature for force-coupling of the pelvic floor muscle contraction. This decrease in core muscle activation, combined with increased intraabdominal pressure from the growing uterus and fetus, increases a woman's likelihood of developing urinary incontinence during pregnancy. A 2003 study investigated the role of a pelvic floor exercise regimen on the incidence of urinary incontinence in pregnant women [23]. Study participants in the treatment group reported significantly less urinary incontinence than the control group at 36 weeks gestation, as well as 3 months postpartum. In addition to the strain placed on the pelvic floor during gestation, vaginal delivery also presents the opportunity for neuromuscular injury. Prolonged labor, with sustained stretch of the levator ani muscles and the pudendal nerve, increases the likelihood of a woman developing neuropathy, affecting muscle strength and function and contributing to urinary incontinence [23].

Adherence to PFPT is multifactorial and includes attendance at each visit, performance of home exercise program between visits and the long-term adherence to home exercise plan [24]. Despite the efficacy of physical therapy treatment for urinary incontinence, as well as the low-risk nature of the intervention, adherence to PFPT has been reported as lower than 50% [25, 26]. A physician's understanding and support of PFPT and its role in conservative care may improve a patient's motivation to participate in PFPT and thus attaining improve outcomes.

4. The role of physical therapy in treatment of pelvic organ prolapse

Pelvic organ prolapse (POP) is a common issue in women following childbirth, with an estimated 94% presenting with evidence of POP noted during routine annual gynecologic examination (Swift 2000). POP is linked to urinary incontinence and sexual dysfunction and is the cause of approximately 200,000 inpatient surgical repairs in the United States annually [27]. Etiology of POP is multifactorial but generally speaking, involves descent of pelvic organs due to increased abdominal pressure, tissue stretch, and loss of functional support from pelvic floor soft tissue. Risk factors include both increased age and parity, obesity, history of excessive Valsalva maneuvers such as with heavy lifting and repetitive straining associated with chronic constipation. Patients with POP may present with bowel, bladder or sexual dysfunction and multiple studies have determined the efficacy of physical therapy intervention for each of these functions per se. A randomized control trial (RCT) by Breakken in 2010 sought to investigate the role of physical therapy intervention in treatment of POP. The study demonstrated statistically significant difference in bladder and rectal elevation with participation in pelvic floor strengthening exercises in the intervention group compared to the control group [28]. Within the study, conservative management of POP with pelvic floor physical therapy was shown to reduce symptoms of vaginal bulging or heaviness, and improve SUI, urge urinary incontinence and bowel symptoms of flatus and loose stool incontinence. Sexual dysfunction related to POP is typically attributed to vaginal obstruction and laxity, and contributes to sexual avoidance, poor body image, as well as reduced sexual desire and arousal [29, 30]. In another study by Breakken et al., women with stage I, II and III POP who underwent a pelvic floor physical therapy program, in addition to education on lifestyle modification, demonstrated a statistically significant medium association between improvement in sexual function and increase in pelvic floor muscle strength [31]. The author reported "Improvement in sexual function included increased awareness, strength and control of pelvic floor muscles, sensation of a 'tighter vagina', improved self-confidence, libido and orgasms, resolution of pain experienced with intercourse and partner reports of sexual gratification." Physical therapy intervention for POP is aimed at functional restoration of pelvic floor muscles, with treatment addressing strength, endurance and coordination of soft tissue, in order to improve support of the pelvic organs. The POPPY trial in 2014, demonstrated further efficacy of PT intervention [32]. In their multicenter RCT, patients with symptomatic POP were randomized into PFPT intervention and control group, with both receiving lifestyle advice. The women who received pelvic floor physical therapy reported fewer POP symptoms at 12 months than the control group, and 80% of participants in the intervention group continued to perform pelvic floor muscle exercises at 12 months after trial entry. This continued adherence to exercise is important in long-term maintenance and management of symptoms and demonstrates further efficacy of PT intervention.

Surgical management of pelvic organ prolapse is typically necessary in symptomatic cases of grade III-IV and in women with significant negative impact on quality of life. Although most women are pleased with their surgical outcomes following repair, 25% require additional post-operative therapy [33]. Post-operative SUI due to poor pelvic floor muscle recruitment may be due to lack of training and coordination, as the patient most likely has not needed to perform a pelvic floor contraction since her prolapse became obstructive [34]. Post-operatively, lower urinary tract symptoms (LUTS) may also include increased daytime urgency and nocturia, in addition to other voiding or storage symptoms. LUTS caused by levator dysfunction, assessed by internal vaginal assessment, or behavioral factors such as dietary irritants or improper fluid intake volumes, assessed by patient interview and patient's completion of food and fluid diaries, may be addressed by a physical therapist pre-operatively, improving outcomes and patient satisfaction scores following POP repair.

5. The role of physical therapy in treatment of constipation

Constipation is a common impairment in children and adults and affects mental, physical and social functioning [35, 36]. An estimated 10–20% of adults worldwide report symptoms of constipation, which can include having a bowel movement fewer than three times per week, presence of hard, dry, small and difficult to pass stool, and pain with bowel movements [37]. Symptoms of constipation also include straining, bloating and the sensation of a full bowel. As constipation is multifactorial and commonly seen in conjunction with other pelvic disorders, it is important to understand the role of physical therapy interventions and utilize them to supplement care of constipation-related symptoms.

Constipation is generally considered a symptom. Amongst other causes, it can develop through poor dietary habits, slow-transit colon, pelvic floor muscle dysfunction, impaired anorectal angle and/or paradoxical pelvic floor contraction. Pelvic floor physical therapists may improve symptoms of constipation through behavioral modification, such as diet and fluid intake modifications and education on proper toileting habits and positions. Changing the angle of the patient's hips, for example, changes the anorectal angle during defecation, allowing for ease of bowel movement through relaxation of puborectalis. In a 2002 study by Rad et al., the difference in bowel emptying while patients were seated on a European toilet compared to an Iranian-style toilet was investigated [38]. This position change puts the patient in a squatting position in the latter category or toilets. The study suggested complete bowel emptying on the Iranian-style toilet and incomplete bowel emptying while seated on the European-style toilet. Use of assistive devices such as the Squatty Potty ™ and physical therapy to improve hip mobility and pelvic floor muscle function may allow for improved defecatory mechanics. Physical therapists may also offer patients nonpharmaceutical interventions to improve bowel motility, including abdominal massage and dietary modifications. Abdominal massage may stimulate peristalsis, decrease colon transit time, increase frequency of bowel movements and decrease pain and discomfort [39]. Abdominal massage may be performed in clinic and taught to the patient or caregiver for symptom management at home. Physical therapists may also encourage dietary changes as part of patient care. Important behaviors for improved bowel motility include increased water consumption and ensuring adequate fiber intake.

Biofeedback is another important tool in the conservative management of constipation. Biofeedback may be used in-clinic and patients may either purchase or rent a biofeedback unit for at-home use. Biofeedback is helpful in improving pelvic floor muscle strength in patients with low tone but is also used effectively in treatment of anismus or pelvic floor dyssynergia. A 2015 study showed a 48% improvement in patient symptom scores using the patient assessment of constipation-symptoms (PAC-SYM) questionnaire following 6–8 sessions of biofeedback therapy with manual and verbal biofeedback, surface electromyography (EMG), rectal balloon sensory therapy, pelvic floor and abdominal massage and core strengthening to correct dyssynergia [40].

Use of rectal ballooning in improving rectal sensation is a treatment some specially-training pelvic floor physical therapists may offer. Chronic constipation and rectal filling may lead to poor sensation in rectum and poor awareness of bowel movement. Pourmomeny assessed the efficacy of biofeedback and rectal balloon training showing decreased constipation in both groups; however, biofeedback training (79% improvement) was superior to balloon training (52% improvement) and should be implemented prior to balloon training) [41].

An important consideration in the discussion of constipation management is that of opioid-induced constipation [42]. As the health care community becomes more aware of the negative side effects of long-term opioid dependence, it is imperative to seek out other less harmful analgesics. Physical therapy plays a role in pain management and functional restoration pre- or post-surgically, and can even be helpful in the prevention of injury with movement screenings for athletes or with clients prior to initiating an exercise program.

6. Conclusion

In conclusion, pelvic floor dysfunction is a multifactorial condition with significant overlap in causative factors and symptom presentation between sexual dysfunction, urinary incontinence, pelvic organ prolapse and constipation. Utilization of physical therapy intervention improves pelvic floor function and, allowing women to employ their bodies' own supportive structures to decrease impairments and maximize their quality of life.

Author details

Dani Zoorob[1]* and Sara Anderson[2]

*Address all correspondence to: dzobgyn@gmail.com

1 University of Toledo, Toledo, OH, USA

2 ProMedica, Toledo, OH, USA

References

[1] What to Expect at Your 1st Visit for Urinary Incontinence [Internet]. Section on Women's Health. American Physical Therapy Association. 2019. Available from: https://www.womenshealthapta.org/wpcontent/uploads/2013/11/What_to_expect_on_your_first_visit-UI.pdf [Accessed: 18 July 2019]

[2] What is Pelvic Floor Physical Therapy? [Internet]. Sexual Health Q&A. International Society for Sexual Medicine. 2019. Available from: https://www.issm.info/sexual-health-qa/what-is-pelvic-floor-physical-therapy/ [Accessed: 18 July 2019]

[3] Bortolami A, Vanti C, Banchelli F, Guccione A, Pillastrini P. Relationship between female pelvic floor dysfunction: An observational study. Journal of Sexual Medicine. 2015;**12**:1233-1241

[4] Rosenbaum TY. The role of physical therapy in female sexual dysfunction. Current Sexual Health Reports. 2008;**5**(2):97-101

[5] Bonder JH, Chi M, Rispoli L. Myofascial pelvic pain and related disorders. Physical Medicine and Rehabilitation Clinics of North America. 2017;**28**(3):501-515

[6] Bradley MH, Rawlins A, Brinker CA. Physical therapy treatment of pelvic pain. Physical Medicine and Rehabilitation Clinics of North America. 2017;**28**(3):589-601

[7] Stein A, Sauder SK, Reale J. The role of physical therapy in sexual health in men and women: Evaluation and treatment. Sexual Medicine Reviews. 2019;**7**(1):46-56

[8] Fitzgerald MP, Anderson RU, Potts J, Payne CK, Peters KM, Clemens JQ, et al. Randomized multicenter feasibility trial of myofascial physical therapy for the treatment of urological chronic pelvic pain syndromes. The Journal of Urology. 2013;**189**(1 Suppl):S75-S85

[9] Mieritz RM, Thorhauge K, Forman A, Mieritz HB, Hartvigsen J, Christensen HW. Musculoskeletal dysfunctions in patients with chronic pelvic pain: A preliminary descriptive survey. Journal of Manipulative and Physiological Therapeutics. 2016;**39**(9):616-622

[10] Mohktar MS, Ibrahim F, Mohd Rozi NF, Mohd Yusof J, Ahmad SA, Su Yen K, et al. A quantitative approach to measure women's sexual function using electromyography: A

preliminary study of the Kegel exercise. Medical Science Monitor: International Medical Journal of Experimental and Clinical Research. 2013;**19**:1159-1166

[11] Bornstein J, Goldstein AT, Stockdale CK, Bergeron S, Pukall C, Zolnoun D, et al. ISSVD, ISSWSH and IPPS Consensus Terminology and Classification of Persistent Vulvar Pain and Vulvodynia. Obstetrics and Gynecology. 2015, 2016;**127**(4):745-751

[12] Zoorob D, South M, Karram M, Sroga J, Maxwell R, Shah A, et al. A pilot randomized trial of levator injections versus physical therapy for treatment of pelvic floor myalgia and sexual pain. International Urogynecology Journal. Jun 2015;**26**(6):845-852

[13] Ferreira CH, Dwyer PL, Davidson M, De Souza A, Ugarte JA, Frawley HC. Does pelvic floor muscle training improve female sexual function? A systematic review. International Urogynecology Journal. 2015;**26**(12):1735-1750

[14] Pauls RN, Karram MN. Sexual function following anti-incontinence surgery. Minerva urologica e nefrologica—The Italian Journal of Urology and Nephrology. 2008;**60**(2):113-122

[15] Minassian VA, Yan X, Lichtenfeld MJ, Sun H, Stewart WF. The iceberg of health care utilization in women with urinary incontinence. International Urogynecology Journal. 2012;**23**(8):1087-1093

[16] Subak LL, Wing R, West DS, Franklin F, Vittinghoff E, Creasman JM, et al. Weight loss to treat urinary incontinence in overweight and obese women PRIDE. The New England Journal of Medicine. 2009;**360**(5):481-490

[17] Dumoulin C, Hay-Smith EJ, Mac Habee-Seguin G. Pelvic floor muscle training versus no treatment, or inactive control treatments, for urinary incontinence in women. The Cochrane Database of Systematic Reviews. 2014;**5**:Cd005654

[18] Bo K. Pelvic floor muscle training is effective in treatment of female stress urinary incontinence, but how does it work? International Urogynecology Journal and Pelvic Floor Dysfunction. 2004;**15**(2):76-84

[19] McLean L, Varette K, Gentilcore-Saulnier E, Harvey MA, Baker K, Sauerbrei E. Pelvic floor muscle training in women with stress urinary incontinence causes hypertrophy of the urethral sphincters and reduces bladder neck mobility during coughing. Neurourology and Urodynamics. 2013;**32**(8):1096-1102

[20] Yang EJ, Lim JY, Rah UW, Kim YB. Effect of a pelvic floor muscle training program on gynecologic cancer survivors with pelvic floor dysfunction: A randomized controlled trial. Gynecologic Oncology. 2012;**125**(3):705-711

[21] Ptak M, Ciecwiez S, Brodowska A, Starczewski A, Nawrocka-Rutkowska J, Diaz-Mohedo E, et al. The effect of pelvic floor muscles exercise on quality of life in women with stress urinary incontinence and its relationship with vaginal deliveries: A randomized trial. BioMed Research International. 2019;**2019**:5321864

[22] Godec C, Cass AS, Ayala GF. Bladder inhibition with functional electrical stimulation. Urology. 1975;**6**(6):663-666

[23] Morkved S, Bo K, Schei B, Salvesen KA. Pelvic floor muscle training during pregnancy to prevent urinary incontinence: A single-blind randomized controlled trial. Obstetrics and Gynecology. 2003;**101**(2):313-319

[24] Shannon MB, Adams W, Fitzgerald CM, Mueller ER, Brubaker L, Brincat C. Does patient education augment pelvic floor physical therapy preparedness and attendance? A randomized controlled trial. Female Pelvic Medicine & Reconstructive Surgery. 2018;**24**(2):155-160

[25] Sinaki M, Merritt JL, Stillwell GK. Tension myalgia of the pelvic floor. Mayo Clinic Proceedings. 1977;**52**(11):717-722

[26] Aguirre F, Heft J, Yunker A. Factors associated with nonadherence to pelvic floor physical therapy referral for the treatment of female pelvic pain. Physical Therapy. 1 Jul 2019;**99**(7):946-952

[27] Boyles SH, Weber AM, Meyn L. Procedures for pelvic organ prolapse in the United States, 1979-1997. American Journal of Obstetrics and Gynecology. 2003;**188**(1):108-115

[28] Braekken IH, Majida M, Engh ME, Bo K. Can pelvic floor muscle training reverse pelvic organ prolapse and reduce prolapse symptoms? An assessor-blinded, randomized, controlled trial. American Journal of Obstetrics and Gynecology. 2010;**203**(2):170.e1-170.e7

[29] Srikrishna S, Robinson D, Cardozo L, Cartwright R. Experiences and expectations of women with urogenital prolapse: A quantitative and qualitative exploration. BJOG: An International Journal of Obstetrics and Gynaecology. 2008;**115**(11):1362-1368

[30] Knoepp LR, Shippey SH, Chen CC, Cundiff GW, Derogatis LR, Handa VL. Sexual complaints, pelvic floor symptoms, and sexual distress in women over forty. The Journal of Sexual Medicine. 2010;**7**(11):3675-3682

[31] Braekken IH, Majida M, Ellstrom Engh M, Bo K. Can pelvic floor muscle training improve sexual function in women with pelvic organ prolapse? A randomized controlled trial. The Journal of Sexual medicine. 2015;**12**(2):470-480

[32] Hagen S, Stark D, Glazener C, Dickson S, Barry S, Elders A, et al. Individualised pelvic floor muscle training in women with pelvic organ prolapse (POPPY): A multicentre randomised controlled trial. Lancet. 2014;**383**(9919):796-806

[33] Nguyen LN, Gruner M, Killinger KA, Peters KM, Boura JA, Jankowski M, et al. Additional treatments, satisfaction, symptoms and quality of life in women 1 year after vaginal and abdominal pelvic organ prolapse repair. International Urology and Nephrology. 2018;**50**(6):1031-1037

[34] Chen A, McIntyre B, De EJB. Management of postoperative lower urinary tract symptoms (LUTS) after pelvic organ prolapse (POP) repair. Current Urology Reports. 2018;**19**(9):74

[35] Belsey J, Greenfield S, Candy D, Geraint M. Systematic review: Impact of constipation on quality of life in adults and children. Alimentary Pharmacology & Therapeutics. 2010;**31**(9):938-949

[36] Heidelbaugh JJ, Stelwagon M, Miller SA, Shea EP, Chey WD. The spectrum of constipation-predominant irritable bowel syndrome and chronic idiopathic constipation: US survey assessing symptoms, care seeking, and disease burden. The American Journal of Gastroenterology. 2015;**110**(4):580-587

[37] Mugie SM, Benninga MA, Di Lorenzo C. Epidemiology of constipation in children and adults: A systematic review. Best Practice & Research Clinical Gastroenterology. 2011;**25**(1):3-18

[38] Rad S. Impact Of Ethnic Habits On Defecographic Measurements. Archives of Iranian Medicine. 2002;**5**(2):115-117

[39] Sinclair M. The use of abdominal massage to treat chronic constipation. Journal of Bodywork and Movement Therapies. 2011;**15**(4):436-445

[40] Baker J, Eswaran S, Saad R, Menees S, Shifferd J, Erickson K, et al. Abdominal symptoms are common and benefit from biofeedback therapy in patients with dyssynergic defecation. Clinical and translational gastroenterology. 2015;**6**:e105

[41] Pourmomeny AA, Emami MH, Amooshahi M, Adibi P. Comparing the efficacy of biofeedback and balloon-assisted training in the treatment of dyssynergic defecation. Canadian Journal of gastroenterology—Journal canadien de gastroenterologie. 2011;**25**(2):89-92

[42] Muller-Lissner S, Bassotti G, Coffin B, Drewes AM, Breivik H, Eisenberg E, et al. Opioid-induced constipation and bowel dysfunction: A clinical guideline. Pain Medicine. 2017; **18**(10):1837-1863

Chapter 2

Efficacy of Physical Therapy in the Management of Reproductive Disorders

Joseph A. Balogun

Additional information is available at the end of the chapter

http://dx.doi.org/10.5772/intechopen.89808

Abstract

Several textbooks and anecdotal reports exist on the management of reproductive disorders by physical therapy (PHT). However, the recommendations from these sources are often not supported by recent empirical outcome evidence. Thus, there is a need for a comprehensive, up-to-date appraisal of the effectiveness of PHT in the management of reproductive disorders. An exhaustive review of the relevant articles published between 1988 and 2019 was undertaken on the primary electronic databases. The search produced 352 "hits," but only 47 of them met the stated purpose of the review and subsequently classified into nine disease domains. The overwhelming majority (91%) of the 47 articles reviewed found the PHT modalities being investigated to be effective. The credibility of the work ranges from "poor" (for the case reports) to "strong" (for the meta-analysis). The pubococcygeus contraction exercise training (PCET), aka Kegel's exercise, was the most studied modality, followed by aerobic exercise. Although substantial evidence suggests that PCET and transvaginal electrical stimulation are effective for reducing the symptoms of stress urinary incontinence (UI), the data on adjunctive techniques (EMG biofeedback, and vaginal cones) are less consistent. There is presently no reliable evidence to support the use of PCET in combination with EMG biofeedback and electrical stimulation to relieve overactive bladder and improve sexual function in men. The conflicting findings are because many of the published studies are heterogeneous in methodology with variant time frame follow-up; therefore, making firm conclusion difficult. There is a need for more randomized controlled trials (RCT) with adequate sample sizes and the use of sensitive, reproducible, and valid outcome measures. In conclusion, systematic reviews and meta-analyses are needed to bolster the rationale for recommending PHT in the management of chronic pelvic diseases in women. Similarly, RCT is required to support the recommendation for using PCET, electric stimulation, and EMG biofeedback to treat ejaculatory/orgasmic dysfunction, prostatitis, UI and erectile dysfunction in men. The information in this chapter will be useful to physical therapist students, frontline clinicians, and healthcare policymakers.

IntechOpen

© 2019 The Author(s). Licensee IntechOpen. This chapter is distributed under the terms of the Creative Commons Attribution License (http://creativecommons.org/licenses/by/3.0), which permits unrestricted use, distribution, and reproduction in any medium, provided the original work is properly cited.

Keywords: reproductive disorders, obstetrics and gynecology, physical therapy, intervention, efficacy

1. Introduction

Reproductive health is within the purview of obstetrics and gynecology; the clinical specialty that deals with pregnancy, child delivery, and the care of the female reproductive system (breast, vagina, uterus, and ovaries), including the management of the dysfunction of the male prostate and the external structures such as the penis, scrotum, and testicles. Several textbooks [1, 2] and expert opinions [3–12] on the reproductive disorders that are amenable to physical therapy (PHT) intervention have been published previously. However, the recommendations from these sources are often based on clinical opinions and speculations that are not supported by empirically based research. Thus, there is presently a need for a credible reference source that evaluates the literature and provides up to date information on the efficacy of PHT in the management of reproductive disorders in obstetrics and gynecology.

2. Review methodology

An exhaustive search of the pertinent literature on the PUBMED, CINAHL and PsycINFO electronic databases was conducted using the primary keywords: reproductive disorders, PHT, intervention, and efficacy. Subsequently, secondary keywords (urinary and fecal incontinence, chronic pelvic inflammatory diseases, postpartum depression, gestational diabetes mellitus, vestibulodynia, dyspareunia, persistent genital arousal disorder, sexual dysfunction, post-mastectomy complications) were selected individually and used in combination with the primary keywords. Following the literature searches, a total of 352 "hits" emerged. The abstract of each literature search output was assessed for their relevance to the review stated goal. Only 47 of the articles met the purpose of the literature review and were classified into nine disease domains, and the pertinent information on each of them presented in **Table 1**. Subsequently, the full articles were read and evaluated for their weaknesses and strengths [13].

Figure 1 illustrates the credibility rating criteria used to evaluate the 47 articles reviewed. The meta-analysis investigation has the highest credibility and is at the top of the pyramid, while the pre-experimental (case report/series) design has the lowest credibility and is at the bottom of the pyramid. The other research designs (quasi-experimental, randomized controlled trial and systematic review) are in between the apex and base of the pyramid.

In this review, the external validity of the findings from case reports/series are considered "poor," or "limited" and quasi-experimental (cross-sectional) designs ranked as "fair", because a cause and effect conclusion cannot be inferred from these two designs as they fail to control for extraneous factors such as history, repeated testing, maturation, selection bias, experimental mortality, instrumentation, and statistical regression [13]. The credibility of the findings from true experimental designs (also known as randomized controlled trials—RCT) is

http://dx.doi.org/10.5772/intechopen.89808

S./No.	Authors	Year	Physical therapy modalities evaluated[1,2,3,4,5,6,7,8,9,10,11,12]	Gender[13]	Study designs[14]	Outcomes[15]	Finding's credibility
Chronic pelvic inflammatory disease (PID)/salpingo-oophoritis (5 studies—11%)							
1	Balogun and Okonofua	1988	SWD	F	Case report	+	Poor
2	Evseeva et al.	2006	SWD	F	Quasi-experimental	+	Fair
3	Lamina and Hanif	2008	SWD	F	Case series	+	Poor
4	Lamina et al.	2008	SWD	F	RCT	+	Moderate
5	Sonali et al.	2015	SWD/PCET/ADL		RCT	+	Moderate
Urinary and fecal (anal) incontinence (10 studies—22%)							
6	Harvey	2003	PCET	F	Systematic review	—	Substantial
7	McLennan et al.	2006	Knowledge PCET	F	Quasi-experimental	—	Fair
8	Vasconcelos et al.	2006	PCET/EMGB	F	RCT	+	Moderate
9	Kari Bø	2012	PCET	F	Systematic review	+	Substantial
10	Terlikowski et al.	2013	ES/EGMB	F	RCT	+	Moderate
11	Park et al.	2013	PCET	F	Meta-analysis	+	Strong
12	Homsi et al.	2015	PCET	F	Systematic review	+	Substantial
13	Adams et al.	2015	PCET	F	Quasi-experimental	+	Fair
14	Castellani et al.	2016	PCET/ES/EMGB	F	RCT	+	Moderate
15	García-Sánchez et al.	2016	PCET	F	Systematic review		Substantial
16	Liu et al.	2018	ES/EMGB/PCET	F	RCT	+	Moderate
Sexual dysfunction (4 studies—9%)							
17	Brotto et al.	2010	PCET	F	Systematic review	?	Substantial
18	Juraskova et al.	2013	PFRE[4]	F	Quasi-experimental	+	Fair
19	Cohen et al.	2016	PCET	M	Systematic review	+	Substantial
Vestibulodynia and dyspareunia (7 studies—15%)							
20	Bergeron et al.	2002	Manual therapy (stretching), EMGB, ES, PCET[11]	F	Retrospective	+	Fair
21	Murina et al.	2008	TENS	F	RCT	+	Moderate

S./No.	Authors	Year	Physical therapy modalities evaluated[1,2,3,4,5,6,7,8,9,10,11,12]	Gender[13]	Study designs[14]	Outcomes[15]	Finding's credibility
22	Dionisi et al.	2008	EMGB/TENS/ES	F	Quasi-experimental	+	Fair
23	Dionisi and Senatori	2011	PCET/TENS/©DMFSE	F	Quasi-experimental	+	Fair
24	Salvatore et al.	2014	Fractional CO_2 laser therapy[7]	F	Quasi-experimental	+	Fair
25	Davis et al.	2013	PFRE/EMGB[4]	F	Quasi-experimental	+	Fair
26	Brotto et al.	2015	PCET	F	Quasi-experimental	+	Fair
Post-partum depression and obesity prevention (7 studies—15%)							
27	Dennis	2004	Relaxation/massage therapy[9]	NS	Systematic review	—	Substantial
28	Dinas et al.	2011	Aerobic exercise[10]	NS	Systematic review	+	Substantial
29	Josefsson et al.	2014	Aerobic exercise[10]	F	Meta-analysis	+	Strong
30	Kvam et al.	2016	Aerobic exercise[10]	F	Meta-analysis	+	Strong
31	Saligheh et al.	2017	Aerobic exercise[10]	F	Systematic review	+	Substantial
32	Wu et al.	2017	Aerobic exercise[10]	F	Systematic review	+	Substantial
33	Soucy et al.	2017	Aerobic exercise[10]	F	RCT	+	Moderate
Survivors of breast cancer (2 studies—4%)							
34	Juvet et al.	2009	Multimodal—Aerobic exercise[10]	F	Systematic review	+	Substantial
35	Cox et al.	2015	Aerobic exercise[10]	F	Quasi-experimental	+	Fair
Infertility due to adhesive disease (2 studies—4%)							
36	Rice et al.	2015	Manual physical therapy[11]	F	Quasi-experimental	+	Fair
37	Okhowat et al.	2015	Deep relaxation massage[12]	F	Quasi-experimental	+	Fair
Gestational diabetes mellitus prevention (2 studies—4%)							
38	Harrison et al.	2016	Aerobic exercise[10]	F	RCT	+	Moderate
39	Wang et al.	2017	Aerobic exercise[10]	F	RCT	+	Moderate
Mastectomy complications: lymphedema, pain and dermatologic adverse events (7 studies—15%)							
40	Seav et al.	2015	Aerobic exercise[10]/PCET	F	Systematic review	—	Substantial
41	Schmidt et al.	2017	Aerobic exercise[10]	F	RCT	+	Moderate

S./No.	Authors	Year	Physical therapy modalities evaluated[1,2,3,4,5,6,7,8,9,10,11,12]	Gender[13]	Study designs[14]	Outcomes[15]	Finding's credibility
42	Lee	2018	Scrambler therapy[16]	F	Case report	+	Poor
43	Zasadzka et al.	2018	Bandaging & decongestive Rx[17]	M/F	Quasi-experimental	+	Fair
44	Dalenc et al.	2018	Hydrotherapy[18]	F	Quasi-experimental	+	Fair
45	Yeung and Semciw	2018	Hydrotherapy (aquatic vs. land)[18]	F	Systematic review	?	Substantial
46	Duyur et al.	2019	Decongestive therapy[17]	F	Quasi-experimental	+	Fair
47	Panchik et al.	2019	Multimodal—aerobic exercise[10]	F	Meta-analysis	+	Strong

[1]SWD = shortwave diathermy.
[2]EMGB = EMG biofeedback.
[3]PCET = PC exercise (Kegel's) training.
[4]PFRE = pelvic floor muscle relaxation exercise.
[5]ES = electrical stimulation.
[6]TENS = transcutaneous electrical nerve stimulation.
[7]LASER = fractional carbon dioxide laser therapy.
[8]MFSE = Daily myofascial stretching exercises.
[9]Relaxation/massage therapy.
[10]Aerobic exercise.
[11]Manual physical therapy.
[12]Deep relaxation massage.
[13]Gender: F = female, M = male, NR = not reported.
[14]RCT = randomized controlled trial (RCT).
[15]Outcome: + = Effective, − = not effective,? = unclear.
[16]Scrambler therapy.
[17]Compression bandaging and complex decongestive therapy.
[18]Hydrotherapy.

Table 1. The relevant information on the efficacy of physical therapy in the management of reproductive disorders.

considered "moderate"; systematic reviews and meta-analyses as "substantial" and "strong," respectively. The outcomes from RCT, systematic reviews and meta-analyses eliminate selection and confounding factor biases. Therefore, a cause and effect conclusion can be drawn from them [13].

3. Results

All the 47 full length articles reviewed appeared in peer-reviewed journals between 1988 and 2019, and the salient points extracted from them are shown in **Table 1**. Most of the published articles reviewed was a quasi-experimental design. The data for 90% of them were collected from females, less than 4% were from males, and the rest did not specify the gender of the study participants. The most popular area of PHT research in obstetrics and gynecology is urinary and fecal (anal) incontinence (22%), followed by mastectomy complications (sexual

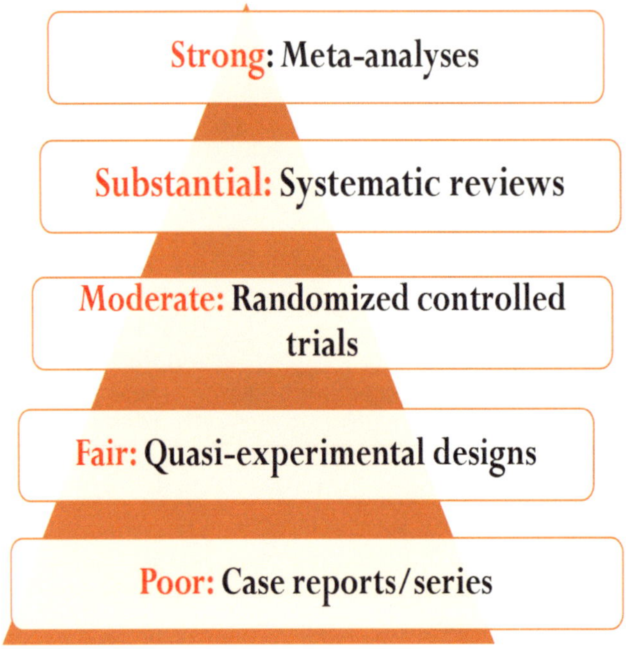

Figure 1. Research credibility pyramid.

dysfunction, lymphedema, pain, and dermatologic adverse events) which accounts for 17%. Vestibulodynia and dyspareunia, post-partum depression, and obesity prevention each accounted for 15% of the PHT research. Chronic pelvic inflammatory disease/salpingo-oophoritis represents 11% and sexual dysfunction was 7% of the published research. The least studied area of women's health PHT (4% each) was the physical/psychological well-being of survivors of breast cancer, including infertility, adhesive disease and gestational diabetes mellitus prevention (**Table 1**).

For historiographic and consistency purposes, the review in each of the nine disease domains was organized in sequential order starting from the oldest to the most recent publications. The aim and major findings for each of the 47 investigations are presented below.

3.1. Chronic pelvic inflammatory disease/salpingo-oophoritis

In 1988, Balogun and Okonofua documented the effectiveness of shortwave diathermy (SWD) while treating a 39-year-old black woman with an eight-year history of chronic PID that is non-responsive to conventional antibiotic therapy [14]. SWD is a deep-heating thermal agent that its use has declined in several countries because of its large size and heavy weight but is enjoying a rebirth due to modern technology that now produced a more compact and light-weight product that can be transported easily within the clinic and use in the home setting. A modified "cross-fire" technique at a thermal dosage level was administered (for each half of the crossfire technique treatment) for 20 and 30 min. At baseline, the patient rated her pain perception on a 10-point visual analog pain scale at the beginning of every treatment session.

After eight sessions of SWD treatment, she was utterly pain-free and remained so for 6 months at follow up.

In three case series, Lamina and Hanif [15] replicated the clinical protocol described earlier by Balogun and Okonofua. Two of the patients in this study had their pain score on the visual analog scale reduced from an average of 6.5 to 0 and remain at 0 levels without any medication 4 months later. The third patient had her pain perception reduced from 6 to 4; and on follow up pain score stay at level three while still on antibiotic treatment.

In a quasi-experimental study, Evseeva et al. investigated the effect of a "low-frequency electrostatic field" for treating chronic salpingo-oophoritis. Sixty-three females with the disorder participated in the study; 52 of them received intensive treatment with the electrotherapy device, while the remaining 11 study participants received a sham treatment. They found the participants who received the "low-frequency electrostatic field" treatment observed significant and long-term pain relief for up to 18 months [16].

In a follow-up RCT, Lamina, Hanif and Gagarawa investigated the effect of SWD in the management of the chronic PID [17]. Thirty-two patients diagnosed with the disorder were assigned randomly to three (SWD, control, and analgesic) groups. The SWD group ($n = 13$) received antibiotics (oral ofloxacin 400 mg twice daily and metronidazole 400 mg twice a day, placebo (sham analgesic) tablets and SWD treatment for 15–20 min on alternate days of the week. The analgesic group ($n = 14$) received antibiotics, analgesics (nonsteroidal anti-inflammatory drugs—oral ibuprofen 400 mg twice daily, and sham SWD, while the control group ($n = 13$) received the same dosage of antibiotics, sham SWD, and placebo tablets. The treatment lasted 30 days, and pain perception was monitored pre-and-post-treatment. The baseline (pretest) pain scores among the groups differ significantly ($F = 4.96$, $p < 0.05$). The pre-and-post-treatment difference observed in the severity of pain was statistically significant ($p < 0.05$) among the groups. The mean pain score of the SWD group compared to the control and analgesics groups was significantly reduced.

In 2015, Sonali et al. investigated the efficacy of SWD in the management of pain associated with chronic PID [18]. They randomly assigned 30 women between 18 and 40 years diagnosed with PID into two groups. The women in group one were treated with medication (antibiotics and analgesics), pubococcygeus contraction exercise training (PCET), aka Kegel's exercise, activities of daily living instruction and SWD. The women in group two received medications, PCET, and activities of daily living instruction, but no SWD. The pre-and-post-intervention visual analog scale and pain disability index were monitored. The result of the investigation showed significant improvement in both outcome measures among the women in group one treated with SWD. The authors concluded that their findings provide a rational basis for recommending SWD instead of analgesics, which often has side effects, during the management of the debilitating pain associated with PID.

In a recent randomized controlled trial, Saif et al. evaluated the effectiveness of SWD and pharmacological agents in the management of the chronic PID [19]. The authors randomly allocated 60 women diagnosed with PID for more than 6 months into three groups; 20 women in each group. The women in group one received both medical (oral doxycycline 100 mg twice daily and metronidazole 500 mg twice daily for 14 days) treatment and SWD. Those in group two received only SWD treatment, and the third group received only medical treatment. The SWD treatment using the crossfire technique was administered for 20 min (split into two sessions of 10 min per session) every alternate day for a total of 15 sessions. At baseline, the gynecologist clinically examined the women, took a cervix biopsy for laboratory analysis and ultrasonography to detect any underlying pathology. Also, the pain level was measured using a 10-point visual analog scale. Post-treatment, after 14 days of treatment for group 1, and the 5th week session for groups 2 and 3, pain score on the 10-point visual analog scale, laboratory (end cervix swab) specimen was taken to examine the number of WBCs, and ultrasonography was also conducted to detect any improvement in previous pathology, self-report of itching, and discharge. A statistically significant ($p < .01$) improvement in itching and discharge was observed among the women in group one when compared to the women in group three; and insignificant differences was obtained between women in groups two and three ($p > .05$). Compared to the baseline, the result revealed a statistically significant difference ($p < .01$) in the visual analog scale pain rating score in the three groups following treatment. No significant difference was observed in the pain rating score when group one was compared with the other two groups ($p > .05$) and insignificant differences was also observed between groups two and three ($p > .05$). There was a statistically significant ($p < .01$) reduction in the number of pus cells in the cervix swab specimen and reduction of fluid in the Douglas pouch for the women in group one compared to the baseline and the other groups. The authors concluded that the most beneficial therapeutic effect is when SWD was used in combination with medical treatment (analgesics and antibiotics).

3.2. Urinary and fecal (anal) incontinence

Harvey investigated the effectiveness of PCET in the prevention of urinary/anal incontinence and prolapse [20]. The major electronic databases were reviewed to identify studies that used prenatal and postpartum PCET. The review yielded 12 investigations on the role of prenatal PCET, which included three RCT which compared PCET for the prevention of UI to controls. Similarly, the authors identified 12 studies that evaluated postpartum PCET for prevention of UI, of which 4 were RCT designs. The author also reviewed five researches that evaluated postpartum PCET for the prevention of anal incontinence; four of the investigations were RCT designs. The analyses revealed that prenatal PCET used in combination with biofeedback does not significantly produce short-term (3 months) decrease in postpartum UI or pelvic floor strength. However, postpartum PCET implemented with vaginal device to provide resistance or feedback, appear to decrease postpartum UI and increase strength. Ongoing reminder and motivational instructions to perform PCET are not effective strategies in preventing postpartum UI. The authors concluded that postpartum PCET does not consistently reduce the incidence of anal incontinence.

A quasi-experimental (cross-sectional) research by McLennan et al. evaluated the knowledge of pregnant women about pelvic floor complications during pregnancy and delivery [21]. A total of 232 women with a mean age of 27 years and the overwhelming majority (85%) had at least grade 12 education participated in the study. A day after delivery, the women completed a 52-item questionnaire that assesses their knowledge of the information provided during routine antenatal care. The research questionnaire intermixed the pelvic floor and general questions. Forty-six percent of the women in the investigation reported that they did not receive any information on PCET; 51% denied receiving information on episiotomy; 47% on UI; 81% fecal incontinence; 73% change in vaginal caliber; and 85% did not receive any information on neuropathy. Education of pregnant women on all these issues occur less frequently ($p < .05$) than counseling on general pregnancy topics. The authors concluded that instruction of pregnant women about pelvic floor risks is very much lacking and advocated the development of educational materials on the issue.

A prospective study by Vasconcelos et al. randomly allocated 56 women (6–15 years old) with dysfunctional elimination syndrome who are nonresponsive to previous therapies into two groups [22]. Both groups received avoiding and drinking schedule, and instruction on adequate toilet posture reinforced through the maintenance of voiding diaries, and PCET intervention but different training sessions and treatment duration. Group one consists of 26 women who received 24 training sessions over 3 months, and Group two which comprised of 30 women also received 16 training sessions of EMG biofeedback therapy offered over 2 months period. Outcome measures (millivoltage recordings of the pelvic floor muscles (PFM) and postvoiding residual urine monitored by dynamic ultrasonography) were monitored at pre-intervention, 1, 6, and 12 months post-intervention time frames. Renal ultrasonography and dynamic ultrasonography were conducted in both groups before and 6 months after the intervention. The data analysis revealed the improvement of urinary continence following training in both groups. Only the patients in group two who received biofeedback training showed a significant decrease in postvoiding residual urine. The authors concluded that their results show that both PCET and biofeedback training modulated episodic UI and urinary tract infection and recommended follow up studies to identify the optimal training parameters, treatment frequency, and duration.

In 2012, Kari Bø analyzed the results of RCT published in English language in the Cochrane reviews. The study reviewed investigated the effectiveness of using PCET to treat stress UI, pelvic organ prolapses, and sexual dysfunction [23]. The author reported Level 1 evidence that PCET is useful in the treatment of stress UI with short-term cure rates between 35 and 80%. Five RCT showed a significant effect of PCET on either pelvic organ prolapse stage, symptoms or PC muscle morphology. The authors found that supervised and more intensive training is more effective than unsupervised training and no adverse effects were reported. None of the RCT addressed the impact of PCET on sexual dysfunction. Based on the findings in the study, the author recommended that PCET should be the first option treatment to manage stress UI and pelvic organ prolapse. The authors cautioned that PCET needs proper instruction and close follow-up for the intervention to be effective.

Using a double-blind, placebo-controlled, randomized design, Terlikowski et al. compared the efficacy of PHT (electrical stimulation and EMG biofeedback) in the treatment of urodynamic stress UI in premenopausal women [24]. The investigators allocated 102 women with stress UI into two groups. Group one ($n = 68$) received the PHT treatment ($n = 68$), and group two received a sham or placebo ($n = 34$) treatment. Both groups had their treatment administered two times per day for 8 weeks. Urinary leakage measured by the standard pad test, voiding diary, urodynamic analysis, and the Incontinence Quality of Life Questionnaire were monitored at three-time frames; before treatment (at baseline), after the intervention (at 8th week) and at 16th weeks follow-up. At the end of the 8th week, the mean urinary leakage was significantly ($p < .0.001$) lower in group one (PHT) than the placebo group (19.5 ± 13.6 vs. 39.8 ± 28.5). The mean urinary leakage was significantly ($p < .0.001$) reduced in group one (PHT) compared to the placebo group at the end of 8th and 16th weeks (8.2 ± 14.8 vs. 14.6 ± 18.9 and 6.1 ± 11.4 vs. 18.2 ± 20.8), respectively. Similarly, there was a statistically significant ($p < .0.001$) improvement in muscle strength, as measured by the Oxford scale, in group one (PHT) compared to the placebo group after 8 and 16 weeks (4.2 vs. 2.6 and 4.1 vs. 2.7), respectively. The urodynamic data for the two groups were not statistically different ($p > .0.05$) at baseline and after treatment. The mean Incontinence Quality of Life Questionnaire score at the end of 8th week, for group one (PHT) compared to the placebo group, was 78.2 ± 17.9 vs. 55.9 ± 14.2 ($p < .0.004$), respectively, and at the end of the 16th week was 80.8 ± 24.1 vs. 50.6 ± 14.9 ($p < .0.001$), respectively. The authors concluded that the combination of electrical stimulation and EMG biofeedback modalities is efficacious in the treatment of premenopausal women's stress UI.

A meta-analysis by Park et al. evaluated published RCT of low-risk obstetric women who received PCET during pregnancy and after delivery to determine whether the training could prevent urinary and fecal incontinence [25]. The authors analyzed articles with high methodological quality published between 1966 and 2012 in the major electronic databases that met the study criteria (n = 14). The meta-analysis of the 14 investigations reviewed included 6454 women, and the result revealed that PCET significantly reduced the development of urinary and fecal incontinence from pregnancy to postpartum.

In 2015, Homsi et al. reviewed the literature on the effects of PFM training on women sexual function using the six major electronic databases for RCT published between 1997 and 2014 [26]. Eight of the RCT met the study criteria, and 1341 women were included in the review. The studies methodological scores range between four and seven and most of them reported a significant improvement in sexual function score after PCET between control and intervention groups. Most of the investigations reviewed found an increase of at least one sexual variable among women with pelvic floor dysfunction, and one study found an improvement in sexual function in women with postpartum selected independently of their continence status.

In a quasi-experimental cohort study, Adams et al. investigated the effectiveness of PCET as primary treatment of women urinary urgency and frequency symptoms [27]. The women (n = 36 out of 57) who met the study inclusion criteria completed 10 weeks of PCET once or twice per week for 10 weeks and symptom assessed by a Pelvic Floor Distress Inventory and Global Patient Impression of Improvement survey, voiding diaries, and subjective measures. At baseline, the women median Pelvic Floor Distress Inventory score was 79.2 (IQR, 53.1–122.9), and decreased to 50.0 (IQR, 25.0–88.5; $p < 0.001$) following PCET; both the urinary and prolapse symptom subscale score on the Pelvic Floor Distress Inventory decreased significantly (from a median of 10.0 voids per day to 8.0 ($p < 0.001$). About 63% of the women reported that they were "much better" or "very much better" on the Patient Global Impression of Improvement survey. The authors concluded that PCET supplemented with myofascial release techniques improves urinary symptoms in the absence of medications and more invasive therapies. The high dropout rates suggest that motivation and logistic factors are needed to ensure the utilization and success of PCET.

A RCT by Castellani et al. compared the relative effectiveness of the combination of PHT (PCET, electrical stimulation, and EMG biofeedback) with medication (intravaginal estriol) to treat the stress UI of postmenopausal women [28]. Sixty-two women diagnosed with the disorder were allocated randomly into two groups. Group one received PHT, and group two received PHT in addition to medication (1 mg intravaginal estriol) for 6 months. Baseline outcome measures were taken at the beginning of the study and 6 months at the end of the study. Pelvic examination, urodynamics, and 24-hour pad tests were also monitored. Urinary incontinence was assessed using the Short Form of the International Consultation on Incontinence questionnaire, and the women's quality of life measured by the Short Form of the Incontinence Impact Questionnaire. At the end of the study, three of the 62 women enrolled in the study dropped out. In Group one, the mean urine leakage decreased from 42.3 ± 20.2 g/die to 31.5 ± 14.2 g/die. And in Group two, the mean urine leakage also decreased from 48.3 ± 19.8 g/die to 22.3 ± 10.1 g/die. The symptoms scores and incontinence status in Group two were significantly better than Group one. The authors concluded that the combination of intravaginal estriol and PHT intervention is a safe and efficient first-line treatment in postmenopausal women with stress UI.

In 2016, García-Sánchez et al. analyzed published work on the effectiveness of PCET in the management of UI [29]. They reviewed the major electronic databases published in Spanish and English over a 10-year period that met the study criteria. Overall, nine full articles and one abstract were reviewed; three of the articles were on UI in female athletes and six on UI in women in general. The nine studies reported an improvement in the disease. The authors concluded that PCET is effective in the management of stress UI.

In a RCT, Liu et al. investigated the efficacy of different treatment methods on stress UI among perimenopausal women [30]. They allocated 72 menopausal women with stress UI into three groups with 24 women in each group. Group one received electrical stimulation treatment combined with biofeedback. Group two received PCET and the women in group three did not receive any treatment (control group). The outcome measures tracked at baseline and after 60-days include clinical parameters of urination, PFM strengths, urine dynamics indexes and Quality of Life Survey scores. Although the women in both groups showed statistically significant (($p < 0.01$) improvement in their UI, PFM strength, leakage times, frequency of urination, urine dynamics index and Quality of Life Survey scores ($P < 0.05$) after 60 days treatment, but the women in group one showed the most significant improvement. The women in the control group showed no significant difference ($p > 0.05$) between the baseline and the post-training 60-day time frame. The authors concluded that both electrical stimulation treatment combined with biofeedback, and PCET could prevent stress UI in perimenopausal women.

3.3. Sexual dysfunction

In 2010, Brotto et al. reviewed the literature over a 7 year period on women's sexual dysfunctions, their diagnostic issues, pathophysiology, assessment, and treatment [31]. They examined the primary research databases, conference proceedings, and lay articles in the press using the keywords of hypoactive sexual desire disorder, female sexual arousal disorder, female orgasmic disorder, and persistent genital arousal disorder. Following the review, the authors recommended assessment of women's sexual dysfunctions using the biopsychosocial clinical interview of the woman and partner (if possible); followed by a physical and psychophysiological examination, patient self-report questionnaires to supplement the interview information and laboratory investigations. At the time when the study was being implemented in the USA, some promising drugs for treating women's sexual dysfunction were undergoing clinical trials. Empirical evidence demonstrating the efficacy of PHT and psychological therapies for women's sexual dysfunction is presently limited. Thus, there is the need for RCT to evaluate the effectiveness of the different treatments recommended to treat women's sexual dysfunction.

A quasi-experimental study by Juraskova et al. evaluated the acceptability, feasibility, and efficacy of using olive oil, vaginal exercise, and moisturize (OVEM)—a polycarbophil-based vaginal moisturizer—to treat sexual dysfunction associated with breast cancer treatment [32]. Twenty-five women with dyspareunia received PHT (PFM relaxation exercises) twice/day for 4 weeks to prevent/manage PFM overactivity. The women were also instructed to apply the OVEM thrice per week to decrease vaginal dryness, use olive oil as a lubricant during sexual intercourse, and complete a weekly compliance diary. During the study, dyspareunia, sexual functioning, quality of life, distress, and PFM functioning were monitored. The outcome measures were tracked at the beginning of the study and the end of the training (fourth week) and at 12 and 26 weeks follow-ups. Each week during the study, the women completed a self-report questionnaire, and the physical therapist recorded objective measures of PFM functioning. The study found significant improvement in dyspareunia, sexual function, and quality of life of the women over time ($p < 0.001$) following the OVEM intervention. The PFM relaxation training also improved dyspareunia, sexual function, and quality of life of the women ($p < 0.001$). The maximum improvements occurred at week 12 follow-up time frame. Most of the women in the study rated PHT (92%), vaginal moisturizer (88%), and olive oil (73%) as helpful and acceptable. Paradoxically, six of the women (11%) had vaginal stenosis during the initial screening, which further confirms the underreporting of sexual problems following breast cancer. The authors concluded that the novel OVEM intervention is acceptable, feasible in a clinical setting and effective in improving dyspareunia and sexual function following breast cancer.

In a systematic review, Seav et al. in 2015 compared the findings of RCT and observational studies on the sexual functioning of women who survived breast cancer [33]. The authors identified 1414 investigations, but only 34 of them met the defined study criteria that used vaginal lubricants (moisturizers, estrogens, dehydroepiandrosterone, testosterone, vibrators, dilators), systemic medications (androgens, anti-depressants, flibanserin, ospemifene), PHT (physical activity, pelvic floor training), counseling and educational interventions on sexual functioning of women with breast cancer. The findings revealed that vaginal moisturizers were effective in improving vaginal dryness, dyspareunia, and sexual satisfaction; educational and counseling interventions showed improvement in various aspects of sexual health. Physical activity, transdermal testosterone or hot flash interventions did not consistently improve the sexual health of the women.

In 2016, Cohen et al., in a systematic review study, evaluated the effect of PCET in the management of male sexual dysfunctions, including erectile dysfunction, ejaculatory/orgasmic dysfunction, prostatitis and chronic pelvic pain syndrome [34]. The authors concluded that PCET is of potential therapeutic benefit for men who suffer from these conditions.

3.4. Vestibulodynia and dyspareunia

In 2002, Bergeron et al. conducted a retrospective study on the effectiveness of PHT (in the form of manual techniques such as stretching, electromyographic biofeedback, electrical stimulation, and PCET home exercises) in improving sexual function and relieving painful intercourse associated with vulvar vestibulitis [35]. Thirty-five women diagnosed with vulvar vestibulitis who received PHT for an average of seven sessions were interviewed on the phone to determine whether PHT or other subsequent treatments had any effect on their pain perception during intercourse and sexual functioning. The length of treatment follow up ranged from 2 to 44 months with a mean of 16 months. Following PHT intervention, 51% of the women in the study showed complete or significant improvement; 20% of them experienced a moderate increase, and 29% observed little to no improvement. The PHT intervention resulted in a significant decrease in pain perception both during intercourse and gynecological examinations; including a substantial increase in the frequency of sex and levels of sexual desire and arousal. The women with favorable outcomes were significantly less educated than those with unfavorable results. The overall findings revealed that dyspareunia associated with vulvar vestibulitis could potentially be managed successfully by PHT.

A double-arm randomized placebo-controlled study by Murina et al. investigated the efficacy of transcutaneous electrical nerve stimulation (TENS) in the treatment of vestibulodynia [36]. Forty women with vestibulodynia were randomly allocated into two groups—active TENS group and sham (placebo) group and each group were treated twice a week for a total of 20 treatment sessions—the treatment with TENS or sham was delivered through a vaginal probe. The outcome measures tracked at baseline, at the end of treatment and 3 months follow up were visual analog scale, the short form of the McGill-Mailsack Pain Questionnaire, the Female Sexual Function Index Questionnaire and the Marinoff Scale for dyspareunia. The baseline visual analog scale and McGill-Melzack Pain Questionnaire scores (6.2 ± 1.9 and 19.5 ± 11.9) significantly decreased (improved) in the TENS group (2.1 ± 2.7, $p = 0.01$) compared to the placebo group (8.5 ± 10.7, $p = 0.001$), respectively. Similarly, the Marinoff dyspareunia scale and the Female Sexual Function Index improved significantly. However, no improvement occurred in the placebo group. The authors concluded that TENS is a simple, effective, safe short-term (3 months) treatment for vestibulodynia.

A quasi-experimental study by Dionisi et al. evaluated the safety, tolerability, and efficacy of a multimodal PHT intervention in the treatment of vulvar pain and vulvar discomfort in women with vulvodynia [37]. One hundred and forty-five women diagnosed with vulvodynia were treated weekly for a total of 10 sessions with EMG biofeedback, TENS, in association with functional electrical stimulation using an intravaginal probe for the treatment, and home program stretching exercise of the PFM. An improvement (decrease) in vulvar pain occurred in 76% of the cases. The authors concluded that the relaxation of the PFM with biofeedback and electroanalgesia is safe and effective in modulating the vulvar pain and dyspareunia in women with vulvodynia.

Another quasi-experimental study conducted by Dionisi and Senatori determined the safety and effectiveness of using intravaginal electrodes TENS for the treatment of vulvar pain and dyspareunia during the postpartum period following perineal trauma caused by episiotomy [38]. Forty-five women with a diagnosis of postpartum dyspareunia from perineal trauma after a vaginal delivery training on how to use the PFM. Also, they were educated on the role of PFM in continuing dyspareunia. Subsequently, they received weekly intravaginal TENS treatment in an outpatient clinic in addition to daily home program myofascial stretching and PCET. Outcome measurements obtained before training (baseline), at the end of the 5th week and 8 months post-training includes the cotton swab test, the Visual Analog Scale, the Marinoff Dyspareunia Scale, and the Anovulvar Distance. The overwhelming majority (85%) of the sample reported an improvement of dyspareunia after five sessions of TENS, and 95% of the women had full remission of the symptoms. All the women were utterly pain-free 8 months following the treatment. The authors concluded that intravaginally applied TENS and pelvic floor relaxation exercises is safe and effective in the relief of vulvar pain and dyspareunia after spontaneous delivery in women with postpartum perineal trauma due to episiorrhaphy.

In 2014, Salvatore et al. conducted a quasi-experimental study to evaluate the efficacy and feasibility of treating vulvovaginal atrophy in postmenopausal women using a fractional carbon dioxide laser therapy [39]. Fifty women (mean age = 59.6; SD = 5.8 years) diagnosed with vulvovaginal atrophy symptoms and who are dissatisfied with previous local estrogen therapies were treated with laser therapy for three sessions over 12 weeks. The women's subjective pain was monitored using the visual analog scale and objectively using the Vaginal Health Index Score inventory; quality of life measured with the SF-12 Standardized Questionnaire at baseline and 12 weeks later. Compared to the baseline measurements, the vulvovaginal atrophy symptoms (vaginal dryness, vaginal burning, vaginal itching, dyspareunia, dysuria), the Vaginal Health Index Score (mean = 13.1; SD = 2.5 at baseline vs. mean = 23.1; SD = 1.9), the physical and mental scores and qualities of life of the women following the laser treatment improved significantly ($p < 0.001$) at the end of the 12-weeks. Eighty-four percent of the women were satisfied with the laser treatment. However, the women reported minimal discomfort at the first fractional carbon dioxide laser application due to the insertion and the movements of the probe. Subsequent treatment from the second application in week four was straightforward to perform in all the women, and no other untoward adverse event recorded during the study. The authors concluded that randomized RCT are needed to confirm the long-term benefits of fractional carbon dioxide laser therapy on vaginal morphology.

A quasi-experimental study by Davis et al. evaluated the changes in pain, depressive symptoms, and sexual outcomes in women with vestibulodynia following PHT (PFM relaxation exercise, EMG biofeedback), sex/psychotherapy, and medical intervention and controls [40]. Two hundred and thirty-nine women with provoked vestibulodynia completed a questionnaire at baseline and 2 years follow up. The questionnaire subscales measured the visual analog scale of genital pain, Global Measure of Sexual Satisfaction, Female Sexual Function

Index, Beck Depression Inventory, Dyadic Adjustment Scale, and sexual intercourse attempts over the past month. The results overall revealed significant improvement on pain ratings, sexual satisfaction and function, and depressive symptoms 2 years post-test. Most of the women received PHT, sex/psychotherapy, and medical treatment; 41% of them did not receive any treatment but improved significantly on pain ratings. None of the single treatment types provided better outcome on any of the outcome measures monitored except depressive symptoms on which women who had surgery were more likely to improve. This study did not demonstrate the superiority of any one treatment over the other and the improvements in the symptoms of vestibulodynia was attributed to natural progression.

A quasi-experimental study by Brotto et al. investigated the efficacy of a multimodal treatment consisting of psychological skills training, PCET and medication management of provoked vestibulodynia [41]. Women (n = 132) with provoked vestibulodynia received the hospital-based treatment for 10-weeks. Of the 132 women, 116 (mean = 28; SD = 7.1 years) provided complete data following the 10 weeks treatment, and 84 women had full data 3–4 months post-test period. At baseline, 38% of the women avoided intimacy, 41% avoided sexual while 50% choose to focus on their partner's sexual arousal and satisfaction. Post-treatment, 54% of the women reported significant improvements in dyspareunia with strong significant effects for the reduction in dyspareunia, sex-related distress, increase sexual arousal and overall sexual functioning ($p < 0.001$). Statistically significant improvements in sexual desire, lubrication, orgasmic function, and sexual satisfaction were observed ($p < 0.05$). Two to three-months post-treatment, all the improvements were still retained. The authors concluded that their study provided strong evidence for the use of multidisciplinary approach in the management of the dyspareunia and sexual dysfunctions experienced by women with provoked vestibulodynia.

3.5. Post-partum depression and obesity prevention

In 2004, Dennis systematically reviewed the major electronic databases from 1966 to 2003 to evaluate the treatment of postpartum depression by non-pharmacological methods [42]. Published studies (n = 21) on interpersonal psychotherapy, cognitive-behavioral therapy, peer and partner support, nondirective counseling, relaxation/massage therapy, infant sleep interventions, infant-mother relationship therapy, and maternal exercise that met the set inclusion criteria were analyzed. The author concluded that he could not ascertain the relative effectiveness of most of the non-pharmacological treatments because of weak and disparate experimental design issues.

Dinas et al. reviewed the publications that investigated the effects of aerobic exercise therapy on acute and chronic depression [43]. The screening criteria used covered several topics such as the "treatment of depression, the link between β-endorphin and exercise, the efficacy of exercise and physical activity as treatments for depression, properties of exercise stimuli used in intervention programs, as well as the efficacy of exercise and physical activity for treating depression in diseased individuals." The result of the analysis revealed that aerobic exercise has salutary effects on depression symptoms; the effects are comparable to those obtained using antidepressant treatments.

A meta-analysis study by Josefsson et al. compared the relative effectiveness of aerobic exercise with no intervention, placebo, and usual care conditions in reducing symptoms of depression among clinically defined adults with depression [44]. After reviewing the major electronic databases, the authors identified 89 articles, but only 15 of them met the inclusion criteria, and 13 reported relevant information needed to calculate effect sizes. The main result showed a significantly large overall effect that favored aerobic exercise intervention. The effect size was even more significant when only designs that had used no intervention or placebo conditions were analyzed. Nevertheless, the effect size was reduced to a moderate level when only the research with high methodological quality were included in the analysis. The authors recommended aerobic exercise therapy for patients with mild to moderate depression who are motivated, and physically healthy to participate in such a program.

Kvam et al. conducted a meta-analysis of RCT published until November 2014 that examined the effectiveness of aerobic exercise in the treatment of unipolar depression, both as an independent and as a combination intervention to antidepressant medication [45]. A total of 23 articles with 977 participants, met the study criteria. The analyses revealed that aerobic exercise had a moderate to a large significant effect on depression score compared to control conditions ($g = -0.68$), but the change was small and not significant at follow-up ($g = -0.22$). Compared to the control group, the aerobic exercise group had a large and significant effect size ($g = -1.24$), and exercise training had a moderate and significant effect compared to usual conventional care ($g = -0.48$). The impact of aerobic exercise was small and not significant when compared to psychological treatment or antidepressant medication ($g = -0.22$ and -0.08, respectively). When aerobic exercise was implemented as an adjunct to antidepressant medication, they yielded a moderate effect ($g = -0.50$) that trended toward statistical significance. The authors concluded that aerobic exercise is an effective treatment for the management of depression, and it is as viable as an adjunct treatment in combination with antidepressants.

A systematic review study by Saligheh et al. evaluated the effectiveness of aerobic exercise on postnatal depression and weight loss. Following data searches of the six major electronic databases, nine of the studies met the stated inclusion criteria [46]. The articles reviewed implemented different exercise therapy modalities (commonly walking), and they incorporated different support strategies to enhance adherence. Two (22%) of the nine studies identified changes in both postnatal depression and weight loss outcomes with small effect sizes. Four of the research (44%) reported a decrease in postnatal depression with variable effect sizes, while three of them (33%) reported no effect. The exercise therapy most likely to reduce postnatal depression and weight loss are those that employ one on one weekly supervision at moderate intensity level and adhered to specific intervention guidelines for over 12 weeks and supplemented by psychosocial strategies such as educational information, advice on exercise therapy, and counseling.

Wu et al. analyzed the English language publications that investigated the effects of physical activity on depressive symptoms in Parkinson disease in the major electronic databases from January 2006 to June 2017 [47]. The authors analyzed 11 of the 769 abstracts that met the eligibility screening criteria and awarded better quality scores ranging from 3 to 8 by the raters.

The research included 342 patients that underwent 17 different kinds of physical activity programs. The results revealed that aerobic exercise training significantly improved the cumulative Parkinson's Disease Rating, Beck Depression Inventory, and the Quality of Life subscale scores. Qigong exercise improved the overall Unified Parkinson's Disease Rating Scale score and decreased incidences of multiple non-motor symptoms and depression. Tai Chi exercises enhanced the postural stability and Quality of Life of the patients.

In 2017, Soucy et al. conducted a RCT to determine the effectiveness of behavioral and aerobic exercise interventions for treating depression [48]. Fifty-nine women with a diagnosis of mild-to-moderate symptoms of depression were assigned randomly to either a behavioral therapy (n = 20), aerobic exercise (n = 19) or a wait-listed control group (n = 20). At pretest, mid-test, immediate post-intervention, and at two-month follow-up time frames, all the women recorded their symptoms. The results revealed that both behavioral and aerobic exercise interventions were significantly more effective in reducing depressive symptoms compared to the control group. The aerobic exercise therapy program significantly involved less treatment time compared to the behavioral therapy program (half the amount of time). The authors concluded that both physical activity at the low-intensity level and behavioral therapy effectively reduce depressive symptoms.

3.6. Survivors of breast cancer in cancer rehabilitation

A systematic review by Juvet et al. evaluated the efficacy of single treatments and the combination of therapies (e.g., rehabilitation programs) on the physical performance and psychological well-being of women following breast cancer treatment [49]. A total of 46 RCT of moderate or high quality were reviewed; seven of the articles were on PHT, 11 examined different types of physical activity, 18 assessed different psychosocial interventions, two of the research were on nutrition, five examined complementary interventions, and three were on a complex rehabilitation program. The research on physical activity showed improved quality of life and decrease fatigue. Three of the investigation revealed that early physical activity was not associated with aggravated lymphedema. Four of the studies showed that cognitive behavior therapy intervention also improved overall quality of life. Based on the findings, the combination of therapies effect cannot be delineated clearly. The authors concluded that there is limited documentation in favor of the efficacy of different rehabilitation interventions for women with breast cancer.

A study by Cox et al. investigated the temporal relationships between several social-cognitive theory constructs and aerobic exercise (physical activity) among women with endometrial cancer receiving aerobic exercise training at four different time frames (T1–T4) [50]. The sedentary women (n = 98) who were at least 6 months posttreatment after endometrial cancer underwent physical activity intervention. The findings revealed that physiological somatic sensations at T2 decreased, self-efficacy at T3 increased, which led to an increase in physical activity at the T4 time frame. The authors posited that self-efficacy is a significant mediator between physiological somatic sensations and physical activity. They concluded that physiological somatic sensations are an important construct that can be used to promote increased physical activity; self-efficacy mediates the relationship between physiological somatic sensations and physical activity, but the timing of the relationship warrants follow-up investigation.

3.7. Infertility due to adhesive disease

A quasi-experimental (retrospective) study by Rice et al. investigated the effectiveness of manual PHT in the management of infertile women with an underlying adhesive disease [51]. The study reviewed the records of 1392 women with diagnoses of infertility, including occluded fallopian tubes, hormonal dysfunction, endometriosis, and those undergoing in vitro fertilization treated at a private PHT practice. All the women had whole-body, patient-centered treatments using manual PHT that focused on restoring mobility and motility to structures affecting reproductive function. Study outcomes measured tubal patency, hormone levels, and pregnancy. The findings revealed a 61% rate of clearing occluded fallopian tubes and a 57% rate of pregnancy. The women with endometriosis had a 43% pregnancy rate. Among women with hormonal dysfunction, the success rate was 49% for lowering elevated levels of follicle stimulating hormone, with a 39% pregnancy rate; and 54% of the women with polycystic ovarian syndrome became pregnant. A 57% pregnancy rate occurred among women who underwent in vitro fertilization after the manual PHT. The authors concluded that manual therapy is an "effective, conservative treatment for women diagnosed as infertile due to mechanical causes, independent of the specific etiology."

Another quasi-experimental (retrospective) study by Okhowat et al. assessed the effectiveness of a deep relaxation massage therapy on invitro fertilization cryo-cycles [52]. Women (n = 267) who received vitrified and warmed blastocysts transfer before embryo transfer participated in the study. The intervention group received a 30-min deep relaxation massage with an oscillating (vibrating) device applied before embryo transfer while the control group did not. The women in the massage therapy group significantly had higher pregnancy rates (58.9% vs. 41.7%, $p < .05$), ongoing pregnancies (53.6% vs. 33.2%, $p < .01$), and birth rates (32.0% vs. 20.3%, $p < .05$) than those in the control group. The women's ages, hormonal substitution protocols, endometrium structures and buildups, quality of transferred embryos, or quality of transfers were not significantly different between the two groups, and no adverse effects occurred in the women who received massage therapy. The authors concluded that receiving massage therapy before blastocyst transfer in a cryo-cycle improves embryo implantation and recommended the use of massage therapy as adjunctive treatment in assisted reproductive technology. The positive outcome was attributed to the reduction in stress level and in uterine contractions, and improvement of blood flow in the abdominal region.

3.8. Gestational diabetes mellitus prevention

A RCT by Harrison et al. investigated the optimal gestational weight gain during early pregnancy among women with higher risk pregnancies [53]. The authors assigned pregnant women (n = 228) at risk of developing gestational diabetes mellitus but receiving standard maternal care to a control (written health information only) or an aerobic exercise program. At 12–15 and 26–28-weeks' gestation period, the women's anthropometric (weight and height), physical activity level (pedometer and International Physical Activity Questionnaire score), risk perception and gestational diabetes mellitus status were monitored. The age and body mass index of the control and intervention groups were similar. At 28 weeks, the gestational weight gain for the control and intervention groups (6.9 ± 3.3 vs. 6.0 ± 2.8 kg) was significantly

($p < 0.05$) different. When the baseline body mass index was stratified, the overweight women in the control group significantly ($p < 0.05$) gained more weight than the overweight women in the intervention group (7.8 ± 3.4 vs. 6.0 ± 2.2 kg); yet in women who are obese, the gestational weight gain was similar in both the control and intervention groups. The physical activity levels declined by the 28 weeks gestation ($p < 0.01$); while the intervention group maintained a 20% higher step count ($p < 0.05$) when compared to the control group (5203 ± 3368 vs. 4140 ± 2420 steps/day). Overall, the gestational diabetes mellitus prevalence rate was 22.8%, with a trend toward fewer cases in the intervention group ($p > .05$). The authors concluded that a low-intensity aerobic exercise program combined with antenatal care promotes healthy gestational weight gain and modulates physical activity decline during early pregnancy. Efficacy in limiting weight gain was highest among women who are overweight and in high-risk women who are ethnically diverse.

A recent RCT by Wang et al. investigated the effects of aerobic exercise on the incidence of gestational diabetes mellitus among pregnant women who are overweight or obese [54]. Singleton women (n = 300) at 10 weeks' gestational age with a pre-pregnancy body mass index of 26.8 ± 2.75 kg/m^2 were assigned randomly to either aerobic exercise or a control group. The women in the exercise group (n = 150) were trained on a cycling ergometer three times per week (at least 30 min/session with a rating of perceived exertion intensity between 12 and 14), while the women in the control group (n = 150) continued their routine daily activities until 37 weeks of gestation. The women in both groups had standard prenatal care. The women in the exercise group had a significantly lower incidence of gestational diabetes mellitus (22% vs. 41%; $p < .001$), fewer gestational weight gain by 25 gestational weeks (4.1 ± 3.0 vs. 5.9 ± 2.58 kg; $p < .001$) and at the end of pregnancy (8.4 ± 3.65 vs. 10.5 ± 3.33 kg; $p < .001$), and reduced insulin resistance levels (2.9 ± 1.27 vs. 3.4 ± 2.00; $p < .05$) at 25 gestational weeks. The aerobic exercise program did not increase the risk of preterm birth nor reduced the mean gestational age at birth.

3.9. Mastectomy complications: lymphedema, pain, and dermatologic adverse events

A RCT by Schmidt et al. investigated the safety and effectiveness of arm crank ergometry in women with lymphedema after axillary lymph node dissection [55]. The women were trained for 12 weeks on the arm crank ergometer twice weekly, and their bioelectrical impedance, arm circumference, muscular strength, quality of life and fatigue were measured and compared with women who received the usual care. The lean body mass and skeletal muscle mass increased and the body fat decreased significantly in the women who trained on the arm crank ergometer. In both groups, the armpit circumference increased substantially during the training period; the increase was higher in the usual care group than the arm crank ergometer group. Similarly, the circumferential measurements obtained in the other regions of the arm decreased significantly in both groups. In both groups, the muscular strength of the upper extremity increased dramatically, with a higher gain obtained in the arm crank ergometer group. The physical functioning, general fatigue and physical fatigue of the women in the arm crank ergometer group improved significantly. In both groups, the investigators found a trend toward improvement in the quality of life, but the gain is not statistically significant. Based on the results, the authors recommended arm crank ergometer training for women with breast cancer following axillary lymph node dissection with the therapeutic goal to improve upper extremity muscle strength, quality of life and reduced arm symptoms.

In 2018, Lee evaluated the effect of Scrambler Therapy (an electrotherapy device use for pain modulation) on the symptoms experienced following breast cancer surgery [56]. A 39-year-old woman after mastectomy had pain and lymphedema of the right upper extremity. She was treated with scrambler therapy for 45 min once a day for 10 days. After 10 sessions of the treatment, the patient pain perception reduced by 6 points on a visual analog pain scale. The patient arm circumference and bioimpedance measurements remained unchanged after 10 treatment sessions. The author concluded that Scrambler Therapy "reduced pain without increased lymphedema."

A quasi-experimental study by Zasadzka et al. in 2018 compared the relative effectiveness of multi-layer compression bandaging and complex decongestive therapy in the treatment of lymphedema [57]. Elderly patients (85 women and 18 men) over 60 years of age with unilateral lower limb lymphedema were recruited and allocated into two groups and treated with complex decongestive therapy (n = 50) and multi-layer compression bandaging (n = 53). The patients' body mass index, and the circumference of the edematous extremities were measured pre-and post-treatment. After 15 treatment sessions, both groups showed a reduction in swelling with a similar decrease in limb volume and circumference, but the multi-layer compression bandaging demonstrated higher efficacy in reducing the limb circumference. The findings in this study suggests that compression bandaging is a treatment of choice in low technology clinical environment because of its low cost and accessibility.

Another quasi-experimental study by Dalenc et al. investigated the effectiveness of hydrotherapy in the management of persistent/long-lasting dermatologic adverse events associated with post-treatment adjuvant therapy and its impact on the quality of life of women with breast cancer [58]. Women with breast cancer but in complete remission after combined standardized (neo) adjuvant chemo, surgical and radiotherapies were assigned into two groups 1–5 weeks post-radiotherapy. The women in the control group (n = 33) received best supportive care while those in the treatment group (n = 35) received three-weeks of hydrotherapy. The women's quality of life, clinical grading of dermatologic adverse events, cancer-related quality of life, dermatologic quality of life and general psychological well-being were monitored. In both groups, significant dermatologic adverse events occurred at the beginning, but the women quality of life (breast, $p < .0001$), systemic therapy side effects ($p < .01$), arm symptoms ($p < .01$), body image ($p < .05$), dermatologic adverse events grading, dermatologic quality of life ($p < .001$) and psychological well-being ($p < .01$) showed significantly greater improvement in the treatment group when compared to the control group. Xerosis (88% of the women at the beginning) completely healed in all the women in the hydrotherapy treatment group. The authors concluded that specific hydrotherapy is an effective supportive care indicated in the management of dermatologic adverse events occurring after early breast cancer therapies.

A systematic review study by Yeung and Semciw evaluated the benefits of hydro (aquatic) therapy in the management of lymphedema by reviewing five electronic databases for RCT which compared aquatic therapy with other lymphedema interventions [59]. In all, six studies met the study criteria; four of them were of moderate quality (average PEDro score 6.5/10) and two of the investigation provided data for inclusion in the meta-analysis. The result revealed there were no significant short-term differences in lymphedema status (measured by lymphedema relative volume) between the women who completed aqua lymphatic therapy compared to land-based standard care (standardized mean difference: 0.14; 95% CI: −0.37 to 0.64, I2 = 0%, p > .59). The authors found low-quality evidence of no significant difference in upper limb physical function (land-based standard care −0.27, 95% CI: −0.78 to 0.23, I2 = 0%, p > .29) between the aqua-lymphatic therapy and standard care. No adverse events were reported in both groups. The authors concluded that aqua lymphatic therapy is not significantly better than standard land-based care in the treatment of the swelling and physical function statuses of women with upper limb lymphedema. To facilitate adherence to treatment, patient preference should guide the choice of treatment.

A recent quasi-experimental study by Duyur et al. compared the long-term effectiveness of complex decongestive therapy used in the treatment of lymphedema [60]. Women with unilateral breast cancer-related lymphedema, (29 women in group one was obese, and 30 women in group two had normal weight or overweight) received manual lymphatic drainage, intermittent pneumatic compression pump, multilayer compression bandaging, lymphedema exercises, and skin care for 1 hour a day, 5 days a week for 3 weeks. The women limb volume was measured before, after and 1 year following complex decongestive therapy. The initial lymphedema volume was 866.3 ± 389.3 mL for the women in group one and 661.8 ± 470.6 mL for the women in group two ($p < 0.05$). The lymphedema severity percentage of the excess volume was 33.4 ± 15.7 for the women in group one and 31.9 ± 19.6 for the women in group two; which was moderate lymphedema. After 15 sessions of therapy, the lymphedema volume of the women in group one decreased to 771.5 ± 389.1 mL ($p < 0.05$), and those in group two also decreased to 468.4 ± 417.4 mL ($p < 0.0001$). Similarly, the percentage of the excess volume of the women in and in group one decreased to 28.5 ± 16.8 ($p < 0.01$), and those in group two declined to 22.1 ± 16.9 ($p < 0.0001$). One-year post-intervention, the volume of the extremities for the women in group one attained the baseline values, but the women in group two maintain the post-treatment volumes of their extremity values. Obesity is a factor known to modulate the efficacy of complex decongestive therapy. Thus, the primary goal in the treatment of breast cancer-related lymphedema is to begin treatment early before the fat accumulation and fibrosis.

Another recent meta-analyses study by Panchik et al. examined the available published research on the effectiveness of aerobic exercise to treat women with, or at risk for breast cancer-related lymphedema [61]. The relevant published articles (n = 807) were retrieved from the major electronic databases, but only 26 of them met the study criteria. The results revealed that conventional aerobic, stretching and resistance exercises, including unconventional exercise approaches such as Yoga, Qigong, and Pilates are safe and effective in the management of the symptoms of the women at risk for and those with breast cancer-related lymphedema. The different forms of exercise improved the women quality of life, body mass index, muscle strength, and mental health and the pain and lymphatic swelling decreased.

4. Discussion

This article provided a comprehensive up to date summary of the outcome research that evaluated the efficacy of PHT in the management of reproductive disorders. The findings summarized in **Table 1** revealed that men's reproductive disorders are understudied. The overwhelming majority (91%) of the 47 studies reviewed found the various PHT modalities evaluated to be effective. The credibility of the articles ranges from "poor" (for the case reports) to "strong" (for the meta-analysis). The PCET used to treat urinary and fecal (anal) incontinence, was the most studied PHT modality, followed by aerobic exercise used for post-partum depression, obesity, gestational diabetes mellitus, and mastectomy complication prevention (**Table 1**). The relevant investigation reviewed indicated that proper instruction and close supervision of the patient are critical for PCET to be effective. At least three systematic reviews and one meta-analysis found PCET to be safe and effective in the management of urinary and fecal incontinence. Based on this strong supporting evidence, it is justified to recommend PCET as a first-line treatment option for the management of voiding dysfunction.

Several of the research reviewed concluded that proper instruction and close supervision of PCET is crucial for the treatment to be effective. The patients who did not improve tend to perform PCET at a low intensity based on their strength. On the other extreme, patients who over work the PFM cause muscle soreness and a decrease in muscle performance; the incontinence may worsen. Therefore, learning the correct protocol [62] is essential for PCET to be effective. Also, the physical therapist must educate the patient to avoid food and drinks that may irritate the bladder and how to change the behaviors that make the symptoms worse by decreasing urinary urge and frequency.

Although the preponderance of the evidence suggests that PCET and transvaginal electrical stimulation are useful for reducing the symptoms of stress UI, data on other adjunctive techniques (EMG biofeedback, and vaginal cones) are less consistent. There is presently no reliable evidence to support the use of PCET in combination with EMG biofeedback and electrical stimulation to relieve overactive bladder and improve sexual function in men. The conflicting findings are because many of the existing studies are heterogeneous in methodology and time frame follow-up; thus, making firm conclusion difficult.

The outcomes of the RCT that evaluated the efficacy of electrical stimulation in the management of stress UI are conflicting [24, 28, 30]. Consequently, there is a need to conduct more RCT with adequate sample sizes and the use of sensitive, reproducible, and valid outcome measures. The optimum electrical parameters for pelvic floor stimulation have not been established currently, but the frequency range of 20–50 Hz is often recommended. The protocol is to apply the electrical stimulation transvaginal for 15–30 min every day at the maximum tolerable intensity for between 4 and 12 weeks.

The use of aerobic exercise to treat post-partum depression, followed by obesity, is the most studied PHT modality followed by the prevention of gestational diabetes mellitus; breast cancer survivor's mental health, sexual dysfunction, lymphedema, pain, and dermatologic adverse events. The evidence for using aerobic exercise as adjunctive treatment in the management of post-partum depression, obesity, and prevention of gestational diabetes is equally convincing; based on positive outcomes from four systematic reviews, two meta-analyses and one RCT [42–47]. The evidence for the use of PHT in the treatment of the mental health, sexual dysfunction, lymphedema, pain, and dermatologic adverse events among women with breast cancer warrant additional systematic reviews and meta-analysis investigations.

Three published RCT [17–19] revealed that when SWD is combined with medication (analgesics and antibiotics), the bimodal treatment is beneficial in the management of PID. Additional RCT with larger sample size, followed by systematic review and meta-analysis investigations are needed to bolster the recommendation to use SWD to treat chronic PID and salpingo-oophoritis.

Two quasi-experimental design study revealed that manual and massage physical modalities hold promise in the management of infertility due to adhesive disease [50, 51]. RCT are urgently needed to substantiate the recommendation. Similarly, the findings from a quasi-experimental study that used fractional carbon dioxide laser therapy to treat vulvovaginal atrophy in postmenopausal women showed great promise [37]. This potentially useful modality is presently underutilized in the treatment of reproductive disorders. Also, the use of TENS in the management of vestibulodynia lacks strong empirical evidence [34–36]. Follow up, RCT are needed to confirm the long-term benefits of fractional carbon dioxide laser therapy on vaginal morphology and for using TENS to treat vulvar pain.

5. Conclusion

This article provided a comprehensive up-to-date review of the relevant studies that evaluated the efficacy of PHT interventions in the management of reproductive disorders. The preponderance of the published research found PHT modalities to be effective. The findings suggest that systematic reviews and meta-analyses are needed to bolster the rationale for recommending PHT in the management of chronic pelvic diseases in women. Similarly, RCT are required to support the recommendation for using PCET, electric stimulation, and EMG biofeedback to treat ejaculatory/orgasmic dysfunction, prostatitis, UI and erectile dysfunction in men. The information in this chapter will be useful to physical therapist students, frontline clinicians, and healthcare policymakers.

Conflict of interest

No conflict of interest to declare.

Author details

Joseph A. Balogun[1,2,3]*

*Address all correspondence to: jbalogun@unimed.edu.ng; jbalogun@csu.edu

1 Research Development and Innovation, University of Medical Sciences, Ondo City, Nigeria

2 Centre of Excellence in Reproductive Health Innovation, University of Benin, Nigeria

3 College of Health Sciences, Chicago State University, USA

References

[1] Mantle J, Haslam J, Barton S. Physiotherapy in Obstetrics and Gynaecology. Elsevier Health Sciences. 2nd ed. Oxford, UK: Butterworth-Heinemann Publishers; 2019

[2] Polden M, Mantle J. Physiotherapy in Obstetrics and Gynecology. Elsevier Health Sciences; Oxford, UK: Butterworth-Heinemann Publishers; 1990

[3] Siegelab AL. Pelvic floor muscle training in males: Practical applications. Urology. 2014;**84**(1): 1-7. Available from: https://www.sciencedirect.com/science/article/pii/S0090429514002738 [Accessed: 25 May 2019]

[4] Rogers G, Story CM. Kegel exercises for men: Do they work? 2016. Available from: https://www.healthline.com/health/kegel-exercises-for-men [Accessed: 25 May 2019]

[5] LaFlamme M, Ellen Ellis M. Prevention of chronic prostatitis. 2016. Available from: https://www.healthline.com/health/chronic-prostatitis [Accessed: 25 May 2019]

[6] Bubnis D, Case L, Goldman C. Exercises to eliminate erectile dysfunction. 2017. Available from: https://www.healthline.com/health/erectile-dysfunction/exercises [Accessed: 25 May 2019]

[7] Pletcher P, Schaefer A. How to last longer in bed. 2015. Available from: https://www.healthline.com/health/mens-health/how-to-last-longer-in-bed [Accessed: 25 May 2019]

[8] Elite Pelvic Rehab. Don't try Kegels until you read this. 2015. Available from: https://elitepelvicrehab.wordpress.com/tag/elite-pelvic-rehab/ [Accessed: 25 May 2019]

[9] Bezner JR. Promoting health and wellness: Implications for physical therapist practice. Physical Therapy. 2015;**95**(1):1433-1444. Available from: https://academic.oup.com/ptj/article/95/10/1433/2686492 [Accessed: 25 May 2019]

[10] Verhagen E, Engbers L. The physical therapist's role in physical activity promotion. British Journal of Sports Medicine. 2009;**43**(2). Available from: https://bjsm.bmj.com/content/43/2/99 [Accessed: 25 May 2019]

[11] American Physical Therapy Association (APTA). Section on Women's Health. 2019. Available from: https://www.womenshealthapta.org/patients/ [Accessed: 25 May 2019]

[12] World Confederation for Physical Therapy (WCPT). Physical therapy and mental health. 2018. Available from: https://www.wcpt.org/sites/wcpt.org/files/files/wptday/18/Booklet/WPTD2018_Booklet_Final.pdf [Accessed: 25 May 2019]

[13] Zimmermann KM. Reproductive system: Facts, functions and disease. Live Science. 2018. Available from: https://www.livescience.com/26741-reproductive-system.html or https://www.newhealthadvisor.com/Female-Reproductive-System-Diseases.html [Accessed: 25 May 2019]

[14] Balogun JA, Okonofua FE. Management of chronic pelvic inflammatory disease with shortwave diathermy. A case report. Physical Therapy. 1988;**68**(10):1541-1545. Available

from: https://www.researchgate.net/publication/20695857_Management_of_Chronic_Pelvic_Inflammatory_Disease_with_Shortwave_Diathermy_A_Case_Report [Accessed: 25 May 2019]

[15] Lamina S, Hanif S. Shortwave in the management of chronic pelvic inflammatory disease: Case reports. Journal of Nigeria Society of Physiotherapy. 2008;**16**(1):31-38. Available from: http://www.jnsp.org/index.php/jnsp/article/viewFile/27/28, https://www.thefreelibrary.com/Shortwave+diathermy+in+the+management+of+chronic+pelvic+inflammatory...-a0190793591 [Accessed: 25 May 2019]

[16] Evseeva CL, Serov VN, Tkachenko NM. Chronic salpingo-oophoritis: Clinical and physiological rationale for therapeutic application of pulse low frequency electro-static field. Vopr Kurortol Lech Fiz Kuit. 2006;**1**:21-24

[17] Lamina S, Hanif S, Gagarawa YS. Short wave diathermy in the symptomatic management of chronic pelvic inflammatory disease pain: A randomized controlled trial. Physiotherapy Research International. 2011;**16**:50-56. © 2010 John Wiley & Sons, Ltd. Available from: http://capenergy.com/assets/files/estudios/52-short-wave-diathermy-in-the-symptomatic.pdf [Accessed: 25 May 2019]

[18] Sonali J, Kaur A, Mitra M. Effect of short-wave diathermy in reducing pain and improving function in patients with pelvic inflammatory diseases. Indian Journal of Physiotherapy and Occupational Therapy. 2015;**9**:20-23. Available from: http://www.indianjournals.com/ijor.aspx?target=ijor:ijpot&volume=9&issue=2&article=005 [Accessed: 25 May 2019]

[19] Saif DS, Fotoh DS, EL Kholy RM, Morsi DI, Farag HM. Combined (physical and medical treatment) therapy versus physical treatment alone and medical treatment alone in the management of chronic pelvic inflammatory disease. Egypt Rheumatology Rehabilitation. 2019;**46**:132. Available from: http://www.err.eg.net/article.asp?issn=1110-161X;year=2019;volume=46;issue=2;spage=132;epage=139;aulast=Saif [Accessed: 25 May 2019]

[20] McLennan MT, Melick CF, Alten B, Young J, Hoehn MR. Patients' knowledge of potential pelvic floor changes associated with pregnancy and delivery. International Urogynecology Journal and Pelvic Floor Dysfunction. 2006;**17**(1):22-26. Available from: https://www.ncbi.nlm.nih.gov/pubmed/16003482 [Accessed: 25 May 2019]

[21] Harvey MA. Pelvic floor exercises during and after pregnancy: A systematic review of their role in preventing pelvic floor dysfunction. Journal of Obstetrics and Gynaecology Canada. 2006;**25**(6):487-498. Available from: https://www.sciencedirect.com/science/article/pii/S1701216316303103?via%3Dihub [Accessed: 25 May 2019]

[22] Vasconcelos M, Lima E, Caiafa L, Noronha A, Cangussu R, Gomes S, et al. Voiding dysfunction in children. Pelvic-floor exercises or biofeedback therapy: A randomized study. Pediatric Nephrology. 2006;**21**(12):1858-1864. Available from: https://link.springer.com/article/10.1007%2Fs00467-006-0277-1 [Accessed: 25 May 2019]

[23] Bø K. Pelvic floor muscle training in the treatment of female stress urinary incontinence, pelvic organ prolapse and sexual dysfunction. World Journal of Urology. 2012;**30**(4):

437-443. Available from: https://link.springer.com/article/10.1007%2Fs00345-011-0779-8 [Accessed: 25 May 2019]

[24] Terlikowski R, Dobrzycka B, Kinalski M, Kuryliszyn-Moskal A, Terlikowski SJ. Transvaginal electrical stimulation with surface-EMG biofeedback in managing stress urinary incontinence in women of premenopausal age: A double-blind, placebo-controlled, randomized clinical trial. International Urogynecology Journal. 2013;**24**(10):1631-1638. Available from: https://www.ncbi.nlm.nih.gov/pmc/articles/PMC3779318/ [Accessed: 25 May 2019]

[25] Park SH, Kang CB, Jang SY, Kim BY. Effect of Kegel exercise to prevent urinary and fecal incontinence in antenatal and postnatal women: Systematic review. Journal of Korean Academy of Nursing. 2013;**43**(3):420-430. Available from: https://www.jkan.or.kr/DOIx.php?id=10.4040/jkan.2013.43.3.420 [Accessed: 25 May 2019]

[26] Homsi C, Ferreira J, Dwyer PL, Davidson M, De Souza A, Alvarez J, et al. Does pelvic floor muscle training improve female sexual function? A systematic review. International Urogynecology Journal. 2015;**26**(12):1735-1750. Available from: https://link.springer.com/article/10.1007/s00192-015-2749-y [Accessed: 25 May 2019]

[27] Adams SR, Dessie SG, Dodge LE, Mckinney JL, Hacker MR, Elkadry EA. Pelvic floor physical therapy as primary treatment of pelvic floor disorders with urinary urgency and frequency-predominant symptoms. Female Pelvic Medicine & Reconstructive Surgery. 2015;**21**(5):252-256

[28] Castellani D, Saldutto P, Galica V, Pace G, Biferi D, Paradiso Galatioto G, et al. Low-dose intravaginal estriol and pelvic floor rehabilitation in post-menopausal stress urinary incontinence. Urologia Internationalis. 2015;**95**(4):417-421. DOI: 10.1159/000381989. Available from: https://www.ncbi.nlm.nih.gov/pubmed/26043913 [Accessed: 25 May 2019]

[29] García-Sánchez E, Rubio-Arias JA, Ávila-Gandía V, Ramos-Campo DJ, López-Román J. The effectiveness of pelvic floor muscle training in treating urinary incontinence in women: A current review. Actas Urológicas Españolas. 2016;**40**(5):271-278. Available from: https://www.ncbi.nlm.nih.gov/pubmed/26614435 [Accessed: 25 May 2019]

[30] Liu L, Zhang Y, Gong J, Chen X, Wu H, Zhu W. Effects of different treatment methods on the clinical and urodynamic state of perimenopausal women with stress urinary incontinence. Iranian Journal of Public Health. 2018;**47**(8):1090-1097

[31] Brotto LA, Bitzer J, Laan E, Leiblum S, Luria M. Women's sexual desire and arousal disorders. Journal of Sexual Medicine. 2010;**7**(1 Pt 2):586-614. 7(2 Pt 1):856. Available from: https://www.ncbi.nlm.nih.gov/pubmed/20092454 [Accessed: 25 May 2019]

[32] Juraskova I, Jarvis S, Mok K, Peate M, Meiser B, Cheah BC, et al. The acceptability, feasibility, and efficacy (phase I/II study) of the OVERcome (Olive Oil, Vaginal Exercise, and MoisturizeR) intervention to improve dyspareunia and alleviate sexual problems in women with breast cancer. Journal of Sexual Medicine. 2013;**10**(10):2549-2558. Available from: https://www.ncbi.nlm.nih.gov/pubmed/23635341 [Accessed: 25 May 2019]

[33] Seav SM, Dominick SA, Stepanyuk B, Gorman JR, Chingos DT, Ehren JL, et al. Management of sexual dysfunction in breast cancer survivors: A systematic review. Womens Midlife Health. 2015;**2**(1):9

[34] Cohen D, Gonzale J, Goldstein I. The role of pelvic floor muscles in male sexual dysfunction and pelvic pain sexual medicine. Review. 2016;**4**(1):53-62. Available from: https://www.sciencedirect.com/science/article/pii/S2050052115000025 [Accessed: 25 May 2019]

[35] Bergeron S, Brown C, Lord MJ, Oala M, Binik YM, Khalifé S. Physical therapy for vulvar vestibulitis syndrome: A retrospective study. Journal of Sex & Marital Therapy. 2002;**28**(3):183-192. Available from: https://www.ncbi.nlm.nih.gov/pubmed/11995597 [Accessed: 25 May 2019]

[36] Murina F, Bianco V, Radici G, Felice R, Di Martino M, Nicolini U. Transcutaneous electrical nerve stimulation to treat vestibulodynia: A randomised controlled trial. BJOG (An International Journal of Obstetrics & Gynaecology). 2008;**115**(9):1165-1170. Available from: https://www.ncbi.nlm.nih.gov/pubmed/18715435 [Accessed: 25 May 2019]

[37] Dionisi B, Anglana F, Inghirami P, Lippa P, Senatori R. Use of transcutaneous electrical stimulation and biofeedback for the treatment of vulvodynia (vulvar vestibular syndrome): Result of 3 years of experience. Minerva Ginecologica. 2008;**60**(6):485-491. Available from: https://www.ncbi.nlm.nih.gov/pubmed/18981976 [Accessed: 25 May 2019]

[38] Dionisi B, Senatori R. Effect of transcutaneous electrical nerve stimulation on the postpartum dyspareunia treatment. Journal of Obstetrics and Gynaecology Research. 2011;**37**(7):750-753. Available from: https://www.ncbi.nlm.nih.gov/pubmed/21395897 [Accessed: 25 May 2019]

[39] Salvatore S, Nappi RE, Zerbinati N, Calligaro A, Ferrero S, Origoni M, et al. A 12-week treatment with fractional CO_2 laser for vulvovaginal atrophy: A pilot study. Climacteric. 2014;**17**(4):363-369. DOI: 10.3109/13697137.2014.899347

[40] Davis SN, Bergeron S, Binik YM, Lambert B. Women with provoked vestibulodynia experience clinically significant reductions in pain regardless of treatment: Results from a 2-year follow-up study. Journal of Sexual Medicine. 2013;**10**(12):3080-3087. Available from: https://www.ncbi.nlm.nih.gov/pubmed/24034424 [Accessed: 25 May 2019]

[41] Brotto LA, Yong P, Smith KB, Sadownik LA. Impact of a multidisciplinary vulvodynia program on sexual functioning and dyspareunia. Journal of Sexual Medicine. 2015;**12**(1):238-247. Available from: https://www.ncbi.nlm.nih.gov/pubmed/25354520 [Accessed: 25 May 2019]

[42] Dennis CL. Treatment of postpartum depression. Part 2: A critical review of nonbiological interventions. The Journal of Clinical Psychiatry. 2004;**65**(9):1252-1265

[43] Dinas PC, Koutedakis Y, Flouris AD. Effects of exercise and physical activity on depression. Irish Journal of Medical Science. 2011;**180**(2):319-325. Available from: https://link.springer.com/article/10.1007%2Fs11845-010-0633-9 [Accessed: 25 May 2019]

[44] Josefsson T, Lindwall M, Archer T. Physical exercise intervention in depressive disorders: Meta-analysis and systematic review. Scandinavian Journal of Medicine & Science in

Sports. 2014;**24**(2):259-272. Available from: https://onlinelibrary.wiley.com/doi/full/10.1111/sms.12050 [Accessed: 25 May 2019]

[45] Kvam S, Kleppe CL, Nordhus IH, Hovland A. Exercise as a treatment for depression: A meta-analysis. Journal of Affective Disorders. 2016;**15**(202):67-86. Available from: https://www.sciencedirect.com/science/article/pii/S0165032715314221?via%3Dihub [Accessed: 25 May 2019]

[46] Saligheh M, Hackett D, Boyce P, Cobley S. Can exercise or physical activity help improve postnatal depression and weight loss? A systematic review. Archives of Women's Mental Health. 2017;**20**(5):595-611. Available from: https://link.springer.com/article/10.1007%2Fs00737-017-0750-9 [Accessed: 25 May 2019]

[47] Wu PL, Lee M, Huang TT. Effectiveness of Physical Activity on Patients with Depression and Parkinson's Disease: A Systematic Review. 2017. Available from: https://journals.plos.org/plosone/article?id=10.1371/journal.pone.0181515 [Accessed: 25 May 2019]

[48] Soucy I, Provencher M, Fortier M, McFadden T. Efficacy of guided self-help behavioural activation and physical activity for depression: A randomized controlled trial. Cognitive Behaviour Therapy. 2017;**46**(6):493-506. Available from: https://www.tandfonline.com/doi/abs/10.1080/16506073.2017.1337806?journalCode=sbeh20 [Accessed: 25 May 2019]

[49] Juvet LK, Elvsaas IKØ, Leivseth G, Anker G, Bertheussen GF, Falkmer U, et al. Rehabilitation of breast cancer patients. In: Report from Norwegian Knowledge Centre for the Health Services. Oslo, Norway: Knowledge Centre for the Health Services at the Norwegian Institute of Public Health, Norwegian Institute of Public Health Systematic Reviews; 2009. p. 02

[50] Cox M, Carmack C, Hughes D, Baum G, Brown J, Jhingran A, et al. Antecedents and mediators of physical activity in endometrial cancer survivors: Increasing physical activity through steps to health. Health Psychology. 2015;**34**(10):1022-1032

[51] Rice AD, Patterson K, Wakefield LB, Reed ED, Breder KP, Wurn BF, et al. Ten-year retrospective study on the efficacy of a manual physical therapy to treat female infertility. Alternative Therapies in Health and Medicine. 2015;**21**(3):36-44

[52] Okhowat J, Murtinger M, Schuff M, Wogatzky J, Spitzer D, Vanderzwalmen P, et al. Massage therapy improves in vitro fertilization outcome in patients undergoing blastocyst transfer in a cryo-cycle. Alternative Therapies in Health and Medicine. 2015;**21**(2):16-22

[53] Harrison CL, Lombard CB, Strauss BJ, Teede HJ. Optimizing healthy gestational weight gain in women at high risk of gestational diabetes: A randomized controlled trial. Obesity (Silver Spring). 2016;**21**(5):904-909

[54] Wang C, Wei Y, Zhang X, Zhang Y, Xu Q, Sun Y, et al. A randomized clinical trial of exercise during pregnancy to prevent gestational diabetes mellitus and improve pregnancy outcome in overweight and obese pregnant women. American Journal of Obstetrics and Gynecology. 2017;**216**(4):340-351

[55] Schmidt T, Berner J, Jonat W, Weisser B, Röcken C, van Mackelenbergh M, et al. Influence of arm crank ergometry on development of lymphedema in breast cancer patients after axillary dissection: A randomized controlled trail. Journal of Rehabilitation Medicine. 2017;**49**(1):78-83

[56] Lee JS. Efficacy of scrambler therapy on breast cancer-related lymphedema. Journal of Physical Therapy Science. 2018;**30**(11):1370-1371

[57] Zasadzka E, Trzmiel T, Kleczewska M, Pawlaczyk M. Comparison of the effectiveness of complex decongestive therapy and compression bandaging as a method of treatment of lymphedema in the elderly. Clinical Interventions in Aging. 2018;**14**(13):929-934

[58] Dalenc F, Ribet V, Rossi AB, Guyonnaud J, Bernard-Marty C, de Lafontan B, et al. Efficacy of a global supportive skin care programme with hydrotherapy after non-metastatic breast cancer treatment: A randomised, controlled study. European Journal of Cancer Care. 2018;**27**(1)

[59] Yeung W, Semciw AI. Aquatic therapy for people with lymphedema: A systematic review and meta-analysis. Lymphatic Research and Biology. 2018;**16**(1):9-19

[60] Duyur Cakıt B, Pervane Vural S, Ayhan FF. Complex decongestive therapy in breast cancer-related lymphedema: Does obesity affect the outcome negatively? Lymphatic Research and Biology. 2019;**17**(1):45-50

[61] Panchik D, Masco S, Zinnikas P, Hillriegel B, Lauder T, Suttmann E, et al. Effect of exercise on breast cancer-related lymphedema: What the lymphatic surgeon needs to know. Journal of Reconstructive Microsurgery. 2019;**35**(1):37-45

[62] Rogers G, Story CM. Kegel exercises for men: Do they work? 2016. Available from: https://www.healthline.com/health/kegel-exercises-for-men [Accessed: 5 May 2019]

Section 2

Musculoskeletal Rehabilitation with Physical Therapy Approaches

Chapter 3

Whole-Body Vibration Exercise as an Intervention to Improve Musculoskeletal Performance

Danúbia da Cunha de Sá-Caputo, Redha Taiar and Mario Bernardo-Filho

Additional information is available at the end of the chapter

http://dx.doi.org/10.5772/intechopen.89372

Abstract

The exposure of individuals to mechanical vibrations produced in vibrating platform can generate whole-body vibration (WBV) exercise. This modality of exercise represents a less tiring alternative to sport, which could benefit mechanical human behavior and prevent sports injuries and musculoskeletal disorders. The specificity of the human body, articulated and connected segments, requires to take into account the biomechanical parameters in protocols involving WBV exercise. Moreover, work time, rest time between the bouts in each session number of sessions, extension of the intervention, and week periodicity must be also well established. Responses to WBV exercise are observed at musculoskeletal, neurological, endocrinological and vascular levels. With respect to the musculoskeletal level, it is verified increase of muscle strength, endurance and power, improvement of the balance, increase of bone mineral density and the decrease of risk of falls. There are several tools to evaluate the responses of the body to WBV exercise. The aim of this chapter is to highlight the relevance of the WBV exercise as an intervention of the physical therapy for the better human optimization.

Keywords: whole-body vibration, human movement analysis, musculoskeletal performance, vibrating platform, clinical effects, biomechanics

1. Introduction

The exposure of individuals to mechanical vibrations produced in vibrating platform can generate whole-body vibration (WBV) exercise when the referred physical agent is transmitted to body of a person that is in contact with the platform. This modality of exercise represents

IntechOpen

© 2019 The Author(s). Licensee IntechOpen. This chapter is distributed under the terms of the Creative Commons Attribution License (http://creativecommons.org/licenses/by/3.0), which permits unrestricted use, distribution, and reproduction in any medium, provided the original work is properly cited. (cc) BY

a less tiring alternative to sport, that could benefit mechanical human behavior and prevent sports injuries, and musculoskeletal disorders [1, 2].

Although, the intervention with WBV is not recent, the way as this procedure is used nowadays, it started in the Soviet Union in the last century to the rehabilitation of astronauts after traveling outside the Earth. In comparison with the astronauts that remained in the Earth, the microgravity or zero gravity has contributed to lead to lack of muscle and bone mass [3]. Unfortunately some conditions in the daily life mimics the microgravity or zero gravity, such as, individuals that (i) have a disease and must be on bed for long time, or (ii) are sedentary and are not stimulated to perform a minimal of physical activity, or (iii) are immobilized due to an accident or (iv) have disability due to muscular or neurological conditions and must be on wheelchair or on bed. Considering these conditions, there is a common finding, that is, the lack of mechanical vibration added to the body. In general, in several simple daily activities, such as walking or running, or practicing sports, as biking, or driving a car, or being in a public transportation, mechanical vibrations are added to the body [1–4].

Naturally, depending on the occupational activity, the individual is also exposed to mechanical vibrations, as the driver of a bus or a truck or an agricultural tractor, the operator of a stone crusher or a drilling machine. These conditions must be also better studied because they might be dangerous to the professionals. Although, these considerations are relevant and must be pointed out due to elevate intensity of the mechanical vibration that can be transmitted to the body of the individual [1, 5, 6].

And, when people cannot do or are not stimulated to perform an activity to add mechanical vibrations to body through a physical activity? There is a simple answer. The individual can be exposed to mechanical vibrations produced in a vibrating platform.

2. Vibrating platform

Considering the movement of the base of the vibrating platform, there are three main types available commercially, as it is illustrated in **Figure 1**. **Figure 1A** represents the vertical vibrating platform, that can be synchronous or triplanar. In the synchronous, the base oscillating uniformly up and down, while in the triplanar, the vibration is applied in anterior/posterior, side to side, and up and down directions. **Figure 1B** shows the side-alternating platform, in which there is reciprocating vertical displacements on the left and right side in relation to a fulcrum, like to a teeterboard. **Figure 1C** indicates the horizontal vibrating platform, in which the base presents movement anterior/posterior alternatively [1, 4, 7].

The mechanical vibration produced in the vibrating platform presents an oscillatory, sinusoidal and deterministic displacement in relation to an equilibrium position. These characteristics are highly desirable and permit the use of this vibratory stimulus in controlled conditions in interventions in health and fitness areas. Nevertheless, the specificity of the human body, articulated and connected segments, requires us to take into account the comportment of biomechanical parameters in protocols involving WBV exercise such as frequency, peak-to-peak displacement and peak acceleration [1, 8].

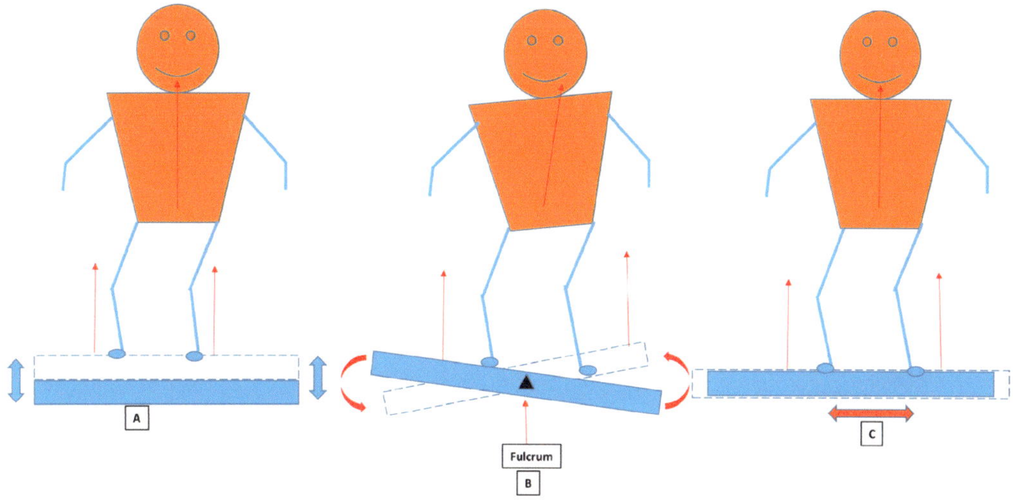

Figure 1. The main available types of vibrating platform: (A) represents the vertical, (B) side alternating and (C) horizontal vibrating platform. The red arrows indicate the movement of the base.

3. Biomechanical parameters of mechanical vibrations

Figure 2 illustrates the displacement of a sinusoidal mechanical vibration and some biomechanical parameters are indicated. It is possible to verify the displacement along of the time in an equilibrium position. The displacement between two successive points, as indicated by the arrows, is defined as the cycle, which is dimensionless parameter. The number of the cycles in the unit of time is the frequency. If it is considered 1 second, the frequency will express in Hertz (Hz) or s^{-1}. It is possible to verify that the displacement of the mechanical vibration has a highest and a lowest peak. This parameter is the peak-to-peak displacement that is measured, for example, in mm. In it, it is found the maximal rate of change in velocity during a cycle. Moreover, it is used to characterize the intensity of the exposition of the magnitude effect. In the highest peak, the highest acceleration, that is, the peak acceleration, measured in m/s^2, or in number of the Earth acceleration (×g) is found. These biomechanical parameters (frequency, peak-to-peak displacement and peak acceleration) are strongly relevant, due to, an individual that is in a vibrating platform will be submitted to them [1, 8].

In **Table 1**, additional information about the biomechanical is indicated of a sinusoidal mechanical vibration.

In addition, some studies with WBV exercise involve also combination intervention with other types of exercises, as the maximal voluntary contraction (MVC). Moreover, the individual can be standing in static position on performing dynamic exercises [9, 10].

Besides the biomechanical parameters, the work and rest time between the bouts in each session, number of sessions, extension of the intervention, week periodicity must be also well established. The biological responses to WBV exercise also depending on these parameters [1, 2, 7].

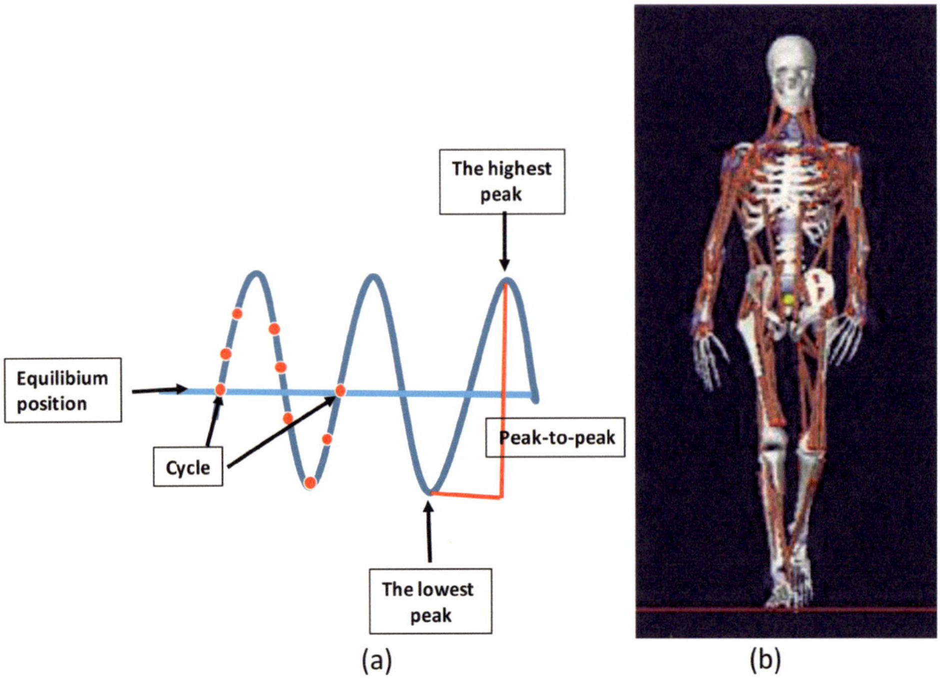

Figure 2. Illustration of a sinusoidal mechanical vibration (a) and articulated human movements (b).

Parameter	Definition	Symbol	Unity (IS)	Formula	Comment
Cycle	Displacement between two sucessive points in the vibration	-	-	-	With repetition of the same characteristics
Frequency	Repetition rate of the cycle	*F*, *v*	Hz (s^{-1})	-	-
Peak-to-peak displacement (Synonymous to peak-to-peak amplitude)	Displacement between the lowest and the highest point of the cycle	*D*	mm	-	Perpendicular distance between the lowest and the highest point of the cycle
Amplitude (Synonymous to Peak Amplitude)	Maximal displacement from the equilibrium position	*A*	mm	A=D/2	-
Peak Acceleration	Maximal rate of change in velocity during a cycle (magnitude effect)	aPeak	$m.s^{-2}$	$aPeak=2x\pi^2xf^2xD$	Often expressed as multiples of Earth's gravity*

*Earth's gravity (commonly symbol: g) is a constant (9.81 ms^{-2}) denotes the nominal acceleration due to gravity at the Earth's surface at sea level (adapted from Rauch et al, 2010 [8])

Table 1. Biomechanical parameters of a sinusoidal mechanical vibration.

4. Biological responses and tools used to evaluate musculoskeletal responses to the WBV

Responses to WBV exercise are observed at musculoskeletal, neurological, endocrinological and vascular levels. In general, related to the musculoskeletal level, increase of muscle strength and of the bone mineral density, endurance and power, improvement of the balance and the decrease of risk of falls have been reported in trained and untrained individuals. These findings can contribute to decrease the possibility of injury, as in the sports, in the improvement of the fitness and on the management of various diseases. WBV exercise can produce beneficial responses, including improvements in muscle strength in trained (athletes) and untrained individuals and in patients with several clinical conditions, such as, chronic obstructive pulmonary disease (COPD), Parkinson's disease (PD), metabolic syndrome (MetS), fibromyalgia (FM) and multiple sclerosis (MS) [11–15]. Moreover, improvements in the walking function, the bone mineral density (BMD) in elderly, the low back pain (LBP), health-related quality of life (QOL), fall risk, balance and gait have been described [1, 7, 16–20].

Considering the musculoskeletal responses to the WBV exercise, several tools have been used in the evaluations, such as the flexibility, the level of pain, rating of perceived effort, recruitment of muscle fibers using electromyography (EMG), infrared thermography (IRT), various Questionnaires and scales and, the human movement analysis [12, 14, 18–21, 23, 24]. These tools can be used by the physiotherapist. Some publications about the WBV exercise responses in various populations and the tools utilized are presented in this chapter. Approaches in rehabilitation considering individuals with several diseases and approaches in healthy (trained and untrained) related to the fitness and wellbeing are discussed.

4.1. Approaches of the whole-body vibration in rehabilitation

Abbasi et al. [19], evaluated the WBV effects (6-week) training on the strength and endurance of core muscles in MS individuals, that were divided in intervention (WBV-G) and no intervention (control-G) groups. Sorensen, flexion, and side bridge endurance tests were used to evaluate the endurance (core muscles), the strength with a dynamometer and the QOL aspects with the quality of life-54 questionnaire (MSQOL-54). The strength, endurance (core muscles) and the MSQOL-54 scores significantly improved in WBV group in comparison to control-G. While the within-group comparison showed significant improvement in the WBV-G, in the control-G, physical and mental components of MSQOL-54 impaired over the investigation. It was concluded that strength and endurance of core muscles as well as QOL of MS patients can be positively influenced by a 6-week WBV training.

Krause et al. [15], investigated if WBV might attenuate the processing functional and neuromuscular degeneration of postural control in MS individuals. Performance in postural control was assessed before and after 6 weeks of a control group (CG) and a WBV intervention period. The center of pressure displacement (COP), muscle activity and co-contraction indices of muscles soleus (SOL), gastrocnemius medialis (GM), tibialis anterior (TA), biceps (BF) and rectus femoris (RF) as well as SOL H/M-ratios were evaluated. In the CG, it was verified that COP enhanced with reduced muscle activity in RF and diminished shank muscle co-contraction. No alterations were found in COP and neuromuscular control after WBV. However, over time, TA activity was diminished, with no changes in muscle activation of SOL, GM and BF or H/M-ratios. It was concluded that in the CG, MS patients experienced substantial deteriorations in postural control which have previously been associated with greater postural instability. No further disease-associated deteriorations were observed following the intervention. Thus, WBV might alleviate neurodegeneration of postural control in people with MS. Abbasi et al. [19] also pointed out that the WBV program was well-tolerated by patients and no adverse event was observed.

Pin et al. [16], in a pilot study examined the feasibility and tolerance of WBV intervention for children and adults with moderate severity of cerebral palsy (CP) being graded as levels III or IV on the Gross Motor Function Classification Scale (GMFCS). Individuals received WBV intervention when standing still on the vibrating platform for three 3-min bouts of vibration (20 Hz, 2 mm amplitude), 4 days/week for 4 weeks. It was carried out assessment at baseline and completion of the intervention included the Gross Motor Function Measure-66 Item Set (GMFM-66 IS), 2-min walk test (2MWT), Timed Up and Go test (TUG) and Pediatric Evaluation of Disability Inventory (PEDI). Fourteen participants (GMFCS level III n = 13, 92%) completed the study. It was concluded that WBV training protocol was feasible, safe and well-tolerated by the individuals with moderate severity of CP, justifying future investigations with larger samples and more rigorous study design. It is also informed that, in this study, the attendance rate was over 90% with no adverse events. All participants tolerated the protocol which was satisfactorily delivered in a clinical setting.

Haas et al. [12] pointed out that is well known that applying vibrations to men influences multiple physiological functions and analyzed post effects of WBV on motor symptoms in PD. They were randomly subdivided into WBV-G and CG. Motor symptoms were assessed by the UPDRS (Unified Parkinson's Disease Rating Scale) motor score. The intervention was with five series of WBV (60 seconds each). On average a significant improvement of 16.8% in the UPDRS motor score was found in the WBV-G. Only marginal changes ($p > 0.05$) were found in the CG. The cross-over procedure showed comparable treatment effects (14.7% improvement after intervention). Considering different symptom clusters, only small changes were observed in limb akinesia and cranial symptoms. Tremor (25%) and rigidity (24%) scores were improved. It was concluded that, considering the structure of symptom changes, it is unlikely that these findings are explainable on peripheral sensory level, exclusively. In addition, considering the results of other investigations one can suppose about alterations in activation of the supplementary motor area and in neurotransmitter functions.

Lee et al. [7] evaluated the effect of WBV in the horizontal direction on balance and gait ability in chronic stroke (CS) survivors, that were randomly allocated into two groups (WBV-G) and CG. In the WBV-G, WBV training in the horizontal direction was conducted for 6 weeks, and a conventional rehabilitation for 30 min, 3 days per week for a 6-week period, was conducted in WBV-G and CG. Outcome variables included the static balance and gait ability measured before training and after 6 weeks. On comparing the outcome variables before and after training in the WBV-G, significant differences were observed in the cadence and single support time of gait ability. However, there were no significant differences in other variables, including velocity, step length, stride length, and double support time. In addition, after training, no significant differences in all variables were observed between the two groups. The results suggest that WBV training in the horizontal direction has few positive effects on balance and gait function in CS survivors.

Huang et al. [22] studied the influence of WBV intervention frequency, amplitude, and body posture on lower limb muscle activation among people with CS. It was also evaluated whether the EMG response to vibration stimulus differed between paretic and non-paretic side and the relationship between muscle activation and WBV transmission. Individuals with CS performed three different exercises on the WBV vertical vibrating platform with various vibration conditions (frequency: 20, 30, 40 Hz; amplitude: 0.8, 1.5 mm), or without vibration. Muscle activity in bilateral vastus medialis (VM), medial hamstrings (MH), TA, and GM was measured by surface EMG. Tri-axial accelerometers were used to measure the acceleration at the platform and bilateral hips and knees. Muscle activity was significantly greater in the bilateral GM, TA, and MH, but not VM, compared with the same exercises without WBV. A great augmentation of muscle activation was observed with WBV with higher amplitude or higher frequency. Leg muscle activation was affected by the body posture. Considering paretic and non-paretic sides, WBV-induced muscle activation was largely similar, except to the TA. The lower WBV transmissibility (measured at the more proximal joints) was related to greater WBV-induced leg muscle activation. It was concluded that adding WBV to exercise significantly increased muscle activation in the GM, TA, and MH on both the paretic and non-paretic sides of CS survivors, and the increase was dependent on the WBV amplitude, frequency, and body posture.

Zheng et al. [18] verified effects of WBV exercise on lumbar proprioception in nonspecific low back pain (LBP) patients that performed an exercise 3 times a week for a total of 12 weeks of WBV exercise. The lumbar proprioception was measured by joint position sense. Outcomes were lumbar angle deviation and visual analogue scale (VAS) score. After the 12-week WBV exercise, lumbar flexion angle deviation was reduced from $3.65 \pm 2.26°$ to 1.90 ± 1.07, and extension angle deviation was reduced from $3.06 \pm 1.85°$ to 1.61 ± 0.75, significantly lower than baseline. After participating in the 12-week WBV exercise, a significant pain reduction was observed. Men in the whole group indicated significantly lower angle deviations in flexion and extension, whereas women indicated significantly lower flexion angle deviation, and no significant difference was found in extension angle deviation. However, by subdividing the entire group into poor and good proprioceptive groups, WBV exercise presented significant enhancement of lumbar proprioceptive ability in the poor flexion proprioception subgroup, poor extension proprioception subgroup, and good extension proprioception subgroup, but not in the subgroup with good flexion proprioceptive ability. It was concluded that lumbar flexion and extension proprioception as measured by joint position sense was significantly enhanced and pain was significantly reduced after 12-week WBV exercise in nonspecific LBP patients. However, the participants with good flexion proprioceptive ability had limited proprioceptive enhancement.

Kim et al. [21] assessed the effect of a 12-week horizontal vibration exercise (HVE) in chronic (LBP) patients as compared to vertical vibration exercise (VVE). Individuals were assigned to the HVE or VVE groups and they performed the intervention (according each group) for 30 min each day, three times a week, for 12 weeks. The level of pain (VAS) and the functionality (Oswestry Disability Index—ODI) were evaluated. The lumbar muscle strength (isokinetic dynamometer), transverse abdominis (TrA) and multifidus muscle thicknesses (ultrasonography), and standing balance (balance parameters) were determined prior to treatment, 6 and 12 weeks after the first treatment, and 4 weeks after the end of treatment (that is, 16 weeks after the first treatment). Significant improvements with time on VAS, ODI, standing balance score, lumbar flexor, and extensor muscle strength without any significant changes in TrA or multifidus muscle thickness were found. No significant differences between HVE and VVE groups according to time in any of the assessments were observed. It is concluded that HVE is as effective as VVE in reducing pain, strengthening the lumbar muscle, and improving the balance and functional abilities of chronic LBP patients. Vibrational exercise increases muscle strength without inducing muscle hypertrophy. Moreover, it was pointed out no adverse events during treatment in either group.

Wang et al. [25] studied effects of WBV exercise for pain intensity and functional disability in individuals with non-specific chronic LBP in a single-blind randomized controlled trial that were randomly allocated to either the intervention group or the CG. The intervention group received WBV exercises and the CG general exercise protocol three times a week for 12 weeks. The pain level (VAS) and functional disability (ODI) were measured. Lumbar joint position sense, QOL (Short Form Health Survey 36) and overall treatment effect (Global Perceived Effect—GPE) were also verified. After the interventions (12 weeks), compared with the CG, the mean VAS and ODI scores significantly decreased by additional 1 point (95% confidence interval (CI) = −1.22 to −0.78), 3.81 point (95% CI, −4.98, −2.63) based on adjusted analysis in the intervention group (WBV exercise). The intervention group provided additional beneficial effects for in terms of lumbar joint position sense, QOL, and GPE. It was concluded that WBV exercise could provide more benefits than general exercise for relieving pain and improving functional disability in patients with non-specific chronic LBP.

Tantawy et al. [26] investigated the effect of WBV exercise on stress urinary incontinence (SUI) after prostate cancer surgery. Individuals with mild SUI after radical prostatectomy were divided in Group 1, who performed pelvic floor muscle training (PFMT) and WBV exercise with a frequency and amplitude of 20 Hz/2 mm for the first two sessions and 40 Hz/4 mm for the rest of the intervention, and Group 2, who performed PFMT training alone. The interventions were conducted three times per week for 4 weeks (both groups). Incontinence VAS (I-VAS) score, International Consultation on Incontinence Questionnaire-Urinary Incontinence-Short Form (ICIQ-UI-SF) score and 24-hour pad test result (24HPT). I-VAS score, ICIQ-UI-SF score and 24HPT results showed significant within-group differences at each assessment (exception of the baseline and post-intervention I-VAS score in Group 2). Group 1 I-VAS score had a median difference of 3.9 cm [95% CI −4.0 to −3.8] from baseline to first follow-up, and a median difference of −2.0 cm (95% CI −2.2 to −1.8) at 4-week follow-up. After 4 weeks of intervention and at follow-up for all measured parameters, comparisons between the groups demonstrated significant differences favoring the Group 1. In conclusion, WBV exercise was an effective modality for treating patients with SUI after prostatectomy.

Sá-Caputo et al. [13] assessed effects of WBV exercise on functional parameters of MetS individuals. The biomechanical parameters of the mechanical vibration were frequency (from 5 up to 14 Hz) and the peak-to-peak displacements (from 2.5 up to 7.5 mm). In each session the individuals performed 1 min-bout of working time with 1 min-bout of passive rest in the peak-to-peak displacements for three-times. The WBV exercise protocol was applied twice per week for 5 weeks. Anterior trunk flexion, gait speed, sit-to-stand test and handgrip strength were investigated. Physiological parameters, as blood pressure and heart rate (HR) were also determined. No significant changes were observed in physiological parameters (arterial blood pressure and HR). Significant improvements were found in trunk flexion, gait speed, sit-to-stand test and handgrip strength after the WBV exercise: It was concluded that WBVE may induce biological responses that improve functional parameters in participants with MetS without interfering in physiological parameters, comparing before and after a 5-week WBV exercise.

Rigamonti et al. [9] evaluated the exercise-induced responses in Growth hormone (GH) isoforms in obese subjects. The acute effects of WBV exercise or maximal voluntary contraction (MVC) alone and the combination of MVC with WBV exercise (MVC + WBVE) on circulating levels of 22 and 20 kDa-GH were evaluated. Considering the stimulation of 22 and 20 kDa-GH secretion, it was found that MVC alone or combined with WBV exercise was significantly effective, but WBV exercise alone was ineffective. Related to the 22 and 20 kDa-GH peaks, after MVC + WBVE and MVC higher values were found in comparison with WBV exercise alone. Moreover, only 22 kDa-GH peak was significantly higher after MVC + WBV than MVC. In addition, the ratio of circulating levels of 22–20 kDa-GH was constant throughout the time window of evaluation after exercise and similar among the three protocols of exercise. It is suggested that the MVC, alone and in combination with WBV exercise stimulated 22 and 20 kDa-GH secretion in obese individuals. Since the ratio of 22–20 kDa-GH is constant after exercise and independent from the interventions in normal-weight subjects; hyposomatotropism (GH deficiency) in obesity does not seem to depend on an unbalance of circulating GH isoforms.

Yang et al. [20] evaluated the effects of WBV exercise on reducing risk of slip-related falls in obese individuals that were randomly assigned in vibration or placebo groups. They received 6-week vibration and placebo intervention on a side-alternating vibrating platform, respectively. Before and after the intervention, isometric knee extensors strength capacity was measured. The individuals (both groups) were also exposed to a standardized slip induced by a treadmill during gait prior to and following the intervention. Dynamic stability (DS) and fall incidences responding to the slip were also evaluated. WBV exercise significantly augmented the muscle strength and improved DS control at recovery touchdown after the slip occurrence. The improved DS could be associated with the enhanced trunk segment movement control, which may be related to the strength increment caused by the WBV exercise. The decrease of the fall rates from the pre-training slip to the post-training slip was greater among the whole-body vibration group than the placebo group (45 vs. 25%). It was concluded that vibration-based training could be a promising alternative or additional modality to active exercise-based fall prevention programs for people with obesity.

Pleguezuelos et al. [11] evaluated cardiac, metabolic, and ventilatory changes during the WBV exercise with three different frequencies in individuals with COPD in a prospective, interventional trial. They completed three sessions of WBV exercise in a vertical platform once a week using frequencies of 35, 25 Hz and no vibration in isometric squatting position. Cardiac, metabolic, and ventilator parameters were monitored (ergospirometer) during the sessions. Changes in oxygen pulse response (VO_2/HR) at the used frequencies were the primary outcome. Compared to the reference of 35 Hz, VO_2/HR at no vibration was 10.7% lower. No significant differences were observed on the comparison between the frequencies of 35 and 25 Hz. The median oxygen uptake (VO_2) was significantly lower 9.43% (25 Hz) and 13.9% (no vibration) in comparison to that was obtained at 35 Hz. The median expiratory volume without vibration was 9.43% significantly lower than the VO_2 at the end of the assessment at 35 Hz vibration. It was concluded that vertical WBV exercise sessions show greater cardiac, metabolic, and respiratory responses compared with the squat position. On comparing the two frequencies used, it was observed that the frequency of 35 Hz provides higher cardiorespiratory adaptation.

Ribeiro et al. [14] characterized the intensity of the WBV stimulation in women diagnosed with FM compared to a CG of healthy women (HW). It was investigated the effect of a single session of WBV intervention on inflammatory responses and the levels of adipokines, soluble tumor necrosis factor receptors (sTNFr1, sTNFr2), and brain-derived neurotrophic factor (BDNF) were determined. Oxygen consumption (VO_2) was estimated (portable gas analysis system), HR was measured (HR monitor), and perceived exertion (RPE) was evaluated (Borg scale of perceived exertion). Acutely mild WBV increased VO_2 and HR similarly in both groups. There was an interaction (disease versus vibration) in RPE, showing a significant higher RPE in FM compared to HW at rest, which further increased in FM after acute WBV, whereas it remained unchanged in HW. A significant interaction (disease vs. vibration) on plasma levels of adiponectin, sTNFR1, sTNFR2, leptin, resistin, and BDNF was found. It was concluded that a single acute session of mild and short WBV can improve the inflammatory status in FM individuals, reaching values close to those of HW at their basal status. Probably, it is possible to speculate that neuroendocrine mechanism seems to be an exercise-induced modulation towards greater adaptation to stress response in these evaluated individuals.

Lai et al. [17] investigated the effect of high-frequency and high-magnitude WBV on the BMD of the lumbar spine in postmenopausal women that were randomized in a WBV group or a CG for a trial of 6 months. The WBV exercise group was exposed to 30 Hz high-frequency and 3.2 g high-magnitude WBV, in a full-standing posture for 5 min, three times per week. The measurement of the lumbar BMD of the two groups before and after the intervention was with dual-energy X-ray absorptiometry. The BMD of the WBV group had significantly increased by 2.032%, while that of the CG had decreased by 0.046% 6 months later. The comparison between the CG and WBV exercise group revealed that the BMD of the WBV exercise group increased significantly. It was concluded that 6 months of high-frequency and high-magnitude WBV yielded significant benefits to the BMD of the lumbar spine in postmenopausal women, and could therefore be provided as an alternative exercise.

4.2. Approaches of the whole-body vibration in fitness of trained and untrained individuals

Chen et al. [27] evaluated how WBV exercise and their interactions influence core muscle activity in healthy young adults. The activities of muscle multifidi (MM), rectus abdominis muscle (RM), erector spinae (ES), abdominis obliquus externus (AOE), and abdominis obliquus internus (AOI) were measured through surface EMG while participants were performing four different exercise forms under three WBV conditions in a vibrating platform generating vertical vibration (condition 1:5 Hz, 2 mm; condition 2: 10 Hz, 2 mm; and condition 3: 15 Hz, 2 mm) and a no-WBV condition in single experimental sessions. WBV frequency of 15 Hz was the best vibration stimulation for core muscles in all the exercises. Single bridge is a better exercise for RM and AOE compared with other exercises, and crunches was the best exercise for MM, AOI, and ES. Significant interaction effect was observed in different frequencies and exercises except for AOI. It is concluded that high vibration frequencies can lead to enhanced exercise benefits within an appropriate frequency range, and different exercises have diverse effects on various muscles.

Oliveira et al. [10] considered that mechanical vibration is a common neuromuscular training technique used in sports training programs to generate acute increases in muscle strength and compared the individual optimal vibration frequency (IOVF) identified by EMG activity and force production in strength training in well-trained volunteers. They performed a familiarization and two interventions sessions, which included MVC (five) of the elbow flexors with a duration of 10 seconds and 5-min intervals between each MVC. Firstly, MVC was performed without mechanical vibration followed by four MVC (randomized) with application of mechanical vibration in the direction of the resultant muscle forces' vector (VDF) or WBV exercise using different frequencies (10, 20, 30, or 40 Hz). Consequently, the mechanical vibration stimulus was superimposed during the MVC. Individual optimal mechanical vibration frequency (identified by EMG) did not coincide with IOVF (identified by force production). Low agreement was observed between the vibration frequencies in generating the higher EMG activity, maximal force, and root mean square of force. These results indicate that the magnitude of the mechanical vibratory stimulus response might be individualized. In conclusion, if the objective is to use acute mechanical vibration in conjunction with strength training, a preliminary mechanical vibration exposure should be performed to determine the individualized mechanical vibratory stimulus of the individual, and, in consequence, the training effects can be optimized.

Moreira-Marconi et al. [23] evaluated the behavior of the skin temperature (Tsk) on regions of the lower limbs from an acute bout of WBV exercise. Using IRT, Tsk and thermal symmetry of the posterior lower extremities (thigh, knee, calf and heel) were examined in healthy participants. IRT was assessed during 60-second WBV exercise (exposures of 0, 30 and 50 Hz generated in a vertical vibrating platform). From the adjusted linear mixed effects model, mechanical vibration frequency, time and regions of the lower extremity were significant. But, as the variable laterality was not significant and it was excluded from the adjusted statistical model. It was verified that the adjusted model was significant and all variables in the model were significant. This indicates that Tsk decreases with the time, independently of the mechanical vibration frequency. The mathematical model of the current study may be useful to justify the patterns observed for all vibration frequencies between and 0 and 50 Hz. It was concluded that the acute exposure of 60-second mechanical vibration has influence on the behavior of Tsk of the posterior region of the lower limbs. Probably, this would be likely associated with a decrease on the blood flow due to WBV exercise. Moreover, it is possible to speculate that during WBV exercise a greater supply of blood would be required where the body responds by shunting blood flow from the skin to working muscle, at least, in the first seconds of the WBV exercise.

Karim et al. [28] examined the immediate effect of WBV exercise on first position sauté height, and on static and dynamic balance professional contemporary dancers. Following instruction, a warm-up, and a training session, participants received a 75-second randomly assigned WBV intervention under four conditions: static demi-plié (0 Hz), static demi-plié (30 Hz), dynamic demi-plié (0 Hz), and dynamic demi-plié (30 Hz). Before and immediately after intervention, participants performed three sautés on the Just Jump® Mat System, provided dynamic balance data via the Star Excursion Balance Test, and static balance data via the Balance Error Scoring System. Dancers from the static first position demi-plié group were found to jump higher than those from the dynamic first position demi-plié group, regardless of WBV frequency. The 30 Hz frequency resulted in significantly improved static balance for both static and dynamic demi-plié. Therefore, the use of WBV exercise is worthy of consideration as a quick method of improving static balance, and use of the static first position demi-plié may be beneficial for improving sauté height.

Wallmann et al. [24] evaluated acute effects of WBV exercise on vertical jump, power, balance, and agility for untrained individuals (who are not collegiate or professional athletes). They were assessed for vertical jump height and power (Myotest accelerometer), balance (NeuroCom Balance Master System), and agility (modified T-test). Each session consisted of (i) five-minutes treadmill warm-up, (ii) practice test, (iii) baseline measurement, (iv) two-minute rest period, (v) WBV exercise at 2 mm and 30 Hz for 60 seconds, and (vi) final measurement. Three different counterbalanced testing sessions were spaced by a minimum of 48 hours between sessions aiming to minimize fatigue. Significant differences were found for both genders for main effect of time for Agility; end point excursion Left; and maximum endpoint excursion Left. Differences for main effect of gender showed females performed better than males in: end point excursion Right; end point excursion Left; maximum endpoint excursion Right; and maximum endpoint excursion Left. Considering the males, they performed better than females in Agility and Power. It was verified a significant interaction between time and gender for vertical jump. Simple main effects showed males jumped higher than females during both pre and post intervention. Females had an important and significant decrease in the vertical jump post intervention. It is concluded that WBV, acutely, would produce significant differences in the main effect of time and agility, and end point and maximum end point excursion Left for both genders. Furthermore, females performed better in balance compared to males and poorer in vertical jump, but males performed better in agility and power.

Zaidell et al. [29] characterized the acceleration transmission and neuromuscular responses to rotational vibration (RV) and vertical vibration (VV) at different frequencies and amplitudes.

Individuals finished two experimental trials (RV versus VV) in which mechanical vibration was delivered during either squatting (30°; RV versus VV) or standing (RV only) with frequencies of 20, 25, and 30 Hz, at peak-to-peak displacement of 1.5 and 3.0 mm. Vibration-induced accelerations were measured with triaxial accelerometers on base of the vibrating platform and bony landmarks at ankle, knee, and lumbar spine. At all frequency/peak-to-peak displacement combinations, accelerations at the ankle were greater during RV with the greatest difference verified at 30 Hz, 1.5 mm. Transmission of RV was also significantly influenced by body posture (standing versus squatting). Irrespective of mechanical vibration type, mechanical vibration transmission to all studied bony landmarks was generally greater at higher peak-to-peak displacement but not at higher frequencies. This was verified mainly above the ankle joint. Acceleration at the lumbar spine increased with greater vibration peak-to-peak displacement but not frequency and was highest with RV during standing. It was concluded that the transmission of the mechanical vibration during WBV is dependent on intensity and direction of mechanical vibration as well as on the body posture. For targeted mechanical vibration loading at the lumbar spine, RV of higher peak-to-peak displacement and lower frequency mechanical vibration while standing is suggested. These findings will contribute to assist with the prescription of WBV to achieve desired levels of mechanical vibration loading at landmarks in the human body.

Yang et al. [30] described that vertical and side-alternating WBV can improve muscle power performance but have a limited efficacy for enhancing change-of-direction (COD) ability. They studied the acute effect of dual- or single-frequency WBV exercise on squat jumps (SJs), countermovement jumps (CMJs), eccentric utilization ratios (EURs), and COD ability in rugby players. Rugby players performed a 4 min partial squat with three types of WBV interventions on a dual-plate WBV machine, including 1 dual-frequency WBV protocol (DFW) with the dominant leg receiving 35 Hz and the non-dominant leg receiving 45 Hz, and 2 single-frequency WBV protocols (SFWs) with 35 or 45 Hz provided to both legs (SFW35Hz and SFW45Hz) in three different days. All the mechanical vibration interventions significantly improved SJ and CMJ performances. However, no significantly change EURs was found. In addition, only the DFW significantly improved COD ability. It was concluded that a 4 min dual-frequency WBV session improved both vertical jumping and COD ability in rugby players, suggesting that this could be a potential warm-up protocol for athletes.

5. Undesirable and unpleasant effects of the whole-body vibration

Despite the positive effects of the WBV exercise that were reported in topics 4.1 and 4.2, undesirable and unpleasant side-effects of these exercises can occur. Crewther et al. [31] verified that untrained participants exposed to acute mechanical vibration frequencies (10, 20 and 30 Hz), amplitudes (1.25, 3.0 and 5.25 mm) and postures (standing, squat) described side-effects, such as hot feet, itching of the lower limbs, vertigo and severe hip discomfort. Moreover, Cronin et al. [32] published that untrained participants suffered side-effects, such as vibration pain of jaw, neck and lower limbs in acute intermittent WBV. Cochrane, [2] discussed that the findings described by Crewther et al. [31] and Cronin et al. [32] are not usual, but it was highlighted the importance of the training of professionals on the use of mechanical vibration technology.

Monteleone et al. [33] published a case of clinical of a significant morbidity following one session of WBV training in a patient with asymptomatic nephrolithiasis. Franchignoni et al. [34] referencied that a healthy elite athlete (steeplechase runner) had two episodes of hematuria after WBV training. Concerning to this, Franchignoni et al. [34] suggested that platforms providing side-alternating vibration may pose some health risks with high amplitudes (the feet are positioned too far from the axis of rotation in this kind of platform).

Hwang et al. [35] applied WBV at different vibration frequencies to CS subjects and examined its immediate effect on their postural sway. The individuals were randomly allocated to one of the two vibration frequency groups (10 and 40 Hz). Before and after the intervention with WBV exercises, the subjects performed quiet standing for 30 seconds. COP parameters (range, total distance, and mean velocity) were analyzed. The 10 Hz WBV exercise did not affect the postural sway of CS subjects, however, the 40 Hz WBV increased postural sway in the ML direction. It was concluded that WBV application to CS individuals in the clinical field may have adverse effects and therefore caution is necessary. In addition, previously, Cochrane [2] pointed out that some of the related side-effects to the use of WBV would be due to lack of familiarization of the participants with the WBV.

6. Conclusion

Considering the findings that were discussed WBV exercise, in general, is a safe, suitable and inexpensive intervention that can be used for the physiotherapists. There is a special relevance the use of WBV exercise in the rehabilitation of individuals with various diseases, but it is also highly relevant in different types of sports and to trained and untrained individuals when the fitness and the wellbeing are considered. Furthermore, it is strongly desired precaution in the use of WBV exercise due to the undesirable and unpleasant side-effects. In consequence, it is relevant to study and to learn more about the parameters used in the protocols with WBV exercise and the clinical conditions of the individuals that will be exposed to mechanical vibrations generated in vibrating platform. It was highlighted the relevance of the WBV exercise as an intervention of the physical therapy for the better human optimization. Putting together, these facts, this chapter was prepared to aid the physiotherapists that have interest in WBV exercise to use properly this intervention.

Acknowledgements

The authors are thankful to *Conselho Nacional de Desenvolvimento Científico e Tecnológico* (CNPq), *Fundação Carlos Chagas Filho de Amparo à Pesquisa do Estado do Rio de Janeiro* (FAPERJ), *Coordenação de Aperfeiçoamento de Pessoal de Nível Superior* (CAPES) and *Programa de Pós-graduação em Ciências Médicas, Universidade do Estado do Rio de Janeiro*, Rio de Janeiro, Brazil, and University of Reims, France.

Conflict of interest

The authors declare no conflict of interest.

Author details

Danúbia da Cunha de Sá-Caputo[1,2], Redha Taiar[3] and Mario Bernardo-Filho[1]*

*Address all correspondence to: bernardofilhom@gmail.com

1 Laboratory of Mechanical Vibration and Integrative Practices, Rio de Janeiro State University, Rio de Janeiro, RJ, Brazil

2 Faculty Bezerra de Araújo, Physiotherapy Course, Rio de Janeiro, RJ, Brazil

3 University of Reims, Reims, France

References

[1] Rittweger J. Vibration as an exercise modality: How it may work, and what its potential might be. European Journal of Applied Physiology. 2010;**108**:877-904

[2] Cochrane DJ. Vibration exercise: The potential benefits. International Journal of Sports Medicine. 2011;**32**:75-99

[3] Hand J, Verscheure S, Osternig L. A comparison of whole-body vibration and resistance training on total work in the rotator cuff. Journal of Athletic Training. 2009;**44**:469-474

[4] Cardinale M, Wakeling J. Whole body vibration exercise: Are vibrations good for you? British Journal of Sports Medicine. 2005;**39**:585-589

[5] Charles LE, Ma CC, Burchfiel CM, Dong RG. Vibration and ergonomic exposures associated with musculoskeletal disorders of the shoulder and neck. Safety and Health at Work. 2018;**9**:125-132

[6] Savage R, Billing D, Furnell A, Netto K, Aisbett B. Whole-body vibration and occupational physical performance: A review. International Archives of Occupational and Environmental Health. 2016;**89**:181-197

[7] Lee G. Whole-body vibration in horizontal direction for stroke rehabilitation: A randomized controlled trial. Medical Science Monitor. 2019;**25**:1621-1628

[8] Rauch F, Sievanen H, Boonen S, Cardinale M, Degens H, Felsenberg D, et al. Reporting whole-body vibration intervention studies: Recommendations of the International Society of Musculoskeletal and Neuronal Interactions. Journal of Musculoskeletal Neuronal Interactions. 2010;**10**:193-198

[9] Rigamonti AE, Haenelt M, Bidlingmaier M, De Col A, Tamini S, Tringali G, et al. Obese adolescents exhibit a constant ratio of GH isoforms after whole body vibration and maximal voluntary contractions. BMC Endocrine Disorders. 2018;**18**(1):96. DOI: 10.1186/s12902-018-0323

[10] Oliveira MP, Menzel HK, Cochrane DJ, Drummond MDM, Demicheli C, Lage G, et al. Individual responses to different vibration frequencies identified by electromyography and dynamometry in different types of vibration application. Journal of Strength and Conditioning Research. 2019. DOI: 10.1519/JSC.0000000000002985

[11] Pleguezuelos E, Casarramona P, Guirao L, Samitier B, Ortega P, Vila X, et al. How whole-body vibration can help our COPD patients. Physiological changes at different vibration frequencies. International Journal of Chronic Obstructive Pulmonary Disease. 2018;**13**:3373-3380

[12] Haas CT, Turbanski S, Kessler K, Schmidtbleicher D. The effects of random whole-body-vibration on motor symptoms in Parkinson's disease. NeuroRehabilitation. 2006;**21**:29-36

[13] Sá-Caputo D, Paineiras-Domingos LL, Francisca-Santos A, Dos Anjos EM, Reis AS, Neves MFT, et al. Whole-body vibration improves the functional parameters of individuals with metabolic syndrome: An exploratory study. BMC Endocrine Disorders. 2019;**19**(1):6. DOI: 10.1186/s12902-018-0329-0

[14] Ribeiro VGC, Mendonça VA, Souza ALC, Fonseca SF, Camargos ACR, Lage VKS, et al. Inflammatory biomarkers responses after acute whole body vibration in fibromyalgia. Brazilian Journal of Medical and Biological Research. 2018;**51**(4):e6775. DOI: 10.1590/1414-431X20176775

[15] Krause A, Lee K, Freyler K, Bührer T, Gollhofer A, Ritzmann R. Whole-body vibration impedes the deterioration of postural control in patients with multiple sclerosis. Multiple Sclerosis and Related Disorders. 2019;**31**:134-140

[16] Pin TW, Butler PB, Purves S. Use of whole body vibration therapy in individuals with moderate severity of cerebral palsy—A feasibility study. BMC Neurology. 2019;**19**(1):80. DOI: 10.1186/s12883-019-1307-5

[17] Lai CL, Tseng SY, Chen CN, Liao WC, Wang CH, Lee MC, et al. Effect of 6 months of whole body vibration on lumbar spine bone density in postmenopausal women: A randomized controlled trial. Clinical Interventions in Aging. 2013;**8**:1603-1609

[18] Zheng YL, Wang XF, Chen BL, Gu W, Wang X, Xu B, et al. Effect of 12-week whole-body vibration exercise on lumbopelvic proprioception and pain control in young adults with nonspecific low back pain. Medical Science Monitor. 2019;**25**:443-452

[19] Abbasi M, Kordi Yoosefinejad A, Poursadeghfard M, Parsaei Jahromi F, Motealleh A, Sobhani S. Whole body vibration improves core muscle strength and endurance in ambulant individuals with multiple sclerosis: A randomized clinical trial. Multiple Sclerosis and Related Disorders. 2019;**32**:88-93

[20] Yang F, Munoz J, Han LZ, Yang F. Effects of vibration training in reducing risk of slip-related falls among young adults with obesity. Journal of Biomechanics. 2017;**57**:87-93

[21] Kim H, Kwon BS, Park JW, Lee H, Nam K, Park T, et al. Effect of whole body horizontal vibration exercise in chronic low Back pain patients: Vertical versus horizontal vibration exercise. Annals of Rehabilitation Medicine. 2018;**42**:804-813

[22] Huang M, Pang MYC. Muscle activity and vibration transmissibility during whole-body vibration in chronic stroke. Scandinavian Journal of Medicine and Science in Sports. 2019;**29**:816-825. DOI: 10.1111/sms.13408

[23] Moreira-Marconi E, Moura-Fernandes MC, Lopes-Souza P, Teixeira-Silva Y, Reis-Silva A, Marchon RM, et al. Evaluation of the temperature of posterior lower limbs skin during the whole body vibration measured by infrared thermography: Cross-sectional study analysis using linear mixed effect model. PLoS One. 2019;**14**(3):e0212512. DOI: 10.1371/journal.pone.0212512

[24] Wallmann HW, Bell DL, Evans BL, Hyman AA, Goss GK, Paicely AM. The effects of whole body vibration on vertical jump, power, balance, and agility in untrained adults. International Journal of Sports Physical Therapy. 2019;**14**:55-64

[25] Wang XQ, Gu W, Chen BL, Wang X, Hu HY, Zheng YL, et al. Effects of whole-body vibration exercise for non-specific chronic low back pain: An assessor-blind, randomized controlled trial. Clinical Rehabilitation. 2019;**33**:1445-1457. DOI: 10.1177/0269215519848076

[26] Tantawy SA, Elgohary HMI, Abdelbasset WK, Kamel DM. Effect of 4 weeks of whole-body vibration training in treating stress urinary incontinence after prostate cancer surgery: A randomised controlled trial. Physiotherapy. 2018. pii: S0031-9406(18)30259-1. DOI: 10.1016/j.physio.2018.07.013

[27] Chen B, Dong Y, Guo J, Zheng Y, Zhang J, Wang X. Effects of whole-body vibration on lumbar-abdominal muscles activation in healthy young adults: A pilot study. Medical Science Monitor. 2019;**25**:1945-1951

[28] Karim A, Roddey T, Mitchell K, Ortiz A, Olson S. Immediate effect of whole body vibration on sauté height and balance in female professional contemporary dancers a randomized controlled trial. Journal of Dance Medicine and Science. 2019;**23**:3-10

[29] Zaidell LN, Pollock RD, James DC, Bowtell JL, Newham DJ, Sumners DP, et al. Lower body acceleration and muscular responses to rotational and vertical whole-body vibration at different frequencies and amplitudes. Dose-Response. 2019;**17**(1):1559325818819946. DOI: 10.1177/1559325818819946

[30] Yang WW, Chou LW, Chen WH, Shiang TY, Liu C. Dual-frequency whole body vibration enhances vertical jumping and change-of-direction ability in rugby players. Journal of Sport and Health Science. 2017;**6**:346-351

[31] Crewther B, Cronin J, Keogh J. Gravitational forces and whole body vibration: Implications for prescription of vibratory stimulation. Physical Therapy in Sport. 2004;**5**:37-43

[32] Cronin JB, Oliver M, McNair PJ. Muscle stiff ness and injury effects of whole body vibration. Physical Therapy in Sport. 2004;**5**:68-74

[33] Monteleone G, De Lorenzo A, Sgroi M, De Angelis S, Di Renzo L. Contraindications for whole body vibration training: A case of nephrolitiasis. The Journal of Sports Medicine and Physical Fitness. 2007;**47**:443-445

[34] Franchignoni F, Vercelli S, Ozçakar L. Hematuria in a runner after treatment with whole body vibration: A case report. Scandinavian Journal of Medicine & Science in Sports. 2013;**23**:383-385

[35] Hwang KJ, Ryu YU. Whole body vibration may have immediate adverse effects on the postural sway of stroke patients. Journal of Physical Therapy Science. 2016;**28**:473-477

Chapter 4

What to Expect: Medical Quality Outcomes and Achievements of a Multidisciplinary Inpatient Musculoskeletal System Rehabilitation

Vincent Grote, Alexandra Unger, Henry Puff and Elke Böttcher

Additional information is available at the end of the chapter

http://dx.doi.org/10.5772/intechopen.89596

Abstract

The incidence of chronic diseases is rising. Rehabilitation plays a vital role in preventing and minimizing the functional limitations associated with chronic conditions and aging. Routine outcome measures include disease-specific and unspecific general health parameters. This study evaluates indicators for medical quality outcomes from 10,373 patients (61.00 ± 13.65 years, 51.7% women) who have undergone orthopedic rehabilitation for three weeks. Inpatient rehabilitation reduces lifestyle-related risk factors, optimizes organ functioning and improves the well-being in the majority of patients (81.3%; SMD = 0.52 ± 0.38). Improvements of unspecific and indication specific outcome parameters can be observed in a comparable magnitude. However, disease specific and unspecific health factors are not directly related to each other (r = 0.19). Age, gender, ICD-classification and time of rehabilitation have an influence on initial values and on indication-specific medical outcomes but are insignificant with regards to improvements in unspecific medical outcome parameters. Inpatient rehabilitation includes two main pathways of medical practice, which can be clearly distinguished in terms of their therapeutic outcome. There are general health interventions, such as lifestyle modifications, diet and physical exercise, and symptom-specific treatments. So multidisciplinary medical rehabilitation improves general well-being and physical functioning as well as reduces risk factors in the majority of patients.

Keywords: inpatient rehabilitation, medical quality outcomes, routine outcome measurement, reference data, rehab success

IntechOpen

© 2019 The Author(s). Licensee IntechOpen. This chapter is distributed under the terms of the Creative Commons Attribution License (http://creativecommons.org/licenses/by/3.0), which permits unrestricted use, distribution, and reproduction in any medium, provided the original work is properly cited. (cc) BY

1. Introduction

The definition of rehabilitation has become more transparent all over the world after the World Health Organization (WHO) published the five health strategies (promotion, prevention, cure, rehabilitation and palliative care) in rehabilitation [1]. Rehabilitation was previously understood as a heterogeneous approach. It was framed as a highly specialized service for athletes, a controlled training intervention or a post-injury service for return-to-work intervention. The definition was standardized through the WHO to a homogenous understanding of rehabilitation as a service to restore functioning, ameliorate the impact of the reduction in capacity and minimize further initial health problems in all stages of health provision [2].

Special care in rehabilitation is given to the ailments of the modern society. As such, especially risk factors like sedentary behavior[1], physical inactivity, overeating causing obesity, alcohol abuse and smoking leading to various chronic diseases that immediately affect the musculoskeletal system [3] are causes for concern. Due to those lifestyle choices that lead to potentially life-threatening conditions, physical activity has become an important therapeutic approach. It is a primary, secondary or tertiary therapeutic approach of chronic diseases over the last decades. Physical activity recommendations are now broadly understood as health-related interventions that propose a minimum dose of physical activity.

The WHO [1] suggests at least 150 minutes of moderate aerobic activity or 75 minutes of vigorous aerobic activity throughout the week for adults. In addition, muscle-strengthening activities should be done involving major muscle groups on two or more days a week and sedentary behavior should be reduced. Small amounts of physical activity already have a positive impact on the health status; however, the strongest effect can be observed in adults that transformed from an inactive to an active lifestyle [4–6].

Medical intervention programs therefore do not only aim to restore physiological functioning, reverse or undo the damage caused by disease or injury, but also rather to optimize the health status by improving strength and aerobic capacity. The amelioration of the physical constitution leads to health-promoting effects like the reduction of high blood pressure, a better glucose profile and reduced blood lipids [7, 8]. Physical activity has a positive impact not only on metabolic and cardiovascular diseases but also on the musculoskeletal system.

Complaints of the musculoskeletal system are most commonly those of inflammatory and degenerative origin. These origins of disease are the cause for chronic pain, painful functional impairment and a reduced quality of life worldwide. Rheumatoid arthritis is found in 3.2% of women and 1.9% of men. Furthermore, another increasing ailment is osteoporosis, which is found in 3.1% of women and 1.9% of men, with a high prevalence from the age of 80 onwards [9].

---

[1]For example, through (screen) workplaces and automation, leisure activities such as video games, social media and television.

The most common symptom of the musculoskeletal system is back pain (60–80% long-time prevalence [10, 11]). The prevalence is dependent on age, with a rise of prevalence with age. The highest prevalence for back pain is set between 40 and 69 years; women are more affected than men [12, 13].

The findings of an analysis by the Austrian Health Survey 2014 [14] report an estimated rate of 24% (about 1.8 Mio individuals) suffering from chronic back pain. Furthermore, 19% claimed about discomfort of the cervical spine. The cervical spine complaint was gender dependent (23% women versus 14% men). Arthrosis was found in 15% of women and 8% of men. The gender difference refers not only to the frequency of the disease but also to the pain perception, due to a higher rate of female pain sensitivity, lower threshold for pain and a lower suspension of pain [15].

Due to the high prevalence of degenerative diseases of the musculoskeletal system, there is also a demand for surgical treatment with endoprosthesis material. The highest operative treatment rates for such procedures worldwide are found in Switzerland, Germany and Austria. In Germany, about 230,000 hip, 170,000 knee and 25,000 shoulder endoprosthesis surgeries were performed in the year 2011 alone [16].

Physiotherapy and physical activity are fundamental components for the process of recovery. The body of available knowledge confirms positive effects of physiotherapy and physical activity throughout all organ systems. It reduces swelling as well as promotes building strength and aerobic capacity. Through the process of physiotherapy and physical activity interventions, a total physiological functionality after surgical treatment can be achieved. Moderate physical activity reduces the risk of osteoporosis and improves the osseointegration of bone substitutes. Almost all musculoskeletal diseases can be treated by therapies including physical activity and strengthening programs [17–20]. Physical activity thus has become the gold standard among medical treatments.

1.1. Orthopedic rehabilitation

Following the WHO definition, the rehabilitative process can be divided into four phases: phase I includes the early mobilization in primary treatment, phase II provides follow-up treatments or post-acute therapy in rehabilitation centers, phase III tries to integrate and stabilize the long-term life modifications and phase IV deals with long-term rehabilitation including a probably outpatient aftercare. The aim of orthopedic inpatient rehabilitation (phase II) is to restore the health status based on the bio-psycho-social health model.

1.1.1. Situation in Austria

Musculoskeletal diseases, caused by inflammatory, degenerative processes or injuries, permit an inpatient orthopedic rehabilitation (WHO, Phase II [21, 22]) over 3–4 weeks for restoring physiological functioning and reintegrating to social and professional life.

Based on historical decisions [23] and Health Technology Assessments (HTA) (e.g., [24]), there is currently a framework of contracts with the federal Austrian social security institutions entities in place[2]. This includes performance agreements for orthopedic rehabilitation (see [25]), based on criteria regarding the quality of processes and treatment outcomes [21]. Criteria include individual detailed results that demand a standardized statistical recording of outcome parameters from admission up to discharge of the rehabilitation program. Furthermore, evaluation and statistical analyses of these medical outcomes are generally not open to the public [26].

1.1.2. Implementation of orthopedic rehabilitation in Austria

There is strong evidence that rehabilitation is necessary as part of the treatments for inflammatory or degenerative diseases, as well as for postoperative conditions or injuries of the musculoskeletal system. The underlying condition's severity and expectancy of the restoration of physical function are requirements for obtaining an inpatient orthopedic rehabilitation. For patients affected by musculoskeletal disease, medical treatment and a large range of rehabilitative treatments are available. The inpatient treatment lasts on average 2–3 hours per day. An individual rehabilitative program consisting of active and passive treatments is provided (see **Table 1**). Active treatments consist of physical activity including gymnastic and individual physiotherapy sessions and the medical training focuses on underwater , ergometer , Nordic walking , strength , balance , relaxation and motion training. Passive treatments contain sessions like massages, thermotherapy, electrotherapy, ultrasound and educational lessons like various lectures, or psychological coaching. Each patient is offered a program of at least 1800 therapy minutes during 3 weeks, split up into approximately 50% active and 50% passive treatments that highly surpass the physical activity guidelines of the WHO (150 minutes workout in moderate intensity and strengthening exercise twice a week).

	Physical exercise	**Medical training**	
Active	Gymnastic	Underwater gym	Approx. 50%
	Individual physiotherapy	Ergometer training	
	Sensomotoric training	Strength training	
	…	Balance & function training	
	(Passive) **Treatments**	**Education**	
Passive	Massages	Health-related talks and trainings	Approx. 50%
	Thermotherapy	Psychological	
	Electrotherapy	Coaching	
	Ultrasound	…	
Required total amount		At least 1800 minutes (within 3 weeks)	

Table 1. Quantity and type of therapies over three weeks.

[2]In particular the pension insurance institution.

Medical rehabilitation is structured in different ways all over the world, although a tendency for a standardization of the social and health system can be observed. In Germany and Austria, the social insurance offers inpatient orthopedic rehabilitation over a period of 3–4 weeks in specialized rehabilitation centers with an interdisciplinary team. Some other countries only provide outpatient rehabilitation [27].

1.2. Efficacy and sustainability of orthopedic rehabilitation

Diseases demand a certain continuity of the therapeutic process for success after rehabilitation. This means that rehabilitative programs should focus not only on physical activity programs during the stay but also on sustainability of physical activity after the rehabilitation. Therefore, an inpatient stay should also lead to a health-related modification in lifestyle. The efficacy of inpatient rehabilitative programs and especially their sustainability over a long period are important research issues. Literature shows that during the rehabilitative stay, pain can be significantly reduced, and a long-term improvement of physiological functionality can be achieved. The success can be measured even after 12–21 months after rehabilitation [28, 29].

The fact remains that physical activity programs have a positive impact on the physiological performance of patients. However, the dropout rate for long-life active and health-related lifestyle change maintenance is high. Findings support the sustained efficacy of an intense, multimodal orthopedic rehabilitation, with moderate evidence, including an improved subjective health status and reduced pain [30]. For rehabilitation treatment after hip and knee endoprosthesis (TEP) [31–34] and chronic back pain [35–37], a level of evidence Ia/Ib is stated. The combination of physiological and psychological training significantly leads to positive changes [18, 38, 39]. The data confirm that a combination of physical activity and psychosocial training-based treatments has an influence on pain reduction and mental well-being.

Studies in other countries state that about 57% of patients in Europe and even 70% of patients in the US are able to restart regular full-time work and show significant improvements of psychosocial, physiological parameters after inpatient rehabilitation [40–43]. An interdisciplinary treatment of medical, physical activity based and psychological therapy ensures a high return to professional life [44, 45].

2. Methods

The medical outcome parameters required by the performance profile of the federal Austrian social security institutions involved in quantifying the quality of rehabilitation outcomes are the basis of this work. We provide descriptive standardized numeric indicators of the rehabilitation process as well as monocentric reference data for a 3-week inpatient orthopedic rehabilitation program. Data collection was performed by doctors and healthcare professionals during routine medical treatment. Standardized clinical characteristics of patients were recorded systematically at the time of admission and discharge. The easily quantifiable medical parameters included general health characteristics such as body measurements and cardiovascular parameters, psychological indicators such as pain and subjective health, as well as specific indicators such as daily activities, motor function and physical performance (see **Table 2**).

These quality-of-outcome measures are to be documented in the discharge report at the beginning and the end of the phase II rehabilitation (this correlates with the methodology of a pre-post comparison). Respectively, data were also summarized using a descriptive evaluation in terms of content and factor analysis. This provides us a simple descriptive evaluation model through independent factors for the sake of a complete evaluation of the outcome quality [26].

2.1. Orthopedic reference sample at the clinical trial center

During the service period from 2016 to 2018, a total of 10,373 patients (61.00 ± 13.65 years, 51.7% women) were enrolled in a specialized interdisciplinary hospital for rehabilitation (Humanomed Center, Austria) (**Table 3**). A categorization of reasons for hospital treatment was based on the admission diagnosis. Reasons for admission were musculoskeletal diseases (M, 85%) or injuries (S, 15%). Categorizations were based on ICD-10. The majority of patients were admitted for rehabilitation due to back pain (29.6%) followed by upper/lower limb joint as well as knee (21.4%), hip (16.3%) and shoulder (12.0%) disorders. About 73.3% of the patients were admitted after surgery (OP)[3]. Just under a half of those patients (42.2%) were treated with an endoprosthesis (EP) (overall, 31.9%). The proportion of EP rehabilitation procedures was 64.7% for knee patients and 84.7% for hip patients. The period between acute care rehabilitation (OP) averaged 8.4 ± 4.0 weeks. However, patients with knee and hip TEP progressed from phase I to phase II earlier (median, 6 weeks)[4].

The average inpatient length of stay was 22.00 ± 2.6 days; 2.2% of all patients discontinued their inpatient treatment prematurely due to a loss of rehabilitation capacity (for example, acute illness) or for private reasons (criterion ≤ 18 treatment days). In 3.8% of the patients, the inpatient stay was 4 weeks.

2.2. Ethical aspects

This study (A retrospective study-Routine Outcome Parameters of an Inpatient Rehabilitation in Austria) was reviewed and approved by an Ethics Committee (Vote by the Ethics Committee of the Medical University of Graz, dated 02.05.2019, EC Protocol Number: 31-321 ex 18/19). Person-related and health-related data were collected as part of routine medical care and quality management at the Humanomed Center Althofen (9330 Althofen, Moorweg 30). Data processing was done according to standard operating procedure by the responsible data processing party: Humanomed Center Althofen GmbH, Data Protection Officer: Mag. Karl Klein, Jesserniggstraße

[3]Corresponds to a follow-up treatment procedure (AHV), which can be used in Austria for three to four months from the grant date (in Germany within 14 days after discharge Phase I). The remaining patients are a (R) HV [(rehabilitation) treatment], where the time limit is 8 to 12 months.

[4]For knee and hip TEP patients in orthopedic rehabilitation, a quasi-experimental control group (waiting group) results from the different onset times [period between acute care (surgery time) and the beginning of the follow-up treatment procedure (AHV)].

http://dx.doi.org/10.5772/intechopen.89596

Orthopedic rehabilitation indicators for medical quality outcomes (MQO, [z*])						
Unspecific general health parameters			**Disease-specific health parameters (indication-specific outcomes)**			
MED1	BMI	[kg/m²]	**ORT1**	Quality of life	EQ-5D	[%]
	Abdominal circumference	[cm]				
	ANATOMY	**[z]**		**ADL** (activities of daily living)		**[z]**
MED2	Blood pressure systolic	[mmHG]	**ORT2**	Motoric function	Roland-Morris	[ ]
	Blood pressure diastolic				WOMAC	[ ]
	Resting heart rate	[bpm]			Constant-Murley	[ ]
	PHYSIOLOGY	**[z]**		**FUNCTION**		**[z]**
MED3	VAS (pain)	[cm; 0–10]	**ORT3**	Walk test	Timed up & go	[sec]
	EQ VAS (self-rated health)	[%; 0–100]			10 m	[sec]
	DISCOMFORT	**[z]**		**PHYSICAL ABILITY**		**[z]**
UH_i	**Unspecific health index** MED1, MED2 & MED3	**[z]**	**SO_i**	**Specific Ortho Index** ORT1, ORT2 & ORT3		**[z]**
MQO	(overall) **Medical quality outcome** UH_i & SO_i					**[z]**

*Standard scores, also called z-values (z), are calculated by subtracting the (population) mean from an individual raw score and then dividing the difference by the (population) standard deviation (here: for all orthopedic patients). As shown in the results section, deviations from zero respectively mean differences of z-values can be interpreted as an effect size (c.f. Cohen's d).

Table 2. Parameters of medical quality outcomes.

Classification according to ICD-10	Number of patients		Age	Women		Endoprosthesis	
Localization/main diagnosis	abs.	%	Mean ± SD	abs.	%	abs.	%
Back (spine)	3067	29.6	57.2 ± 13.3	1509	49.2	12	0.4
M41, M43, M48, M50, M51, M53, M54, S32, S22, S12							
Knee	2220	21.4	64.7 ± 12.5	1225	55.2	1437	64.7
M17, M23, S83							
Hip	1688	16.3	67.1 ± 11.0	928	55.0	1429	84.7
M16							
Shoulder	1249	12.0	57.8 ± 11.3	562	45.0	32	2.6
M75, S42, S43, S46							
Lower leg and thigh	723	7.0	62.1 ± 16.5	414	57.3	103	14.2
S82, S86, S72							
Other arthritis	400	3.9	62.7 ± 13.4	219	54.8	139	34.8
M19, M25							
Other	330	3.2	60.7 ± 14.4	173	52.4	141	42.7
T84, S52, M79, M77, M87, S92, M06							
Other diseases (musculoskeletal system)	696	6.7	55.3 ± 15.4	338	48.6	17	2.4
ICD-10Kat < n = 20							
Total	10373	100.0	61.0 ± 13.6	5368	51.7	3310	31.9

Table 3. Sample number of patients undergoing rehabilitation of the musculoskeletal system.

9, 9020 Klagenfurt. The data from the hospital information system upon which the publication is based were compiled in compliance with all regulations of the Austrian Privacy Act and the Declaration of Helsinki in its current version. Data collection was done also in accordance with national legalization (hospital statutes, contracts with insurance-authorized institutions, etc.) through the rational of mainly collecting scientific data in the public interest.

2.3. Medical outcome quality

Medical outcome quality is defined as the "measurable change in the profession-ally assessed state of health, the quality of life and the satisfaction of a patient" (see Austrian Federal Quality of Healthcare Act, GQG). The outcomes become visible by "the difference between the initial state and the state at treatment end" (c.f. [46]).

The outcome measurement in rehabilitation can be based on various methodological approaches, such as questionnaires, performance tests, equipment measurements and functional physical examinations. The outcome quality measurement, "the outcome," includes features on health (e.g., symptoms and pain), functional levels (e.g., performance) and educational levels. In addition to the patient's subjective assessment ("patient-reported outcomes (PRO)"), medical, diagnostic and other relevant outcome measures/criteria (e.g., ICF) are documented by healthcare professionals.

The aim of the present work is to provide a valid basis for routinely assessing the quality of medical outcomes (routine outcome measurement) based on common data acquisition. The focus therefore is on general (nonspecific, body constitution based) and indication-specific parameters. Continuously collected medical reference values have diverse potential benefits in quality assurance, awareness raising, goal setting and decision-making. The data are also important for evaluation of different care models.

2.3.1. Quantifying "medical outcome quality"

In addition to the descriptive analysis of single indicators, the analysis evaluates the effects of inpatient rehabilitation stay and the medical quality outcome (MQO). This is calculated on the basis of representative monocentric normative data (N = 10,373; see **Table 3**). The selection of clinical parameters follows the requirements of federal social security instate in the performance profiles of accredited Austrian institutions for outcome analysis, which should guarantee a comparable medical service quality standard. A success index is calculated by summarizing the compulsory basic clinical data of the patients (see **Table 2** and [26]).

1. The "Unspecific Health Index" is the arithmetic mean of three independent areas of measurement: body measurements (BMI and abdominal circumference), cardiovascular parameters (blood pressure and resting heart rate), discomfort (visual analogue scales (VAS pain, [47]) and subjective health status (EQ-VAS, [48])). These parameters should provide a simple and quick overview of "unspecific" effectiveness of a rehabilitative stay.
2. The "Specific Ortho Index" corresponds to a z-normalized mean of "activities of daily living" (EQ5D), "function" (Roland-Morris, WOMAC or Constant-Murley, depending on the affected body region) and the "physical ability" (walking tests).

The Unspecific Health Index can be interpreted as an indicator of general health status or the current body constitution, whereas the Specific Ortho Index corresponds to a disease-specific health parameter (indication-specific outcome). Both indexes together form the "medical quality outcome" in equal parts.

2.3.2. *Statistical methods*

Based on the value distributions, the individual outcome parameters were transformed into z-values, which allowed a conversion into percentiles. By means of the z-standardization, different scaled quantities can be summarized and changes can be uniformly quantified [standardized mean differences (SMD)]. A value of 50% (median) or a z-value of zero corresponds-given a normal distribution-to the representative mean of admission and discharge data of all patients at the clinical trial center. A z-value of 1, corresponds to a deviation from the mean by one standard deviation. Z-differences with no significant changes are in a range of 0.00 ± 0.20. Changes from admission to discharge are illustrated by effect sizes. In addition, the number of patients (relative frequency in %) is stated, which could improve clinically (categorical representation: better, equal, and worse). The threshold used is an average z-difference (~SMD) >0.20 (MED 1–3, ORT 1–3) or >0.33 (unspecific Health Index, Specific Ortho Index, and overall medical quality outcome). Alternatively, the average (percentile) change compared to the time of admission is calculated and, if necessary, treated according to the indication.

Statistical data processing was performed using IBM® SPSS® Statistics (version 22). In addition to descriptive methods, statistical analysis included parametric methods such as multifactorial variance analyses for repeated measures [(M)AN(C)OVA; between-effects: gender (2), covariate: age, within-effect: rehabilitation course (2)], regression analysis and Pearson correlations. Individual missing values were not replaced for statistical analysis. The specification of p-values was omitted, instead effect sizes were used [partial Eta^2 and standardized mean differences (Cohen's d or z-values/-differences, SMD)]. The representation of the partial Eta^2 (η^2) was chosen because even the very small numerical differences became statistically significant even if they were not relevant in terms of content and clinical relevance. A η^2 between 0.01 and 0.06 corresponds to a small effect. Occurrences of 0.06–0.14 correspond to a middle effect and values >0.14 to a large effect [49]. The application of multivariate variance analyses (MANOVA) and a factor-analytical reduction of the basic clinical data to individual factors or a total value (MQO) follow substantive, statistical considerations for better clarity.

3. Results

The effect of the rehabilitation stay and the change between the initial state and the discharge state differ between the individual success factors for medical rehabilitation (see **Tables 4, 6** and **7**). Specific and unspecific outcomes show a comparable change in sensitivity ($\eta^2_{\text{unspecific}} = 0.522$ [UH_i] vs. $\eta^2_{\text{specific}} = 0.540$ [SO_i]). The relationship between specific and unspecific outcome characteristics (changes) is small ($r < 0.20$, see **Figure 1** and **Table 5**), which is reflected in a multivariate analysis of temporal changes in the variance ($\eta^2_{unifactorial} = 0.654$ [MQO_i]).

The nonspecific overall score-the "Health Index (UH_{Index})"-shows that 72.5% of patients benefit directly from the rehabilitation stay. About 21.8% of the patients remain unchanged and 5.8% worsen between the beginning and the end of the rehabilitation (see **Table 4**). The detailed analysis of average improvement in general health features by 13.58 percentile points shows that anatomical features, such as body mass index and abdominal circumference, remain unchanged over the 3 weeks in the majority (86.4%). By contrast, cardiovascular features such as blood pressure and resting heart rate are directly influenced by inpatient rehabilitation, with an average improvement of 11.5 percentile points. The most pronounced effects of inpatient rehabilitation can be seen in the symptoms of complaints, where almost every rehabilitation (84.9%) reported a significant improvement. A similarly positive change can be seen in the ADL score (+17.6 percentile points), motor function (+22.2 percentile points) and physical performance, where 2/3 (67.5%) of patients can improve markedly.

[%]	better	equal	worse	Ø-improvement*
MED1: Anatomy (BMI, AC)	11,2	86,4	2,4	*MED1: +1,33*
MED2: Physiology (BP, RHR)	56,5	15,7	27,8	*MED2: +11,50*
MED3: Discomfort (VAS, SHS)	84,9	9,9	5,2	*MED3: +27,89*

BMI... Body Mass Index, AC ... Abdominal Circumference, BP... Blood Pressure, RHR... Resting Heart Rate, VAS... Visual Analog Skale (pain), SHS... Subjective Health Status (EQ-VAS); Threshold for classification: MED1-3: 0,20 (z-difference);

Achievements of an multidisciplinary inpatient musculoskeletal system rehabilitation

[relative frequency in %]	better	equal	worse	Ø-improvement*
Unspecific Health Index	72,5	21,8	5,8	UH_{Index}: +13,58
Specific Ortho Index	77,0	19,0	4,0	SO_{Index}: +17,70
Overall Medical Quality Outcome	**81,3**	**16,4**	**2,3**	$\mathbf{MQO_{Index}}$**: +15,62**

**. Average improvement (percentiles) from admission to discharge;*
Threshold for classification Unspecific Health, Specific Ortho & overall Medical Quality Outcome Indices ~0,33 SMD;

[%]	better	equal	worse	Ø-improvement*
ORT1: ADL (EQ5D)	58,6	33,1	8,3	*ORT1: +17,57*
ORT2: Function (RM, WOMAC or CM)	76,3	18,0	5,6	*ORT2: +22,17*
ORT3: Physical Ability (WT)	67,5	30,7	1,8	*ORT3: +12,96*

ADL... Activities of Daily Living, RM... Roland Morris, CM... Constant Murley, WT... Walking Tests;
Threshold for classification: ORT1-3: 0,20 (z-difference);

Table 4. Overview of medical quality outcomes.

Almost all considered medical factors (MED, ORT) provide a comparable contribution to the overall success (MQO, all $r \geq 0.40$, except for MED1: $r = 0.11$). The correlation between Unspecific Health Index and Specific Ortho Index is relatively low ($r = 0.19$; see **Figure 1** and **Table 5**). Therefore, immediate changes in unspecific health scores are not directly associated with improvements in (indication-) specific functional characteristics. One exception is the (subjective) complaints (MED 3), which are related to specific outcome changes ($r = .34$).

However, the extent of improvement in medical outcome and the effect size are similar in all areas (see **Tables 4**, **6** and **7** and **Figure 1**). Just the anatomy factor (MED 1) changed only slightly during rehabilitation ($\eta^2_{MED1} = 0.072$; **Tables 6** and **7**). The individual parameters for all patients are presented in **Tables 6** and **7** below.

3.1. Output values and descriptive data for individual measurements

The starting point (initial) values of rehabilitation clearly show the deficits of the affected patients (see **Tables 6** and **7**). The average BMI is 28.9 ± 5.4 units (37.0% of patients have a BMI > 30) and 77.3% of patients have "high-normal" or "hypertonic" blood pressure. The perceived pain (VAS; 0–10) of patients is 3.8 ± 2.1 and the subjective health status (EQ-VAS; 0–100) is estimated to be 63.7 ± 16.6% on average.

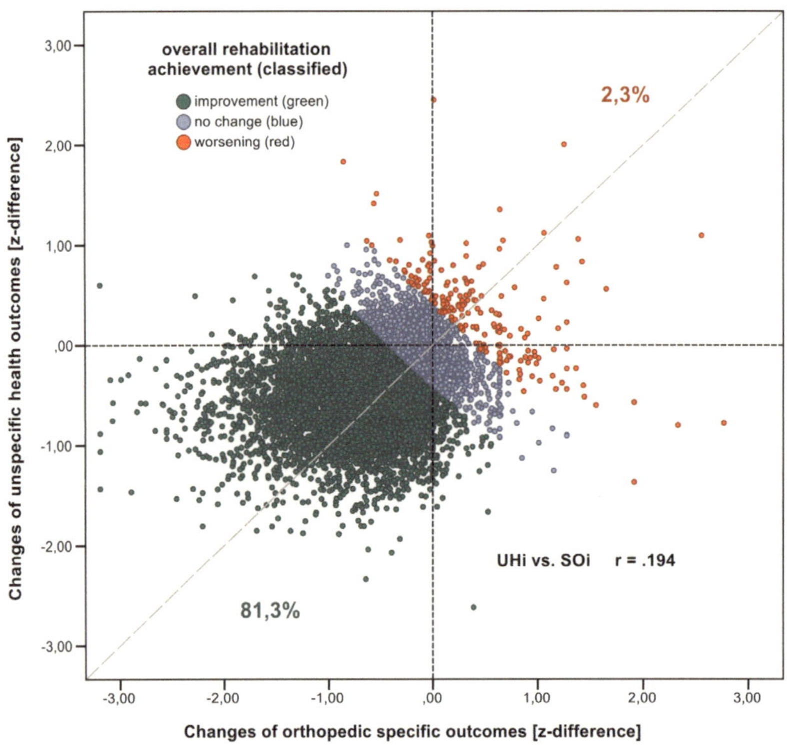

Figure 1. A value of zero (± 0.20 [z]) stands for no significant changes from admission to discharge (blue dots). The mean for UHi is −0.45 ± 0.43 and for SOi −0.59 ± 0.55. The overall MQOi (mean of UHi & SOi) is −0.52 ± 0.38 (centroid).

http://dx.doi.org/10.5772/intechopen.89596

Correlation of changes in medical factors [Pearson]		MED 1 (Anatomy)	MED 2 (Physiology)	MED 3 (Discomfort)	UH_i (Unspecific health ind.)	Overall MQO (medical quality outcome)
ORT 1 (ADL)	r	0.000	−0.007	0.285	0.162	**0.671**
	p	0.982	0.496	0.000	0.000	0.000
ORT 2 (Function)	r	0.012	−0.006	0.314	0.183	**0.638**
	p	0.288	0.620	0.000	0.000	0.000
ORT 3 (Physical ability)	r	−0.020	−0.011	0.072	0.033	**0.399**
	p	0.113	0.406	0.000	0.010	0.000
SO_i (Specific Ortho Index)	r	−0.002	−0.009	0.340	0.194	**0.833**
	p	0.878	0.385	0.000	0.000	0.000
Overall MQO (medical quality outcome)	r	**0.107**	**0.444**	**0.579**	**0.704**	1
	p	0.000	0.000	0.000	0.000	

Bold values show the correlation of each health parameter with the overall medical quality outcome.

Table 5. Correlations between changes in MQO factors.

MQO indicators & factors	Initial values (beginning of rehabilitation; prae)		Change from admission (prae) to discharge (post)				
Measure	**Mean ± standard deviation (SD)**		**Mean diff. (post-prae) ±SD**		**(z) Normalized difference ± SD**		**part. Eta^2**
BMI [kg/m^2]	28.89	5.38	−0.15	1.45	−0.03	0.27	0.011
Abdominal circumference [cm]	100.24	13.71	−0.99	2.78	−0.07	0.20	0.114
MED 1: Anatomy [z]	**0.10**	**0.97**	**−0.05**	**0.18**	**−0.05**	**0.18**	**0.072**
RRsys [mmHG] (blood pressure systolic)	130.74	11.30	−4.78	13.00	−0.37	1.02	0.119
RRdia [mmHG] (blood pressure diastolic)	76.87	7.45	−2.28	9.44	−0.29	1.19	0.055
heart rate [bpm]	78.74	11.67	−1.41	12.13	−0.12	1.01	0.014
MED 2: Physiology [z]	**0.14**	**0.89**	**−0.37**	**1.01**	**−0.37**	**1.01**	**0.120**
VAS [cm; 0–10] (pain)	3.75	2.14	−1.68	1.69	−0.70	0.70	0.501
self-rated health [%; 0–100] (EQ-VAS)	63.70	16.60	13.79	14.84	−0.80	0.86	0.465
MED 3: Discomfort [z]	**0.45**	**0.92**	**−0.91**	**0.75**	**−0.91**	**0.75**	**0.598**
UH: unspecific health Index [z] MED1, MED2, MED3	**0.23**	**0.59**	**−0.45**	**0.43**	**−0.45**	**0.43**	**0.522**

Bold values show summarized factors of outcome measures from unspecific general health parameters (see **Table 2**).

Table 6. Starting point values and changes in individually measures quantities.

http://dx.doi.org/10.5772/intechopen.89596

MQO indicators & factors	Initial values (beginning of rehabilitation; prae)		Change from admission (prae) to discharge (post)				
Measure	**Mean ± standard deviation (SD)**		**Mean diff. (post - prae) ± SD**		**(z) Normalized difference ± SD**		**part. Eta^2**
ORT 1: ADL [0-100 & z] (activities of daily living; EQ5D)	**68.36**	**24.36**	**9.22**	**13.20**	**−0.59**	**0.84**	**0.361**
Roland-Morris [0–24]	8.42	5.26	−3.16	3.92	−0.59	0.73	0.394
WOMAC [Sum; 0–240]	73.70	42.17	−32.54	32.26	−0.77	0.77	0.504
Constant-Murley [Sum; 0–100]	41.09	17.19	17.98	11.53	−0.91	0.58	0.709
ORT 2: Function [z]	**0.36**	**0.97**	**−0.73**	**0.73**	**−0.73**	**0.73**	**0.475**
Time up & go [sec]	11.04	6.49	−2.62	3.30	−0.46	0.58	0.393
10m [sec]	9.55	5.23	−1.95	2.88	−0.43	0.63	0.327
ORT 3: Physical ability [z]	**0.22**	**1.11**	**−0.44**	**0.55**	**−0.44**	**0.55**	**0.403**
SO: specific ortho index [z] ORT1, ORT2 & ORT3	**0.31**	**0.83**	**−0.59**	**0.55**	**−0.59**	**0.55**	**0.583**

Bold values show summarized factors of outcome measures from disease-specific health parameters (see **Table 2**).

Table 7. Initial values and changes in individual measurements.

Unspecific and indication-specific outcome data (see **Tables 6** and **7**) show clear success during the rehabilitation stay, with complaints (MED 3, η^2 = 0.598) and motor function (ORT 2, η^2 = 0.478) improving markedly within the 3 weeks.

Based on the subsample survey of knee and hip TEP patients, it can be seen that changes occur in the nonspecific factors independent of the time of rehabilitation (interaction: time x post-op week: η^2 = 0.001). This result is in contrast to (disease-specific) outcome characteristics (SOi) where the time of onset (post-op week) plays a more important role (interaction: η^2 = 0.061; see **Table 9** (cf. [26]).

3.2. Comparison of outcomes based on ICD-classification

If one considers the initial medical evaluation values and changes there of as a result of the inpatient rehabilitation stay, we need to evaluate also the initial severity and admission diagnosis. The admission diagnosis was evaluated based on the standardized ICD-10 classification ("ICD") (see **Tables 8** and **9**). This classification shows that knee patients have worse MED 1 (Anatomy) values at the beginning of rehabilitation (0.36 ± 0.96). In back pain patients, especially negative MED 3 initial medical evaluation values (Discomfort) are prominent (MED 3: η^2 = 0.068). The symptom-specific characteristics (ORT, SO_i) and their differences in initial values were somewhat less pronounced (SO_i: η^2 = 0.010 vs. UH_i: η^2 = 0.017; see **Table 9**).

Overall adding up the MQO factors, the initial medical evaluation values are comparable between the ICD diagnostic groups (η^2_{MQOi} = 0.004), but in individual cases, they certainly play an important role ($\eta^2_{multivariat}$ = 0.080, see **Table 9**).

3.3. Influencing factors of age, gender and initial values

Depending on further grouping characteristics (between factors), it is shown that gender ($\eta^2_{multivariat}$ = 0.076) and age ($\eta^2_{multivariat}$ = 0.067) contribute a significant amount to initial values, which is lower within unspecific than in specific parameters (see **Table 9**; (cf. [26]). Additionally, medical initial values are influenced by the factor injuries (*S*) vs. chronic conditions (*M*; $\eta^2_{multivariat}$ = 0.058), as well as the symptom presentation "ICD" ($\eta^2_{multivariat}$ = 0.080).

Potential success through rehabilitation with unspecific outcome indicators (changes of condition pre and post, see also **Table 4**) can be observed within all grouping characteristics of a similar magnitude (interaction time x between factor: η^2_{UHi} < 0.003 see **Table 9**). In contrast, age, ICD, postOP and initial value of MQO play a role for alterations in specific outcome indicators (Age: η^2_{OHi} = 0.039, ICD: η^2_{OHi} = 0.040, postOP: η^2_{OHi} = 0.061 and initial MQO value: η^2_{OHi} = 0.143). All these factors influence the specific outcome significantly. Older patients (>61 years of age), patients with knee and hip issues, patients who enter phase 2 earlier after surgery (<6 weeks) and particularly patients with worse medical initial values show a more advantageous rehabilitation outcome for symptom-specific indicators (not shown).

http://dx.doi.org/10.5772/intechopen.89596

MQO indicators & factors		Initial values (beginning of rehabilitation; prae)		Change from admission (prae) to discharge (post)		
Classification according to ICD-10 (cf. Table 3)		**Mean* ± standard deviation (SD)**		**Mean diff.** (post - prae) ± SD**		**part. Eta²**
MED 1: anatomy	hip	0.15	0.94	−0.05	0.17	0.069
	knee	0.36	0.96	−0.06	0.18	0.086
	back (spine)	0.06	0.97	−0.05	0.19	0.058
	total	**0.18**	**0.97**	**−0.05**	**0.18**	**0.068**
MED 2: physiology	hip	0.19	0.90	−0.38	1.02	0.120
	knee	0.18	0.84	−0.34	1.00	0.107
	back (spine)	0.13	0.93	−0.40	1.03	0.129
	total	**0.16**	**0.89**	**−0.37**	**1.01**	**0.116**
MED 3: discomfort	hip	0.07	0.90	−0.83	0.68	0.600
	knee	0.38	0.86	−0.91	0.73	0.610
	back (spine)	0.65	0.92	−0.99	0.79	0.610
	total	**0.43**	**0.93**	**−0.92**	**0.74**	**0.596**
UHi: unspecific health Idx	hip	0.14	0.57	−0.42	0.40	0.517
	knee	0.31	0.57	−0.44	0.42	0.516
	back (spine)	0.28	0.61	−0.48	0.44	0.538
	total	**0.26**	**0.59**	**−0.45**	**0.43**	**0.515**
ORT 1: ADL	hip	0.37	1.09	−0.84	0.95	0.437
	knee	0.34	0.96	−0.69	0.86	0.390
	back (spine)	0.23	0.97	−0.52	0.80	0.295
	total	**0.30**	**1.00**	**−0.66**	**0.87**	**0.378**
ORT 2: function	hip	0.25	0.99	−0.78	0.77	0.507
	knee	0.37	0.96	−0.78	0.76	0.507
	back (spine)	0.27	0.97	−0.61	0.73	0.411
	total	**0.30**	**0.97**	**−0.71**	**0.76**	**0.473**

MQO indicators & factors		Initial values (beginning of rehabilitation; prae)		Change from admission (prae) to discharge (post)		
Classification according to ICD-10 (cf. Table 3)		**Mean* ± standard deviation (SD)**		**Mean diff.** (post - prae) ± SD**		**part. Eta^2**
ORT 3: physical ability	hip	0.37	0.93	−0.53	0.53	0.505
	knee	0.24	0.84	−0.47	0.47	0.498
	back (spine)	-0.07	0.98	−0.31	0.43	0.339
	total	**0.15**	**0.94**	**−0.42**	**0.48**	**0.456**
SOi: specific ortho Idx	hip	0.32	0.81	−0.72	0.55	0.633
	knee	0.32	0.73	−0.64	0.49	0.630
	back (spine)	0.16	0.78	−0.48	0.46	0.513
	total	**0.26**	**0.77**	**−0.60**	**0.51**	**0.597**
MQOi: overall idx	hip	0.23	0.56	−0.57	0.37	0.703
	knee	0.31	0.54	−0.54	0.36	0.697
	back (spine)	0.22	0.58	−0.48	0.36	0.641
	total	**0.25**	**0.56**	**−0.52**	**0.36**	**0.677**

*Positive (z-) values show a bad initial state at the beginning of rehabilitation.
**Negative (z-normalized) differences show an improvement from admission to discharge.
Bold values show overall means of summarized medical quality factors for the three most common orthopedic diagnoses.

Table 8. Symptom-specific (ICD) MQO.

Factors (main effects)	Unifactorial part. Eta^2 for initial values (prae)*					Unifactorial part. Eta^2 for changes (prae-post; interaction)**					
Between factors:	Sex	Age	Type	ICD***	Post-OP	Sex	Age	Type	ICD	Post-OP	Initial value$_{MQO}$
MQO variables	f/m	4-stage	M/S	**h/k/b**	5-stage	f/m	4-stage	M/S	h/k/b	5-stage	3-stage
MED 1: anatomy	0.018	0.023	0.024	**0.013**	0.001	0.004	0.005	0.000	0.001	0.001	0.006
MED 2: physiology	0.018	0.003	0.001	**0.000**	0.003	0.002	0.001	0.000	0.000	0.001	0.023
MED 3: discomfort	0.013	0.007	0.001	**0.068**	0.016	0.005	0.002	0.000	0.007	0.002	0.042
Unspecif. health$_{Idx}$	**0.007**	**0.011**	**0.007**	**0.017**	**0.007**	**0.000**	**0.001**	**0.001**	**0.003**	**0.001**	**0.061**
ORT 1: ADL	0.028	0.041	0.011	**0.003**	0.012	0.006	0.021	0.000	0.022	0.033	0.055
ORT 2: function	0.012	0.029	0.003	**0.002**	0.005	0.005	0.009	0.000	0.012	0.021	0.085
ORT 3: physical ability	0.032	0.161	0.027	**0.042**	0.020	0.009	0.041	0.005	0.040	0.048	0.094
Specific ortho$_{Idx}$	**0.036**	**0.103**	**0.018**	**0.010**	**0.015**	**0.013**	**0.039**	**0.001**	**0.040**	**0.061**	**0.143**
MQO$_i$: overall$_{idx}$	**0.009**	**0.061**	**0.003**	**0.004**	**0.004**	**0.006**	**0.021**	**0.000**	**0.011**	**0.033**	**0.168**
Multivariate (Pillai's trace)	**0.076**	**0.067**	**0.058**	**0.080**	**0.016**	**0.022**	**0.020**	**0.006**	**0.040**	**0.020**	**0.103**

Between factor: sex (female, male), age (quantile; ≤ 52, 53–61, 62–72, 73+), type (disease [M], injury [S]), ICD (hip, knee, back/spine), post-OP (period between surgery and rehabilitation; ≤ 6 weeks, 43–70 days, 71–105 days, 106–366 days, >1 year), initial value MQO (tertile); A part. Eta2 ($\eta 2$) between 0.01–0.06 corresponds to a small effect, occurrences of 0.06–0.14 a middle effect and values >0.14 a large effect.
*Initial state at the beginning of rehabilitation.
**Differences (improvements) from admission to discharge (corresponds to the interaction: time x factor).
***C.f. **Table 8**.
Bold values show the influence (effect size) of the approval diagnosis on baseline values and the impact of other moderating variables on summarized unspecific and specific health factors.

Table 9. MQO and potential influence factors.

4. Discussion

In times of dwindling resources, evidence-based justifications of medical measure effectiveness are gaining ever more practical and healthcare economic importance. New possibilities of medical treatment measures and constantly changing framework conditions are a challenge for quality assurance management, which uses structural, process and outcome characteristics to evaluate the degree to which predefined goals have been achieved. Potential environmental influences or a change of framework conditions can also be evaluated with regard to the MQO. The recorded routine data are used both as an evaluation criterion and as comparison data of the expected MQO or output values.

Current treatment paths emphasize a stratified approach, active therapies and educational measures, whereby evidence of effectiveness and clinical practice still clearly diverge [28, 50, 51].

Based on presented clinical observations through routine operating procedures of a multidisciplinary inpatient musculoskeletal system rehabilitation, evaluation can be performed. The evaluation takes into account facility and patient comparisons and is based on standardized assessments of different treatment options as well as factors of outcome quality. Existing performance profiles have a certain amount of latitude to focus on treatment or to apply promising therapeutic options. Such differentiated treatment pathways are necessary for efficient and successful treatment so that individual patients or specific patient groups can be addressed.

A physician/therapist or facility can use the results presented to make an evidence-based decision relatively quickly on whether the treatment process is proceeding to their satisfaction. Orthopedic patients receive a realistic assessment of what and how much they will improve their physical abilities through the 3-week inpatient medical treatment.

The selection of outcome parameters follows evidence-based and economic considerations that should guarantee a comparable standard of quality medical treatment. Indication-specific characteristics (ORT, SO_i) are at the center of the rehabilitative treatment, to restore the ability to function and work or to reintegrate into the social and professional environment. Another focus is on nonspecific health features such as individuals that are overweight, have high blood pressure or are physically inactive. These characteristics are associated with poorer health, cardiovascular disease and metabolic disorders. They are among the most important variable risk factors for chronic diseases and premature death [52].

An important task in inpatient rehabilitation is, in addition to the individual symptomatic treatment of a patient, to sustainably reduce these risk factors. Quality of life and functioning are characterized by positive lifestyle modifications, for example, an increase in physical activity. A reduction in the recorded basic clinical parameters such as BMI, abdominal circumference, blood pressure, heart rate and pain [53–56] is therefore also highly relevant in the inpatient rehabilitation of degenerative and inflammatory disorders of the musculoskeletal system [57, 58]. A mathematical comparison with "healthy" patient reference data underlines the importance of the MQO factors presented in this work, which deviate in the order of about one standard deviation of healthy individuals.

In order to work meaningfully and deductively, it is helpful to reduce the abundance of partially redundant information to a manageable, uniform level. An additive summary of independent medical areas (factors) to a key figure (UH_i or SO_i and overall MQO) is to be discussed in terms of content and statistics. These key figures give a simple and quick overview of the "unspecific" effectiveness of the rehabilitative stay for certain healthcare teams or treatment programs.

4.1. Nonspecific quality of outcomes

When assessing the effectiveness of inpatient rehabilitation based on the nonspecific health outcome characteristics, it is not so important to use grouping characteristics such as symptoms. Grouping based on gender and age is here too of minor importance. Comparing the values at discharge with the initial medical evaluation data shows that 72.5% of patients benefit directly from inpatient rehabilitation (see **Table 4**). Significant interactions with grouping features are present but can be classified as "small" compared to the main effects ($\eta^2 < 0.003$; see **Table 9**). The observed strong rehabilitation effect is similar for all subgroups ($\eta^2 > 0.500$; see **Tables 6** and **8**). This unspecific success is probably attributable to all inpatient rehabilitation stays and to the preventive effect of activity or movement in the rehabilitation setting.

The change in the nonspecific MQO is independent of the time of rehabilitation, the post-OP week ($\eta^2_{UHi} < 0.001$; see **Table 9**). In an untreated "real" control group without rehabilitation, therefore, no positive change in the constitutional state of health is to be expected.

In contrast, the importance of early inpatient rehabilitation as early as possible is revealed in disease-specific outcome characteristics such as function or physical ability ($\eta^2_{OHi} = 0.061$). This underlines the importance of a multidimensional view of specific and nonspecific outcome quality, describing two independent (active) components of rehabilitation (see **Figure 1** and **Table 5**).

4.2. Specific quality of outcomes

The most pronounced effects of inpatient rehabilitation are seen in the complaint (MED 3) and indication-specific characteristics (ORT 2, ORT 3 and SO_i). More than 2/3 of patients experience significant improvement of symptoms and specific characteristics (see **Table 4**). About 77.0% of patients show indication-specific improvement of outcomes in inpatient rehabilitation. However, 19.0% did not show significant changes and 4.0% showed worsening from rehabilitation beginning to rehabilitation end. Therefore, it is important to remember that not all patients can directly benefit from treatment. In sum, (overall MQO) improvement is achieved, in the vast majority (81.3%, SMD = 0.52 ± 0.38; see **Figure 1**). Improvement of unspecific and indication-specific outcome parameters is achieved in a comparable magnitude.

Unlike nonspecific health scores, moderating factors play a more important role in the specific outcome quality. In particular, patients who enter Phase II earlier (<6 weeks) after surgery and patients with worse initial medical evaluation show better rehabilitation success in symptom-specific characteristics (see **Table 9**).

4.3. The applicability of our results in rehabilitative clinical practice

Despite large international differences in healthcare teams and treatment measures in rehabilitation, the observed effect sizes can support individual evaluation but cannot replace it. In addition to case by case evaluation, it is important to consider the medical focus, the rehabilitative practice and performance profiles, as documented outcomes come about through different treatment programs and the associated different use of healthcare resources.

Absolute values and individual profiles of the MQO should always be evaluated according to the given setting and at the doctor's discretion. Single measurements are subject to a variety of moderating influences and measurement errors. The presented continuous measures of MQO have advantages in terms of their (scale) properties and sensitivity to frequently applied categorical criteria.

When using the presented clinical reference values of the MQO for orthopedic rehabilitation (WHO phase II) in Austria, apart from the reference sample, the monocentric character of the work has to be considered. The need for adjusting for different facility comparisons cannot be definitively answered. Different individual starting values must always be taken into account, as worse outcome parameters at the beginning of rehabilitation are accompanied by a greater potential for improvement (e.g., $r_{MQO} = -0.461$). Due to the prescribed performance profiles and the centrally controlled assignment modalities by the insurers, however, it can be assumed that the initial values presented and especially the changes in the MQO are representative of the inpatient rehabilitation of the musculoskeletal system in Austria.

The presented results and experiences of the clinical trial center suggest that the expected rehabilitation effects in the MQO factors are universal. Risk adjustment or indication- and group-specific modeling does not seem necessary. A closer characterization of nonresponders and types is still pending.

4.4. Limitation

The practical significance of the MQO outcomes or relationships with external criteria (endpoints), such as the incapacity for work, remains to be tested. Especially the global evaluation between MQO and sociomedical relevant external criteria is a potential further route for development. It is to be clarified which of the observed changes in MQO have significance for the sustainability of rehabilitative measures and to what extent optimized treatment pathways can influence them. Improvements in one outcome may well be accompanied by deterioration in other outcomes. Therefore, multidimensional approaches to the quality of results are always the methods of choice.

5. Conclusions

In addition to the usual "primary patient-oriented" assessment of quality of outcomes, the subjective assessment and satisfaction through self-reporting of patients as well as quality registers on surgical frequencies, length of stay and complications, these factors present a

http://dx.doi.org/10.5772/intechopen.89596

valuable addition to the medical outcome quality evaluation. These can be essential for decision-making or can contribute to the design processes and further developments of quality assurance in rehabilitation facilities.

Acknowledgements

The authors would like to thank the HUMANOMED Group and their colleagues and the Medical University of Graz for the support in the development and execution of this research.

Conflict of interest

The authors declare no conflict of interest.

Author details

Vincent Grote[1,2,3], Alexandra Unger[2,4], Henry Puff[1] and Elke Böttcher[1]*

*Address all correspondence to: elke.boettcher@humanomed.at

1 Humanomed Center Althofen, Austria

2 Lifestyle-Related Diseases (LIFEMED), Medical University of Graz, Austria

3 Otto Loewi Research Center, Division of Physiology, Medical University of Graz, Austria

4 University College of Teacher Education (UCTE) Carinthia, Viktor Frankl University College (UC), Austria

References

[1] Global Recommendations on Physical Activity for Health. Geneva: WHO; 2010. Available from: https://www.ncbi.nlm.nih.gov/pubmed/26180873. ISBN: 978 92 4 159 997 9

[2] Stucki G et al. Rehabilitation: The health strategy of the 21st century. Journal of Rehabilitation Medicine. 2018;**50**(4):309-316

[3] Lewis R et al. Strategies for optimising musculoskeletal health in the 21(st) century. BMC Musculoskeletal Disorders. 2019;**20**(1):164

[4] Warburton DE et al. A systematic review of the evidence for Canada's physical activity guidelines for adults. International Journal of Behavioral Nutrition and Physical Activity. 2010;**7**:39

[5] Katzmarzyk PT et al. Sedentary behavior and health: Update from the 2018 physical activity guidelines advisory committee. Medicine and Science in Sports and Exercise. 2019;**51**(6):1227-1241

[6] King AC, Powell KE, Kraus WE. The US physical activity guidelines advisory committee report-introduction. Medicine and Science in Sports and Exercise. 2019;**51**(6):1203-1205

[7] Stefani L, Galanti G. Physical exercise prescription in metabolic chronic disease. Advances in Experimental Medicine and Biology. 2017;**1005**:123-141

[8] Pedersen BK, Saltin B. Exercise as medicine - evidence for prescribing exercise as therapy in 26 different chronic diseases. Scandinavian Journal of Medicine & Science in Sports. 2015;**25**(Suppl 3):1-72

[9] Fuchs J, Rabenberg M, Scheidt-Nave C. Prevalence of selected musculoskeletal conditions in Germany: Results of the German health interview and examination survey for adults (DEGS1). Bundesgesundheitsblatt, Gesundheitsforschung, Gesundheitsschutz. 2013;**56**(5-6):678-686

[10] Edwards J et al. Prevalence of low back pain in emergency settings: A systematic review and meta-analysis. BMC Musculoskeletal Disorders. 2017;**18**(1):143

[11] Palazzo C et al. The burden of musculoskeletal conditions. PLoS One. 2014;**9**(3):e90633

[12] Hartvigsen J et al. What low back pain is and why we need to pay attention. The Lancet. 2018;**391**(10137):2356-2367

[13] Hoy D et al. A systematic review of the global prevalence of low back pain. Arthritis and Rheumatism. 2012;**64**(6):2028-2037

[14] Klimont J et al. Österreichische Gesundheitsbefragung 2014. Hauptergebnisse des Austrian Health Interview Survey (ATHIS) und Methodische Dokumentation. Wien: Statistik Austria; 2015

[15] Bartley EJ et al. Enhanced pain sensitivity among individuals with symptomatic knee osteoarthritis: Potential sex differences in central sensitization. Arthritis Care & Research (Hoboken). 2016;**68**(4):472-480

[16] OECD. Health at a Glance 2017. 2017

[17] Masaracchio M et al. Timing of rehabilitation on length of stay and cost in patients with hip or knee joint arthroplasty: A systematic review with meta-analysis. PLoS One. 2017;**12**(6): e0178295

[18] Kamper SJ et al. Multidisciplinary biopsychosocial rehabilitation for chronic low back pain: Cochrane systematic review and meta-analysis. BMJ. 2015;**350**:h444

[19] Goh SL et al. Efficacy and potential determinants of exercise therapy in knee and hip osteoarthritis: A systematic review and meta-analysis. Annals of Physical and Rehabilitation Medicine. 2019;**62**(5):356-365

[20] Artz N et al. Effectiveness of physiotherapy exercise following total knee replacement: Systematic review and meta-analysis. BMC Musculoskeletal Disorders. 2015;**16**:15

[21] Gyimesi M et al. Rehabilitationsplan 2016. Hauptverband der österreichischen Sozialversicherungsträger. Vienna; 2016. p. 273

[22] Rehabilitation after cardiovascular diseases, with special emphasis on developing countries. Report of a WHO expert committee. World Health Organization Technical Report Series. 1993;**831**:1-122

[23] Pacher A. Die Geschichte der Kur. Natürliche Heilvorkommen und Kurorte in Österreich. In: Marktl W, editor. Natürliche Heilvorkommen und Kurorte. Vienna: Österreichischer Heilbäder- und Kurorteverband (OHKV); 2014. pp. 104-106

[24] Wilbacher I, Maringer B. Orthopädische Rehabilitation in verschiedenen Settings - Nach großen Operationen an Hüfte oder Knie und mit Fokus auf ältere Personen. Hauptverband der österreichischen Sozialversicherungsträger; 2014. p. 77

[25] Deutsche Rentenversicherung. Reha-Therapiestandards Hüft- und Knie-TEP für die medizinische Rehabilitation der Rentenversicherung, Geschäftsbereich Sozialmedizin und Rehabilitation - Bereich Reha-Wissenschaften. Berlin: DRV; 2016. p. 36

[26] Grote V et al. Medizinische Ergebnisqualität: Unspezifische Outcome-Parameter einer stationären Rehabilitation des Stütz- und Bewegungsapparates in Österreich. Physikalische Medizin, Rehabilitationsmedizin, Kurortmedizin. 2019;**29**(02):104-117

[27] Medizinische Rehabilitation in Deutschland und im restlichen Europa. Die Rehabilitation. 2018;**57**(06):341-341

[28] Meyer C, Denis CM, Berquin AD. Secondary prevention of chronic musculoskeletal pain: A systematic review of clinical trials. Annals of Physical and Rehabilitation Medicine. 2018;**61**(5):323-338

[29] Knaller C, Eisenmann A, Pertl D. Wirksamkeit der stationären rehabilitation für Erwachsene nach zwölf Monaten. Wien: Gesundheit Österreich Forschungs- und Planungs GmbH; 2012. p. 403

[30] Bethge M, Müller-Fahrnow W. Wirksamkeit einer intensivierten stationären Rehabilitation bei muskuloskelettalen Erkrankungen: Systematischer Review und Meta-Analyse. Rehabilitation. 2008;**47**(4):200-209

[31] Di Monaco M, Castiglioni C. Which type of exercise therapy is effective after hip arthroplasty? A systematic review of randomized controlled trials. European Journal of Physical and Rehabilitation Medicine. 2013;**49**(6):893-907. quiz 921-3

[32] Lin PC. An evaluation of the effectiveness of relaxation therapy for patients receiving joint replacement surgery. Journal of Clinical Nursing. 2012;**21**(5-6):601-608

[33] Mak JC et al. Evidence-based review for patients undergoing elective hip and knee replacement. ANZ Journal of Surgery. 2014;**84**(1-2):17-24

[34] Brem MH et al. Stop of loss of cognitive performance during rehabilitation after total hip arthroplasty-prospective controlled study. Journal of Rehabilitation Research and Development. 2010;**47**(9):891-898

[35] Bystrom MG, Rasmussen-Barr E, Grooten WJ. Motor control exercises reduces pain and disability in chronic and recurrent low back pain: A meta-analysis. Spine (Phila Pa 1976). 2013;**38**(6):E350-E358

[36] Cherkin DC et al. A comparison of the effects of 2 types of massage and usual care on chronic low back pain: A randomized, controlled trial. Annals of Internal Medicine. 2011; **155**(1):1-9

[37] Henschke N et al. Behavioural treatment for chronic low-back pain. Cochrane Database of Systematic Reviews. 2010;**7**:CD002014

[38] Linton SJ, Nordin E. A 5-year follow-up evaluation of the health and economic consequences of an early cognitive behavioral intervention for back pain: A randomized, controlled trial. Spine (Phila Pa 1976). 2006;**31**(8):853-858

[39] Malfliet A et al. Best evidence rehabilitation for chronic pain part 3: Low Back pain. Journal of Clinical Medicine. 2019;**8**(7)

[40] Caby I et al. A controlled and retrospective study of 144 chronic low Back pain patients to evaluate the effectiveness of an intensive functional restoration program in France. Healthcare (Basel). 2016;**4**(2)

[41] Marin TJ et al. Multidisciplinary biopsychosocial rehabilitation for subacute low back pain. Cochrane Database of Systematic Reviews. 2017;**6**:CD002193

[42] Hazard RG et al. Functional restoration with behavioral support. A one-year prospective study of patients with chronic low-back pain. Spine (Phila Pa 1976). 1989;**14**(2):157-161

[43] Håland Haldorsen EM et al. Is there a right treatment for a particular patient group? Comparison of ordinary treatment, light multidisciplinary treatment, and extensive multidisciplinary treatment for long-term sick-listed employees with musculoskeletal pain. Pain. 2002;**95**(1):49-63

[44] Schwarz B et al. Multiprofessional teamwork in work-related medical rehabilitation for patients with chronic musculoskeletal disorders. Journal of Rehabilitation Medicine. 2015; **47**(1):58-65

[45] Momsen AM et al. Multidisciplinary team care in rehabilitation: An overview of reviews. Journal of Rehabilitation Medicine. 2012;**44**(11):901-912

[46] Donabedian A. The quality of care. JAMA. 1988;**260**(12):1743

[47] Keilani M et al. Assessment in der Physikalischen Medizin und Rehabilitation. Physikalische Medizin, Rehabilitationsmedizin, Kurortmedizin. 2014;**24**(05):A6

[48] Moock J. Präferenzbasierte Lebensqualitätsmessung: Der EQ-5D Fragebogen. Physikalische Medizin, Rehabilitationsmedizin, Kurortmedizin. 2008;**18**(05):245-249

[49] Cohen J. Statistical Power Analysis for the Behavior Science. 2nd ed. Hillsdale, New Jersey: Lawrence Erlbaum Associates; 1988

[50] Foster NE et al. Prevention and treatment of low back pain: Evidence, challenges, and promising directions. Lancet. 2018;**391**(10137):2368-2383

[51] Shiri R, Coggon D, Falah-Hassani K. Exercise for the prevention of low Back pain: Systematic review and meta-analysis of controlled trials. American Journal of Epidemiology. 2018;**187**(5):1093-1101

[52] Mathers C et al, editor. Global Health Risks: Mortality and Burden of Disease Attributable to Selected Major Risks. Geneva, Switzerland: World Health Organization; 2009

[53] Bundy JD et al. Systolic blood pressure reduction and risk of cardiovascular disease and mortality: A systematic review and network meta-analysis. JAMA Cardiology. 2017;**2**(7): 775-781

[54] Seccareccia F et al. Heart rate as a predictor of mortality: The MATISS project. American Journal of Public Health. 2001;**91**(8):1258-1263

[55] Geneen LJ et al. Physical activity and exercise for chronic pain in adults: An overview of Cochrane reviews. Cochrane Database of Systematic Reviews. 2017;**4**(4):CD011279

[56] Papathanasiou G et al. Association of high blood pressure with body mass index, smoking and physical activity in healthy young adults. Open Cardiovascular Medicine Journal. 2015;**9**:5-17

[57] Hurley M et al. Exercise interventions and patient beliefs for people with hip, knee or hip and knee osteoarthritis: A mixed methods review. Cochrane Database of Systematic Reviews. 2018;**4**(4):CD010842

[58] Zheng H, Chen C. Body mass index and risk of knee osteoarthritis: Systematic review and meta-analysis of prospective studies. BMJ Open. 2015;**5**(12):e007568

Section 3

Neurophysiological Aspects and Physical Therapy Interventions

Chapter 5

Effectiveness of Motor Imagery on Physical Therapy: Neurophysiological Aspects of Motor Imagery

Yoshibumi Bunno

Additional information is available at the end of the chapter

http://dx.doi.org/10.5772/intechopen.90277

Abstract

Immediate enrollment in physical therapy and facilitation of the spinal motor neuron excitability are very important. We previously suggested that the F-wave parameters were significantly increased during motor imagery. Thus, motor imagery is a beneficial method to facilitate the spinal motor neuron excitability for patients with various motor dysfunctions. We also indicated that the imagined muscle contraction strength may not affect the spinal motor neuron excitability. Additionally, kinesthetic imagery can more facilitate the spinal motor neuron excitability; however, longer duration of motor imagery may decrease the spinal motor neuron excitability. Thus, when applying motor imagery to physical therapy, slight imagined muscle contraction strength may be sufficient to facilitate the spinal motor neuron excitability, and the duration and strategy of imagery should be considered.

Keywords: motor imagery, F-wave, muscle contraction strength, duration, strategy

1. Introduction

Motor imagery (MI) is the mental representation of a movement in the absence of any actual overt movement. It is a cognitive process creating specific motor actions within the working memory [1]. MI may be a beneficial tool to improve various motor functions for patients with stroke-induced motor deficits [2–5]. Decline of motor evoked potential (MEP) amplitude, an index of corticospinal excitability obtained when transcranial magnetic stimulation is applied to the primary motor cortex, can be observed post-stroke [6]. Additionally, a significant reduction of spinal motor neuron excitability has been shown in the post-stroke acute phase [7]. Thus, corticospinal excitability, including that of spinal motor neurons, would be reduced

IntechOpen

© 2019 The Author(s). Licensee IntechOpen. This chapter is distributed under the terms of the Creative Commons Attribution License (http://creativecommons.org/licenses/by/3.0), which permits unrestricted use, distribution, and reproduction in any medium, provided the original work is properly cited.

post-stroke. Corticospinal excitability is considered to be an index of functional motor recovery [8], and immediate enrollment in rehabilitation for stimulation of corticospinal and spinal motor neuron excitability may be important to achieve better outcomes.

Neuroimaging studies show that MI activates motor-related brain regions, including the primary motor cortex, supplementary motor area, premotor area, prefrontal cortex, somatosensory area, parietal lobe, cingulate gyrus, cerebellum, and basal ganglia [9, 10]. Similarly, these regions have been shown as activated during motor execution [9, 10]. Furthermore, the MEP amplitude was shown as significantly increased during MI [11–13]. Thus, MI may stimulate the central nervous system. Various patterns of spinal motor neuron excitability have been observed during MI [14–16]. The F-wave is one of the indices of spinal motor neuron excitability. It is a compound action potential resulting from re-excitation (backfiring) at spinal anterior horn cells by an antidromic impulse following the distal electrical stimulation of motor nerve fibers [17–19]. The F-wave amplitude increases when the corticospinal descending volley collides with the antidromic peripheral volley [20]. Additionally, the F-wave is a reliable index of spinal motor neuron excitability, even when motor output is extremely low, as is the case during MI [21].

As described previously in this chapter, stimulating spinal motor neuron excitability would improve motor function. Our final goal is to find the most beneficial approach by which MI can increase the spinal motor neuron excitability. In the following sections, we introduce our research on spinal motor neuron excitability under various MI conditions. At the end of the chapter, we discuss the application of MI to physical therapy from a neurophysiological perspective.

2. The spinal motor neuron excitability during MI under different imagined muscle contraction strengths

2.1. Purpose

We previously reported that the spinal motor neuron excitability increased significantly when participants performed MI of isometric thenar muscle activity under 50% maximal voluntary contraction (MVC) [22]. However, it was unclear whether the magnitude of the imagined muscle contraction strength affects the spinal motor neuron excitability. Therefore, we used F-wave measurements to investigate the spinal motor neuron excitability during MI of isometric thenar muscle activity under various imagined muscle contraction strengths. Specifically, we adopted the 10, 30, 50, 70, and 100% MVC for imagined muscle contraction strength [23–25].

2.2. Materials

We conducted two experiments to assess the spinal motor neuron excitability during MI under different imagined muscle contraction strengths. Firstly, we measured the F-wave during MI under 10, 30, 50, and 70% MVC for 10 healthy volunteers (5 males, 5 females; mean age = 28.7 ± 4.5 years). Secondly, we measured the F-wave during MI under 50 and 100% MVC for 15 healthy volunteers (13 males, 2 females; mean age = 25.3 ± 5.0 years). All participants provided informed consent before study commencement. This research was approved by the

Research Ethics Committee at Kansai University of Health Sciences. All recordings were conducted in accordance with the Declaration of Helsinki.

2.3. Methods

A Viking Quest electromyography (EMG) machine ver. 9.0 (Natus Medical Inc., USA) was used for the F-wave recording. A pair of silver disc electrodes (10 mm diameter, Natus Medical Inc., USA) were placed over left thenar eminence and base of the first dorsal metacarpal bone. The skin was cleaned with an abrasive gel, and then impedance was maintained below 5 kΩ. The F-wave was evoked from the left thenar muscles by delivering supramaximal electrical stimuli, 0.2 ms in duration and 0.5 Hz in frequency, to the median nerve at the left wrist. Supramaximal stimuli were determined 20% higher than the maximal stimulus intensity required to elicit the largest compound muscle action potential (M-wave). The sensitivity for the F-wave was set at 200 μV/division and a sweep of 5 ms/division. The bandwidth filter range was 20 Hz–3 kHz.

Participants were placed in the supine posture on a bed and instructed to fix their eyes on the display of a pinch meter (Digital Indicator F304A, Unipulse Corp., Japan) throughout the F-wave recording. To determine the baseline of spinal motor neuron excitability, the F-wave was measured during relaxation for 1 min (rest). Thereafter, participants exerted isometric left thenar muscle contraction at 50% MVC (i.e., participants pressed the sensor of the pinch meter using their thumb and index finger at 50% MVC) for 1 min with visual feedback. For the MI trial, participants performed MI of isometric thenar muscle activity under 50% MVC for 1 min (50% MI). Immediately after the 50% MI trial, the F-wave was recorded during relaxation for 1 min (post). There were 30 supramaximal electrical stimuli delivered during each trial for the F-wave recording. The above process was defined as the MI at 50% MVC condition (50% MI condition). This protocol was repeated for conditions of 10, 30, 70, and 100% MI. Each condition was performed randomly on different days.

2.4. F-wave data analysis

All measured F-wave data were analyzed with respect to two parameters: persistence and the F/M amplitude ratio. The minimum F-wave peak-to-peak amplitude was 20 μV [26]. The persistence was represented as the percentage of detected F-wave responses out of 30 supramaximal electrical stimuli. It reflects the number of backfiring spinal anterior horn cells [17, 19]. The F/M amplitude ratio was obtained as the mean of the ratios of each detected F-wave response amplitude divided by the corresponding M-wave amplitude; it reflects the number of backfiring spinal anterior horn cells and individual spinal anterior horn cell excitability [19]. Therefore, the persistence and F/M amplitude ratio are considered indices of spinal motor neuron excitability.

2.5. Statistical analysis

2.5.1. The F-wave during MI under 10, 30, 50, and 70% MVC

Because the Shapiro-Wilk test did not confirm the normality of the F-wave data, a nonparametric method was used for statistical analysis. The persistence and F/M amplitude ratio among the three trials (rest, MI, and post) under each MI condition (10, 30, 50, and 70% MI) were compared using the Friedman test and Scheffe's post hoc test.

We also calculated the relative value obtained by dividing the F-wave data during MI under the four MI conditions by that at rest and compared the results using the Friedman test. SPSS Statistics ver. 19 software (IBM Corp., USA) was used for statistical analysis. The threshold for statistical significance was set at $p < 0.05$.

2.5.2. The F-wave during MI under 50 and 100% MVC

The persistence and F/M amplitude ratio among three trials (rest, MI, and post) under each MVC MI conditions were compared using the Friedman test and Scheffe's post hoc test. The relative values between the two MI conditions were compared using the Wilcoxon signed rank test.

2.6. Results

2.6.1. The F-wave during MI under 10, 30, 50, and 70% MVC

The persistence during MI under all MI conditions was significantly higher than that at rest (10% MI vs. rest and 70% MI vs. rest, $p < 0.01$; 30% MI vs. rest and 50% MI vs. rest, $p < 0.05$) (**Tables 1–4**). The F/M amplitude ratio during MI under 10, 30, and 50% MI conditions was significantly higher than that at rest (10% MI vs. rest and 50% MI vs. rest, $p < 0.01$; 30% MI vs. rest, $p < 0.05$) (**Tables 1–3**). The F/M amplitude ratio during MI under the 70% MI condition tended to be more increased than that at rest ($p = 0.082$) (**Table 4**). The F/M amplitude ratio immediately after MI under all MI conditions was reduced to the rest level (**Tables 1–4**).

The relative values of the persistence and F/M amplitude ratio did not show significant differences among all MI conditions (**Table 5**).

	rest	10% MI	post
Persistence (%)	61.8 ± 12.6	91.9 ± 9.70**	73.1 ± 20.7
F/M amplitude ratio (%	0.90 ± 0.35	2.46 ± 2.61**	1.18 ± 0.67
Latency (ms)	25.3 ± 0.98	25.2 ± 1.25	25.5 ± 0.99

Mean ± SD.

**$p < 0.01$; significant difference between rest and 10% MI trial.

10% MI: Motor imagery of isometric opponens pollicis activity at 10% MVC

Table 1. The F-wave under 10% MI condition.

	rest	30% MI	post
Persistence (%)	61.2 ± 19.5	88.0 ± 12.2*	60.0 ± 18.7
F/M amplitude ratio (%	1.00 ± 0.94	2.92 ± 2.95*	1.11 ± 0.52
Latency (ms)	24.9 ± 1.16	24.6 ± 0.99	24.9 ± 1.14

Mean ± SD.

**$p < 0.05$; significant difference between rest and 30% MI trial.

30% MI: Motor imagery of isometric opponens pollicis activity at 30% MVC

Table 2. The F-wave under 30% MI condition.

	rest	50% MI	post
Persistence (%)	62.7 ± 22.3	94.0 ± 9.40*	65.5 ± 27.0
F/M amplitude ratio (%	1.08 ± 0.28	2.60 ± 2.30**	0.98 ± 0.40
Latency (ms)	24.5 ± 1.61	24.3 ± 1.82	24.5 ± 1.58

Mean ± SD.
*$p < 0.05$; significant difference between rest and 50% MI trial.
**$p < 0.01$; significant difference between rest and 50% MI trial.
50% MI: Motor imagery of isometric opponens pollicis activity at 50% MVC

Table 3. The F-wave under 50% MI condition.

	rest	70% MI	post
Persistence (%)	55.9 ± 17.6	88.1 ± 10.8**	65.3 ± 19.9
F/M amplitude ratio (%	0.94 ± 0.33	1.79 ± 1.23	1.11 ± 0.44
Latency (ms)	24.4 ± 1.37	24.1 ± 1.27	24.3 ± 1.15

Mean ± SD.
**$p < 0.01$; significant difference between rest and 70% MI trial.
70% MI: Motor imagery of isometric opponens pollicis activity at 70% MVC

Table 4. The F-wave under 70% MI condition.

	10% MI condition	30% MI condition	50% MI condition	70% MI condition
relative values of persistence	1.53 ± 0.31	1.58 ± 0.61	1.78 ± 0.93	1.69 ± 0.45
relative values of F/M amplitude rati	2.40 ± 1.38	3.31 ± 0.56	2.52 ± 1.96	2.10 ± 1.37
relative values of latency	0.99 ± 0.02	0.99 ± 0.02	0.99 ± 0.03	0.99 ± 0.02

Mean ± SD.
MI: Motor imagery

Table 5. Relative values of the F-wave under 10% MI, 30% MI, 50% MI, and 70% MI condition.

	rest	50% MI	post
Persistence (%)	50.8 ± 21.7	88.2 ± 13.2**	48.3 ± 19.9
F/M amplitude ratio (%	1.71 ± 0.89	3.96 ± 4.56**	1.29 ± 0.56
Latency (ms)	25.5 ± 1.40	24.9 ± 1.91	25.3 ± 1.29

Mean ± SD.
**$p < 0.01$; significant difference between rest and 50%MI trial.

Table 6. The F-wave under 50% MI condition.

2.6.2. The F-wave during MI under 50 and 100% MVC

The persistence during MI under the 50% MI and 100% MI conditions was significantly higher than that at rest (50% MI vs. rest and 100% MI vs. rest, $p < 0.01$; **Tables 6** and **7**), and the F/M amplitude ratio during MI under 50% and 100% MI conditions was significantly higher than

	rest	100% MI	post
Persistence (%)	60.8 ± 24.9	91.9 ± 7.58**	60.7 ± 21.5
F/M amplitude ratio (%	1.32 ± 1.12	3.57 ± 4.67**	1.39 ± 1.25
Latency (ms)	25.2 ± 1.32	24.8 ± 1.31	25.2 ± 1.40

Mean ± SD.

**p < 0.01; significant difference between rest and 100% MI trial.

Table 7. The F-wave under 100% MI condition.

	50% MI condition	100% MI condition
relative values of persistence	2.04 ± 1.17	2.06 ± 1.71
relative values of F/M amplitude ratio	2.75 ± 2.04	2.53 ± 1.76
relative values of latency	0.98 ± 0.06	0.99 ± 0.03

Mean ± SD.

MI: Motor imagery

Table 8. Relative values of the F-wave under 50% MI and 100% MI condition.

that at rest (50% MI vs. rest and 100% MI vs. rest, $p < 0.01$; **Tables 6** and **7**). The F/M amplitude ratio immediately after MI (at post) under the 50% and 100% MI conditions did not show any significant differences compared with that at rest (**Tables 6** and **7**).

The relative values of the persistence and F/M amplitude ratio did not show significant differences between two MI conditions (**Table 8**).

2.7. Discussion

2.7.1. The spinal motor neuron excitability during MI of isometric thenar muscle activity

Both the persistence and the F/M amplitude ratio were significantly increased during MI under 10, 30, 50, 70, and 100% MVC. Previous research has demonstrated that the activation of various brain regions contributes to motor preparation and planning during MI [9, 10]. Thus, it is considered that the activation of the central nervous system that contributes to motor preparation and planning during MI is responsible for the observed increase in spinal motor neuron excitability via the descending pathways, such as the corticospinal and extrapyramidal tracts.

Furthermore, all participants in our previous studies performed MI while holding the sensor of the pinch meter. Mizuguchi et al. [27] reported that while holding an object, the corticospinal excitability during MI was modulated by a combination of tactile and proprioceptive inputs. Thus, it is plausible that holding the pinch meter sensor during MI caused tactile and proprioceptive perceptions to cooperatively increase the spinal motor neuron excitability along with the MI-activated pathways.

2.7.2. The spinal motor neuron excitability during MI under different imagined muscle contraction strengths

Relative values of the persistence and F/M amplitude were similar among all MI conditions. This result indicated that the magnitude of imagined muscle contraction strength may not affect spinal motor neuron excitability. Bonnet et al. [28] reported that the H-reflex amplitude during MI was similar between 2 and 10% MI conditions. Hale et al. [29] also reported that the H-reflex amplitude during MI of ankle plantar flexion was similar among five (i.e., 20, 40, 60, 80, and 100% MVC) MI conditions. Similarly, Aoyama and Kaneko [30] reported that the H-reflex amplitude during MI was similar between 50 and 100% MI conditions. MI is the mental representation of a movement in the absence of any overt movement [1]. The neural mechanism that inhibits actual movement and muscle contraction during MI may be involved in this result. Park et al. [31] reported that the MEP amplitude during MI was similar among all six (i.e., 10, 20, 30, 40, 50, and 60% MVC) MI conditions. Furthermore, the magnitude of primary motor cortex activity during MI did not correlate with that of the imagined muscle contraction strength, although the activities of the supplementary motor and premotor area during MI were strongly correlated with it [32]. The supplementary motor and premotor areas play crucial roles in larger force generation [33], motor planning, preparation, and inhibition [34, 35]. Thus, these areas may inhibit the actual muscle contraction depending on the magnitude of the muscle contraction strength. These areas are also directly connected to the primary motor cortex, and inhibitory inputs from them may suppress additional primary motor cortex excitation conferred by MI with high imagined contraction strengths. Therefore, the degree of spinal motor neuron excitability during MI at various imagined muscle contraction strengths may be modulated by both excitatory and inhibitory inputs from the central nervous system.

2.8. Conclusion

Our previous research has shown significant facilitation of the spinal motor neuron excitability during MI of isometric thenar muscle activity. The imagined muscle contraction strength may not be affected by the spinal motor neuron excitability. Thus, MI of isometric thenar muscle activity under slight MVC (i.e., 10% MVC) could substantially facilitate the spinal motor neuron excitability.

3. Does the duration of motor imagery affect the spinal motor neuron excitability?

3.1. Purpose

We previously reported that MI can increase the spinal motor neuron excitability and that the magnitude of imagined muscle contraction strength may not affect spinal motor neuron excitability [23–25]. In these studies, the duration of each MI session was 1 min. Driskell et al. [36] suggested that longer MI sessions do not always prove beneficial; they recommended a duration of approximately 20 min for an MI training session. Another study suggested that MI for 10–15 min elicited the most significant effect on performance [37]. Moreover, Twinning et al. [38] suggested that 5 min is the temporal limit beyond which it is difficult to concentrate and perform MI. As described previously, stimulation of spinal motor neuron excitability may be important for post-stroke rehabilitation; however, time-dependent changes in spinal motor neuron excitability during MI have not yet been investigated. Additionally, MI ability has a significant effect on brain activation [39] and corticospinal excitability [40]. In this study, we used F-waves to investigate whether the duration of MI and MI ability affects the spinal motor neuron excitability [41].

3.2. Materials

Eleven healthy volunteers participated in this research (8 males, 3 females, mean age = 26.4 ± 6.0 years). All participants gave written informed consent before study commencement. The study was approved by the Research Ethics Committee at the Graduate School of Kansai University of Health Sciences. All recordings were conducted in accordance with the Declaration of Helsinki.

3.3. Methods

The environment and F-wave recording conditions were set as previously described [23–25]. For the rest trial (rest), the F-wave was measured during relaxation for 1 min. Subsequently, participants learned the isometric thenar muscle activity at 50% MVC for 1 min with visual feedback. For the MI trial, participants performed the MI of isometric thenar muscle activity under 50% MVC for 5 min. F-waves were measured at 1, 3, and 5 min after the beginning of MI (1-, 3-, and 5-min MI, respectively). Immediately after MI, the F-wave was measured again during relaxation (post). After F-wave recordings, participants were asked to evaluate their vividness of MI, how vividly they could imagine isometric thenar muscle activity at 50% MVC, at 1, 3, and 5-min using a seven-point Likert scale ranging from 1 (very difficult to perform MI vividly) to 7 (very easy to perform MI vividly).

Background electromyography (EMG) was recorded using telemetry EMG (MQ-8, Kissei Comtec Co., Ltd., Japan) and EMG recording software (Vital Recorder 2, Kissei Comtec Co., Ltd.). Surface EMG signals were recorded for 5 min from the left thenar muscles to confirm no muscle contractions during MI. A pair of disposable Ag/AgCl electrodes (Blue Sensor N-00-S, Ambu A/S, Denmark) were placed over the muscle surface with an inter-electrode distance of 20 mm. EMG signals were recorded at rest; at 1, 3, and 5 min of MI; and post-trial. The recorded EMG data were analyzed using a multi-purpose biological information analysis system (BIMUTAS-Video, Kissei Comtec Co., Ltd.) after analog to digital conversion at a sampling frequency of 1 kHz. The root mean square values of the EMG data in each trial were then calculated.

3.4. Statistical analysis

We used a nonparametric method because the normality of F-wave data was not confirmed using the Shapiro-Wilk test. The persistence and F/M amplitude ratio among five trials (rest, 1, 3, 5-min MI, and post, respectively) were compared using the Friedman test and Scheffe's post hoc test. The rating scores of MI vividness at 1, 3, and 5-min MI were compared using the Friedman test and Scheffe's post hoc test. The SPSS statistics ver. 19 (IBM Corp., USA) was used for statistical analysis. The threshold for statistical significance was set at $p = 0.05$.

3.5. Results

In **Figure 1** it is possible to verify that persistence and F/M amplitude ratio were significantly facilitated until 3 min from the beginning of MI task.

The score of MI vividness at 5-min MI was significantly decreased compared to 1-min MI (*$p < 0.05$; **Table 9**).

There were no significant differences in the RMS data among five trials, and thus there was no measurable muscle activity during MI for 5 min.

3.6. Discussion

Both persistence and F/M amplitude ratio were significantly higher until 3 min from the beginning of MI. This result may suggest that participants could perform MI for at least 3 min without much difficulty. However, there were no significant differences in persistence and F/M amplitude ratio between the at rest and 5-min MI conditions. Additionally, the F/M amplitude ratio for the 5-min MI conditions was significantly lower than that for 1- and 3-min conditions. These findings may be due to mental fatigue; in one study, mental fatigue was found to have altered the maximal force production of the elbow flexor [42]. It also made it difficult for participants to maintain their focus on imagined movement [43]. Furthermore, repetitive MI of a handgrip movement decreased the MEP amplitude more than that at rest [44]. Thus, mental fatigue caused by sustained mental activity may have induced a decline of the spinal motor neuron excitability.

Furthermore, a decline of spinal motor neuron excitability can be also explained by MI habituation. MI is closely related to attentional processing [45]. Brain activation decreases by habituation after performing a cognitive motor task for 10 min. Furthermore, the corticospinal excitability was also decreased by habituation [46]. Specifically, brain activity showed

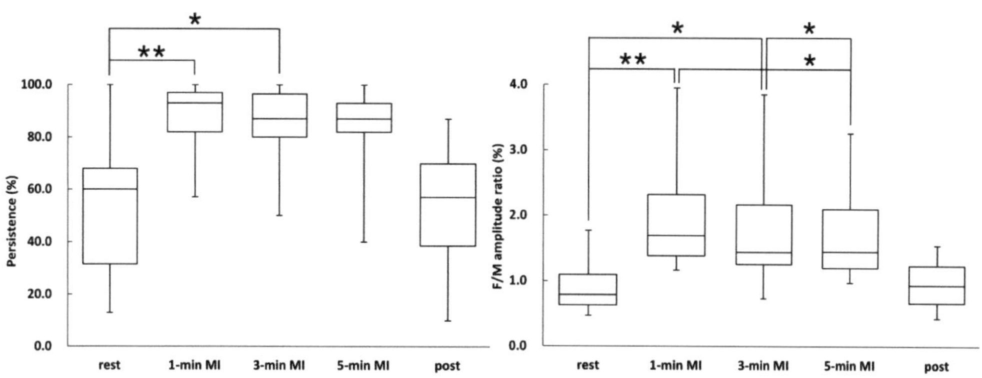

Figure 1. Changes in persistence and F/M amplitude ratio during MI for 5 min (*$p < 0.05$, **$p < 0.01$). The persistence at 1 and 3 min MI was significantly higher than that at rest. The F/M amplitude ratio at 1 and 3 min MI was significantly higher than that at rest. Additionally, the F/M amplitude ratio at 5 min MI was significantly smaller than that at 1 and 3 min MI.

	1-min MI	3-min MI	5-min MI
Rating score of MI vividness	5.71 ± 0.76	3.57 ± 0.53	2.29 ± 0.76*

Mean ± SD.
*p < 0.05; significant difference between 1-min and 5-min MI

Table 9. Rating scores of MI vividness at 1-min MI, 3-min MI, and 5-min MI.

an increase at 2 min before the onset of the task; however, after 4–6 min, activity decreased. Additionally, at the spinal level, the T-reflex amplitude, another index of the spinal motor neuron excitability, was significantly decreased due to habituation following sustained mental work for 20 min [47]. Our results also seemed to indicate that habituation to MI might occur approximately 4 min after its initiation and suggested that longer excitation times during MI might not be required for habituation of the central nervous system and spinal motor neurons.

Finally, practice time and MI ability were considered as possible factors affecting spinal motor neuron excitability. Regarding clinical use of MI for motor skill learning, Twining et al. [38] indicated that participants found it difficult to concentrate and perform MI for more than 5 min. Mental chronometry measured similar times for actual performance and MI [48]. Specifically, participants experienced difficulties in performing MI accurately beyond the practice time. In our study, the practice time for the motor task was only 1 min; thus, 1 min of practice time may be insufficient to continue performing MI for 5 min. Indeed, the vividness of MI tended to decrease with MI time. Furthermore, the vividness of MI at 5 min post MI initiation was significantly decreased relative to that at 1 min post MI initiation.

3.7. Conclusion

The persistence and F/M amplitudes at 1- and 3-min MI were significantly increased; however, the persistence and the F/M amplitude ratio at 5-min MI were reduced to rest levels. Thus, MI for 1–3 min may positively affect the spinal motor neuron excitability. In physical therapy, the duration of MI should be considered. As described in the Discussion section, matching the time of task practice to that of MI might be important. However, in this study, we did not investigate time-dependent changes of the spinal motor neuron excitability after motor learning for 5 min. Therefore, further research is required to resolve this issue. A limitation of this research is that differences in the brain activity during MI under 10, 30, 50, 70, and 100% MVC were not evaluated. Further study would be required to resolve this issue.

4. Imagery strategy affects the spinal motor neuron excitability: using kinesthetic and somatosensory imagery

4.1. Purpose

Previous research has demonstrated that MI increases the spinal motor neuron excitability and that the magnitude of imagined contraction strength may not affect it [23–25]. Additionally, the duration of MI should be considered in physical therapy [41].

MI includes various components of perception that can be associated with actual movement [49], which is why the effects of MI may differ depending on the choice of sensory modality. Here, we used F-wave and MI ability to investigate whether the choice of imagery strategy affects the spinal motor neuron excitability [50].

4.2. Materials

Fourteen healthy volunteers participated in this research (10 males, 4 females, mean age = 23.4 ± 4.8 years). All participants gave written informed consent before study commencement. The study was approved by the Research Ethics Committee at the Graduate School of Kansai University of Health Sciences. All recordings were conducted in accordance with the Declaration of Helsinki.

4.3. Methods

The environment and F-wave recording conditions were set as previously described [23–25, 41]. To determine the baseline of the spinal motor neuron excitability, the F-wave was measured during relaxation for 1 min (rest). Subsequently, participants exerted isometric left thenar muscle contraction at 50% MVC for 1 min with visual feedback. Simultaneously, participants were instructed to learn the two imagery strategies: somatosensory (tactile and pressure perception of thumb finger pulp during pressing of the sensor of the pinch meter) and kinesthetic (thenar muscle contraction during pressing of the sensor of the pinch meter at 50% MVC). After learning each imagery strategy, participants performed somatosensory imagery (SI), kinesthetic imagery (KI), and combined somatosensory and kinesthetic imagery (SKI) randomly for 1 min. In SKI trial, participants performed kinesthetic and somatosensory imagery simultaneously. After all the F-wave recording, participants were asked to evaluate difficulty of each imagery strategies by using a 5-point Likert scale, ranging from 1 (very hard to image vividly) to 5 (very easy to image vividly).

Background electromyography (EMG) was recorded during rest and three imagery trials.

4.4. Statistical analysis

We used a nonparametric method because the normality of F-wave data was not confirmed using the Shapiro-Wilk test. The persistence and F/M amplitude ratio among four trials (rest, SI, KI, and SKI, respectively) were compared using the Friedman test and Scheffe's post hoc test. The rating scores of each imagery strategies (SI, KI, and SKI, respectively) were compared using the Friedman test and Scheffe's post hoc test. The background EMG data were compared using the Friedman test. The SPSS statistics ver. 19 (IBM Corp., USA) was used for statistical analysis. The threshold for statistical significance was set at $p = 0.05$.

4.5. Results

The persistence during SI and KI were significantly higher than that at rest ($^{**}p < 0.01$; **Figure 2**). The persistence during SKI was tended to be increased than that at rest ($p = 0.097$; **Figure 2**). The F/M amplitude ratio during KI was significantly higher than that at rest ($^{*}p < 0.05$; **Figure 2**).

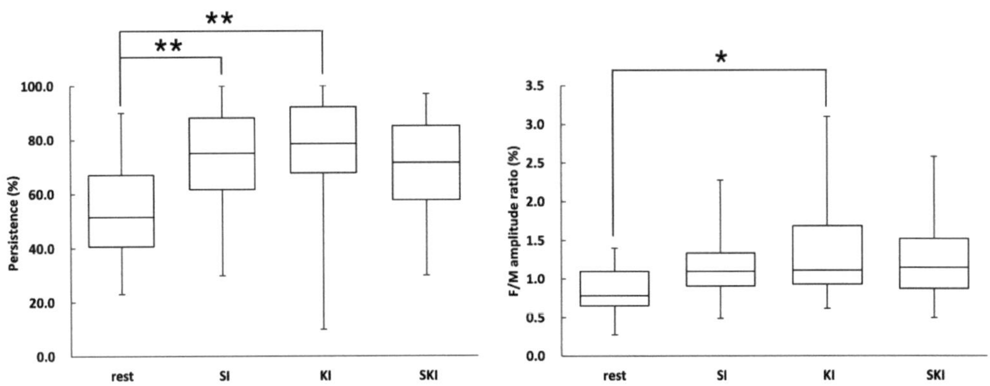

Figure 2. Changes in persistence and F/M amplitude ratio during SI, KI, and SKI (*$p < 0.05$, **$p < 0.01$). The persistence during SI and KI was significantly higher than that at rest. The persistence during SKI was tended to be increased than that at rest. The F/M amplitude ratio during KI was significantly higher than that at rest.

	SI	KI	SKI
Rating score of MI vividness	3.64 ± 0.63	3.86 ± 0.95	3.21 ± 0.89*
Mean ± SD.			
*p < 0.05; significant difference between KI and SKI trial			
SI, somatosensory imagery; KI, kinesthetic imagery; SKI, combined somatosensory and kinesthetic imagery			

Table 10. Rating scores of MI vividness during SI, KI, and SKI.

The rating score of SKI vividness was significantly lower than that at rest (*$p < 0.05$; **Table 10**).

There were no significant differences in the background EMG data among four trials (rest, SI, KI and SKI, respectively), and thus there was no measurable muscle contraction during three imagery trials.

4.6. Discussion

Both persistence and F/M amplitude ratio were significantly higher than the corresponding at-rest values. Previous neurophysiological studies reported that various regions of the brain related to motor functions were activated [9, 10] and that the MEP amplitude was significantly increased during KI [11, 13]. Thus, it seems that the central nervous system can better stimulate spinal motor neuron excitability via the descending pathways.

The persistence during SI was significantly higher than that at rest. This result was unexpected. We previously hypothesized that the spinal motor neuron excitability would remain unchanged because there are no motor-related factors in SI. Furthermore, there are no previous reports of tactile and proprioceptive perception SI increasing the corticospinal excitability including that of the primary motor cortex. Thus, it may be difficult to increase the spinal motor neuron excitability by SI. However, it is possible for SI to include kinesthetic components. Participants in this research were asked to imagine tactile and pressure perception while holding the pinch meter sensor between their thumb and index finger. Thus, they might have unintentionally imagined tactile and pressure perception along with thenar muscle activity.

The persistence during SKI tended to be increased as compared to that at rest. The rating score of SKI vividness was the lowest among the three imagery strategies. These results indicate that participants may not be able to perform SKI as vividly as the other two strategies. In this study, participants were required to pay attention to kinesthetic and somatosensory perceptions simultaneously. The decline in the amount of attention that can be allocated to each imagery strategy may have made it difficult for the participants to perform SKI vividly. Indeed, there was a positive correlation between the corticospinal excitability and MI vividness [40].

4.7. Conclusion

From the result of this research, KI may be a more effective imagery strategy, which can increase the spinal motor neuron excitability. Thus, the imagery strategy should be considered in physical therapy. Also, the spinal motor neuron excitability during SI was significantly increased. However, the mechanism that SI increases spinal motor neuron excitability is unclear. As a limitation of this research, we did not investigate brain activity during SI. Further research will be required to resolve this limitation.

5. How to use MI in physical therapy?

Our research indicates that MI of the isometric thenar muscle activity can increase spinal motor neuron excitability [22–25, 41, 50]. After a stroke or a spinal cord injury, the excitability of the central nervous system decreases due to various factors, including the damage of neural substrates, loss of sensory inputs, and disuse of affected limbs [51]. Additionally, corticospinal excitability decreases following a decline in the size and number of corticospinal neurons [52]. Furthermore, decline of spinal motor neuron excitability was shown in the post-stroke acute phase [7, 53]. Thus, it may be important to stimulate corticospinal excitability, including that of the spinal motor neurons, as soon as possible. Patients in an early postoperative and post-stroke stage have difficulties in performing physical activities. However, considering the characteristics of MI, it can be a beneficial method to stimulate spinal motor neuron excitability without any overt movement and muscle contraction.

Furthermore, MI can improve not only the spinal motor neuron excitability but also various motor functions. Yue et al. [54] indicated that MI under 100% MVC for 4 weeks can increase the muscle strength of little finger abduction. Additionally, Sidaway et al. [55] indicated that MI under 100% MVC for 4 weeks can increase muscle strength of ankle dorsiflexion. About these results, Grosprêtre et al. [56] considered that MI may strengthen brain-to-muscle communication, including the enhanced recruitment of spinal motor neurons and involvement of the descending command. Although other groups [54, 55] adopted maximal imagined muscle contraction strengths for MI training, our results [23–25] revealed that the magnitude of imagined muscle contraction strength did not affect spinal motor neuron excitability. Thus, low (i.e., 10% MVC) imagined muscle contraction strengths might be sufficient for stimulation of spinal motor neuron excitability and muscle strength. Our research [25, 41, 50] also revealed that kinesthetic imagery can better stimulate spinal motor neuron excitability and that spinal motor neuron excitability remained higher than the at-rest value until 3 min after MI initiation. Therefore, to increase the effects of MI, kinesthetic perception should be chosen as the imagery strategy. Additionally, the duration of each MI session should be less than 3 min.

In conclusion, MI can increase the spinal motor neuron excitability, and its effect would be changed depending on the duration and strategy of imagery. Thus, the duration and strategy of imagery should be considered in clinical settings.

Acknowledgements

The author would like to thank Prof. Toshiaki Suzuki from Graduate school of Kansai University of Health Sciences for helpful comments on this manuscript.

Conflict of interest

There is no conflict of interest.

Author details

Yoshibumi Bunno[1,2]*

*Address all correspondence to: bunno@kansai.ac.jp

1 Graduate School of Health Sciences, Graduate School of Kansai University of Health Sciences, Sennan, Osaka, Japan

2 Clinical Physical Therapy Laboratory, Faculty of Health Sciences, Kansai University of Health Sciences, Sennan, Osaka, Japan

References

[1] Guillot A, Di Rienzo F, Maclntyre T, Moran A, Collet C. Imagining is not doing but involves specific motor commands: A review of experimental data related to motor inhibition. Frontiers in Human Neuroscience. 2012;**6**:247. DOI: 10.3389/fnhum.2012.00247

[2] Jackson PL, Lafleur MF, Malouin F, Richards C, Doyon J. Potential role of mental practice using motor imagery in neurologic rehabilitation. Archives of Physical Medicine and Rehabilitation. 2001;**82**:1133-1141. DOI: 10.1053/apmr.2001.24286

[3] López ND, Monge Pereira E, Centeno EJ, Miangolarra Page JC. Motor imagery as a complementary technique for functional recovery after stroke: A systematic review. Topics in Stroke Rehabilitation. 2019;**26**:1-12. DOI: 10.1080/10749357.2019.1640000

[4] Paolucci T, Cardarola A, Colonnelli P, Ferracuti G, Gonnella R, Murgia M, et al. Give me a kiss! An integrative rehabilitative training program with motor imagery and mirror therapy for recovery of facial palsy. European Journal of Physical and Rehabilitation Medicine. 2019. DOI: 10.23736/S1973-9087.19.05757-5

[5] Kawasaki T, Tozawa R, Aramaki H. Effectiveness of using an unskilled model in action observation combined with motor imagery training for early motor learning in elderly people: A preliminary study. Somatosensory & Motor Research. 2018;**35**(3-4):204-211. DOI: 10.1080/08990220.2018.1527760

[6] Foltys H, Krings T, Meister IG, Sparing R, Boroojerdi B, Thron A, et al. Motor representation in patients rapidly recovering after stroke: A functional magnetic resonance imaging and transcranial magnetic stimulation study. Clinical Neurophysiology. 2003;**114**(12):2404-2415. DOI: 10.1016/S1388-2457(03)00263-3

[7] Drory VE, Neufeld MY, Korczyn AD. F-wave characteristics following acute and chronic upper motor neuron lesions. Electromyography and Clinical Neurophysiology. 1993;**33**(7):441-446

[8] Triggs WJ, Calvanio R, Levine M. Transcranial magnetic stimulation reveals a hemispheric asymmetry correlate intermanual differences in motor performance. Neuropsychologia. 1997;**35**(10):1335-1363. DOI: 10.1016/S0028-3932(97)00077-8

[9] Hanakawa T, Dimyan MA, Hallett M. Motor planning, imagery, and execution in the distributed motor network: A time-course study with functional MRI. Cerebral Cortex. 2008;**18**:2775-2788. DOI: 10.1093/cercor/bhn036

[10] Hanakawa T. Organizing motor imageries. Neuroscience Research. 2016;**104**:56-63. DOI: 10.1016/j.neures.2015.11.003

[11] Fourkas AD, Ionta S, Aglioti SM. Influence of imagined posture and imagery modality on corticospinal excitability. Behavioural Brain Research. 2006;**168**(2):190-196. DOI: 10.1016/j.bbr.2005.10.015

[12] Fadiga L, Buccino G, Craighero L, Fogassi L, Gallese V, Pavesi G. Corticospinal excitability is specifically modulated by motor imagery: A magnetic stimulation study. Neuropsychologia. 1998;**37**(2):147-158. DOI: 10.1016/S0028-3932(98)00089-X

[13] Stinear CM, Byblow WD. Modulation of corticospinal excitability and intracortical inhibition during motor imagery is task-dependent. Experimental Brain Research. 2004;**157**(3):351-358. DOI: 10.1007/s00221-004-1851-z

[14] Taniguchi S, Kimura J, Yamada T, Ichikawa H, Hara M, Fujisawa R, et al. Effect of motion imagery to counter rest-induced suppression of F-wave as a measure of anterior horn cell excitability. Clinical Neurophysiology. 2008;**119**(6):1346-1352. DOI: 10.1016/j.clinph.2007.11.179

[15] Kasai T, Kawai S, Kawanishi M, Yahagi S. Evidence for facilitation of motor evoked potentials (MEPs) induced by motor imagery. Brain Research. 1997;**744**(1):147-150. DOI: 10.1016/S0006-8993(96)01101-8

[16] Oishi K, Kimura M, Yasukawa M, Yoneda T, Maeshima T. Amplitude reduction of H-reflex during mental movement simulation in elite athletes. Behavioural Brain Research. 1994;**62**(1):55-61. DOI: 10.1016/0166-4328(94)90037-X

[17] Fisher MA. F-waves-physiology and clinical uses. The Scientific World Journal. 2007;**7**(1): 144-160. DOI: 10.1100/tsw.2007.49

[18] Kimura J. F-wave velocity in the central segment of the median and ulnar nerves. A study in normal subjects and in patients with Charcot-Marie-Tooth disease. Neurology. 1974;**24**(6):539-546. DOI: 10.1212/WNL.24.6.539

[19] Mesrati F, Vecchierini MF. F-waves neurophysiology and clinical value. Neurophysiologie Clinique. 2004;**34**(5):217-243. DOI: 10.1016/j.neucli.2004.09.005

[20] Mercuri B, Wassemann EM, Manqanotti P, Ikoma K, Samii A, Hallett M. Cortical modulation of spinal excitability: An F-wave study. Electroencephalography and Clinical Neurophysiology. 1996;**101**:16-24. DOI: 10.1016/0013-4694(95)00164-6

[21] Rossini PM, Rossi S, Pasqualetti P, Tacchio F. Cortical excitability modulation to hand muscles during movement imagery. Cerebral Cortex. 1999;**9**:161-167. DOI: 10.1093/cercor/9.2.161

[22] Suzuki T, Bunno Y, Onigata C, Tani M, Uragami S. Excitability of spinal neural function during several motor imagery tasks involving isometric opponens pollicis activity. NeuroRehabilitation. 2013;**33**(1):171-176. DOI: 10.3233/NRE-130942

[23] Bunno Y, Yurugi Y, Onigata C, Suzuki T, Iwatsuki H. Influence of motor imagery of isometric opponens pollicis activity on the excitability of spinal motor neurons: A comparison using different muscle contraction strengths. Journal of Physical Therapy Science. 2014;**26**(7):1069-1073. DOI: 10.1589/jpts.26.1069

[24] Bunno Y, Onigata C, Suzuki T. The imagined muscle contraction strengths did not affect the changes of spinal motor neurons excitability. Journal of Novel Physiotherapies. 2016;**S3**:008. DOI: 10.4172/2165-7025.S3-008

[25] Bunno Y, Fukumoto Y, Todo M, Onigata C. The effect of motor imagery on spinal motor neuron excitability and its clinical use in physical therapy. In: Suzuki T, editor. Neurological Physical Therapy. Rijeka: IntechOpen; 2017. pp. 29-50. DOI: 10.5772/67471

[26] Panayiotopoulos CP, Chroni E. F-waves in clinical neurophysiology: A review, methodological issues and overall value in peripheral neuropathies. Electroencephalography and Clinical Neurophysiology. 1996;**101**:365-374. DOI: 10.1016/0924-980X(96)95635-0

[27] Mizuguchi N, Sakamoto M, Muraoka T, Nakagawa K, Kanazawa S, Nakata H, et al. The modulation of corticospinal excitability during motor imagery of action with objects. PLoS One. 2011;**6**(10):e26006. DOI: 10.1371/journal.pone.0026006

[28] Bonnet M, Decety J, Jeannerod M, Requina J. Mental simulation of an action modulates the excitability of spinal reflex pathways in man. Cognitive Brain Research. 1997;**5**(3):221-228. DOI: 10.1016/S0926-6410(96)00072-9

[29] Hale BS, Raglin JS, Koceja DM. Effect of mental imagery of a motor task on the Hoffmann reflex. Behavioural Brain Research. 2003;**142**(1-2):81-87. DOI: 10.1016/S0166-4328(02)00397-2

[30] Aoyama T, Kaneko F. The effect of motor imagery on gain modulation of the spinal reflex. Brain Research. 2011;**1372**(1):41-48. DOI: 10.1016/j.brainres.2010.11.023

[31] Park WH, Li S. No graded responses of finger muscles to TMS during motor imagery of isometric finger forces. Neuroscience Letters. 2011;**494**(3):255-259. DOI: 10.1016/j.neulet.2011.03.027

[32] Romero DH, Lacourse MG, Lawrence KE, Schandler S, Cohen MJ. Event-related potentials as a function of movement parameter variations during motor imagery and isometric action. Behavioural Brain Research. 2000;**117**(1-2):83-96. DOI: 10.1016/S0166-4328(00)00297-7

[33] Oda S, Shibata M, Moritani T. Force-dependent changes in movement-related cortical potentials. Journal of Electromyography and Kinesiology. 1996;**6**(4):247-252. DOI: 10.1016/S1050-6411(96)00010-7

[34] Nakata H, Sakamoto K, Ferretti A, Perrucci MG, Gratta CD, Kakigi R, et al. Somato-motor inhibitory processing in humans: An event-related functional MRI study. Neuroimage. 2008;**39**(4):1858-1866. DOI: 10.1016/j.neuroimage.2007.10.041

[35] Watanabe J, Sugiura M, Sato K, Sato Y, Maeda Y, Matsue Y, et al. The human prefrontal and parietal association cortices are involved in NO-GO performances: An event-related fMRI study. NeuroImage. 2002;**17**(3):1207-1216. DOI: 10.1006/nimg.2002.1198

[36] Driskell J, Copper C, Moran A. Does mental practice enhance performance? Journal of Applied Psychology. 1994;**79**:481-492. DOI: 10.1037/0021-9010.79.4.481

[37] Hinshaw KE. The effects of mental practice on motor skill performance: Critical evaluation and meta-analysis. Imagination, Cognition and Personality. 1991;**11**:3-35. DOI: 10.2190/X9BA-KJ68-07AN-QMJ8

[38] Twining WE. Mental practice and physical practice in learning a motor skill. Research Quarterly. 1949;**20**:432-435

[39] Lorey B, Pilqramm S, Bischoff M, Stark R, Vaitl D, Kindermann S, et al. Activation of the parieto-premotor network is associated with vivid motor imagery—A parametric fMRI study. PLoS One. 2011;**6**:e20368. DOI: 10.1371/journal.pone.0020368

[40] Williams J, Pearce AJ, Loporto M, Morris T, Holmes PS. The relationship between corticospinal excitability during motor imagery and motor imagery ability. Behavioural Brain Research. 2012;**226**:369-375. DOI: 10.1016/j.bbr.2011.09.014

[41] Bunno Y. Does the duration of motor imagery affect the excitability of spinal anterior horn cells? Somatosensory & Motor Research. 2018;**35**(3-4):223-228. DOI: 10.1080/08990220.2018.1538963

[42] Bray SR, Graham JD, Martin Ginis KA, Hicks AL. Cognitive task performance causes impaired maximum force production in human hand flexor muscles. Biological Psychology. 2012;**89**:195-200. DOI: 10.1016/j.biopsycho.2011.10.008

[43] Rozand V, Lebon F, Stapley PJ, Papaxanthis C, Lepers R. A prolonged motor imagery session alter imagined and actual movement durations: Potential implications for neurorehabilitation. Behavioural Brain Research. 2016;**297**:67-75. DOI: 10.1016/j.bbr.2015.09.036

[44] Kluger BM, Palmer C, Shattuck JT, Triggs WJ. Motor evoked potential depression following repetitive central motor initiation. Experimental Brain Research. 2012;**216**:585-590. DOI: 10.1007/s00221-011-2962-y

[45] Decety J. The neurophysiological basis of motor imagery. Behavioural Brain Research. 1996;**77**:45-52. DOI: 10.1016/0166-4328(95)00225-1

[46] Tana MG, Montin E, Cerutti S, Bianchi AM. Exploring cortical attentional system by using fMRI during a Continuous Performance Test. Intelligence and Neuroscience. 2010:329213. DOI: 10.1155/2010/329213

[47] Brunia CH, Zwaga HJ, van Boxtel A. Tendon reflex amplitude with increasing task difficulty. Ergonomics. 1973;**16**:495-499. DOI: 10.1080/00140137308924538

[48] Guillot A, Collet C. Duration of mentally simulated movement: A review. Journal of Motor Behavior. 2005;**37**:10-20. DOI: 10.3200/JMBR.37.1.10-20

[49] McNorgan C. A meta-analytic review of multisensory imagery identifies the neural correlates of modality-specific and modality-general imagery. Frontiers in Human Neuroscience. 2012;**6**:285. DOI: 10.3389/fnhum.2012.00285

[50] Bunno Y. Imagery strategy affects spinal motor neuron excitability—Using kinesthetic and somatosensory imagery. Neuroreport. 2019;**30**(7):463-467. DOI: 10.1097/WNR.0000000000001218

[51] Liepert J, Bauder H, Miltner WHR, Taub E, Weiller C. Treatment-induced cortical reorganization after stroke in humans. Stroke. 2000;**31**:1210-1216. DOI: 10.1161/01.STR.31.6.1210

[52] Wrigley PJ, Gustin SM, Macey PM, Nash PG, Gandevia SC, Macefield VG, et al. Anatomical changes in human motor cortex and motor pathways following complete thoracic spinal cord injury. Cerebral Cortex. 2009;**19**:224-232. DOI: 10.1093/cercor/bhn072

[53] Naseri M, Petramfar P, Ashraf A. Effect of motor imagery on the F-wave parameters in hemiparetic stroke survivors. Annals of Rehabilitation Medicine. 2015;**39**:401-408. DOI: 10.5535/arm.2015.39.3.401

[54] Yue G, Cole KJ. Strength increases from the motor program: Comparison of training with maximal voluntary and imagined muscle contractions. Journal of Neurophysiology. 1992;**67**(5):1114-1123. DOI: 10.1152/jn.1992.67.5.1114

[55] Sidaway B, Trzaska AR. Can mental practice increase ankle dorsiflexor torque? Physical Therapy. 2005;**85**(10):1053-1060. DOI: 10.1093/ptj/85.10.1053

[56] Grosprêtre S, Jacquet T, Lebon F, Papaxanthis C, Martin A. Neural mechanisms of strength increase after one week motor imagery training. European Journal of Sport Science. 2017;**18**(2):209-218. DOI: 10.1080/17461391.2017.1415377

Chapter 6

Parkinson's Disease Rehabilitation: Effectiveness Approaches and New Perspectives

Luciana Auxiliadora de Paula Vasconcelos

Additional information is available at the end of the chapter

http://dx.doi.org/10.5772/intechopen.89360

Abstract

Parkinson's disease has been considered one of the most important and common neurodegenerative diseases in the world. Its motor and nonmotor signs determine a huge functional loss, leading the individuals to lose their independence. Although the treatment requires a pharmacological approach, physical therapy has confirmed its importance in this process. Today, neurorehabilitation is indispensable to increase many of the cardinal signs of the disease. Using traditional or technological approaches, physical therapy has reached good results in improving motor and nonmotor functions, as well as the quality of life of Parkinsonians. However, it is important to develop and to fortify the physical therapy approach so that we can provide stronger evidence about our practice.

Keywords: Parkinson's disease, rehabilitation, physical therapy

1. Introduction

In this chapter, we will discuss some important topics about Parkinson's disease (PD), a progressive and neurodegenerative disease, that is characterized by many motor and nonmotor symptoms and with wide-reaching implications for patients and their families [1, 2]. It is neuropathologically characterized by nigrostriatal cell loss and the presence of intracellular a-synuclein-positive inclusions called Lewy bodies [3].

It is the most common movement disorder with approximately 1–2% of the population over 65 years of age suffering from PD. This percentage increases in people of 85 years of age and older, about 3–5% [3]. According to the World Health Organization, 6.1 million individuals have Parkinson's disease globally [4]. Some authors have shown that the burden of Parkinson's

IntechOpen

© 2019 The Author(s). Licensee IntechOpen. This chapter is distributed under the terms of the Creative Commons Attribution License (http://creativecommons.org/licenses/by/3.0), which permits unrestricted use, distribution, and reproduction in any medium, provided the original work is properly cited.

disease has more than doubled over 26 years worldwide, from 2.5 million patients in 1990 to 6.1 million patients in 2016. So, we can expect that the trend will continue in the next 30 years having approximately more than 12 million individuals suffering from PD [5]. In 2016, there were 211,296 estimated deaths caused by Parkinson's disease [4].

PD is characterized mainly by four motor symptoms: resting tremor, bradykinesia, rigidity, and postural instability [1] with balance decrements and gait disruption [2]. It may present problems in performing personal activities of daily living, such as eating, drinking, cutting food, walking in the neighborhood, and writing [6].

The diagnosis of PD is based on medical history and a neurological examination since there are no blood tests, laboratory tests, or imaging examinations that have been proven to help in diagnosing PD [7], and its treatment is based on a pharmacological approach. The main therapy is based on levodopa and dopamine agonists and is very successful in the early stages of the disease, when dopaminergic symptoms and signs are predominant and long-term motor complications still have not developed [8].

The traditional classification and disease progression of Parkinson's disease (PD) orient toward disease milestones that can be most obviously followed along motor domains. However, diverse nonmotor domains, quality of life, psychosocial burden, and stigma have been used as important domains for the course of PD and the outcome parameters of clinical trials [9].

At present, there is no cure for PD, but a variety of medications provide relief from the symptoms. Individuals who are affected usually are given levodopa combined with carbidopa. Levodopa helps in at least three-quarters of Parkinsonian cases; however, not all symptoms respond equally to the drug. Bradykinesia and rigidity respond best, while tremor may be only marginally reduced. Problems with balance and other symptoms may not be alleviated at all [7].

In this scenario, physiotherapy has a significant importance in a multidisciplinary team focused on the rehabilitation of individuals with PD, with the purpose of maximizing functional ability and minimizing secondary complications through movement rehabilitation within a context of education and to support the person as a whole [10].

The main focuses of physiotherapy for individuals with PD are transfers, posture, upper limb function, balance (and falls), gait, and physical capacity and activity. Physiotherapy also uses cueing strategies, cognitive movement strategies, and exercises to maintain or to increase independence, safety, and quality of life. The traditional and new strategies will be addressed in this chapter [10].

2. Pathophysiology of PD

Physiologically, the symptoms associated with Parkinson's disease are the result of the loss of a number of neurotransmitters, most notably dopamine. It is characterized neuropathological by nigrostriatal cell loss and the presence of intracellular a-synuclein-positive inclusions called Lewy bodies [3, 11]. All these alterations change the function of the basal ganglia system, resulting in Parkinson's main movement disorders.

http://dx.doi.org/10.5772/intechopen.89360

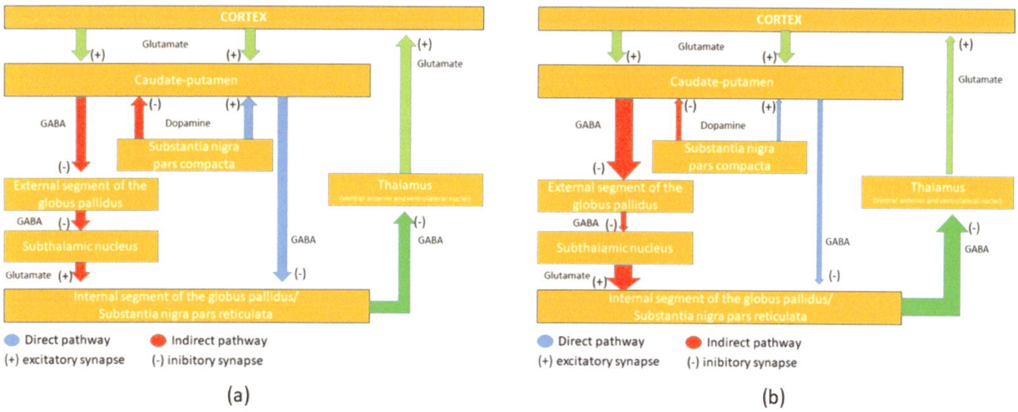

Figure 1. A schematic view of the functional anatomy of the basal ganglia. There are the normal direct and indirect pathways (panel a) and the alteration of direct and indirect pathways in Parkinson's disease (panel b). Modified from Magrinelli et al. [8] and Nitrini and Bacheschi [12].

Cell loss in the substantia nigra occurs in a region-specific manner, with the lateral ventral tier of the pars compacta being most affected. It is estimated that at least 50% of the nigral neurons must degenerate to produce symptoms, and, at autopsy, most cases show more than 80% reduction [8].

The basic basal ganglia circuitry and the balance between the direct and indirect striatal pathways provide a simple heuristic model for PD's main signs. According to this model, the pathophysiological hallmark of PD, hypokinetic signs are the prevalence of the indirect pathway over the direct one, consequently, resulting in increased neuronal firing activity in the output nuclei of the basal ganglia and leading to excessive inhibition of thalamocortical and brainstem motor systems, interfering with normal speed of onset movement and execution. On the other hand, overactivity in the direct pathway and imbalance with the indirect one may cause reduced inhibitory basal ganglia output and result in reduced basal ganglia filtering and parallel facilitation of multiple movement fragments. (See **Figure 1**) [8].

Another important region that has been linked to physiopathology of PD is the cerebellum. Its reciprocal connections with basal ganglia, especially with striatum and external segment of the globus pallidus, strengthens the hypothesis that it plays a role in the pathogenesis of some PD symptoms and signs [8].

Histopathology alterations can be described in this pathophysiological situation. There usually can be seen some histological characteristics not just in nerve tissue. The most important marker is called Lewy bodies. They are made of a protein called alpha-synuclein, which, in a healthy brain, plays a number of important roles in neurons, especially at synapses [13].

Lewy bodies can be found in many regions of the brain and some reports have suggested that the substantia nigra is not the first place where they form in Parkinson's disease [14].

Neither cell loss nor the formation of Lewy bodies is absolutely specific for PD, but both are required for a diagnosis of PD under current definitions. Additionally, it's necessary to consider that not all affected neurons in PD are dopaminergic. An example to be cited is the cholinergic neurons from the dorsal vagal nucleus. This variety of regions has been suggested to be responsible for the complex clinical picture in PD [13].

This pathophysiological situation seems to be multifactorial. It can be considered by genetic factors, inflammation, immune response, and environmental elements [14].

While having a family member with PD may increase a person's risk, PD is not normally considered a genetic disease. Variants in three genes (SNCA, UCHL 1, and LRRK 2) have been reported in familial PD. Mutations in three other genes (PARK 2, PARK 7, and PINK 1) have been found in sporadic PD [14, 15].

On the other hand, large population studies have suggested that individuals taking nonsteroidal anti-inflammatory drugs (NSAIDs) have less risk of developing idiopathic PD, which suggests that anti-inflammatory drugs may be a promising disease-modifying treatment for Parkinsonian patients [16].

Some reports have provided direct evidence of interactions between α-synuclein and environmental agents. Some options described in the literature are heavy metals (iron, copper, manganese, lead, and mercury), pesticides (including insecticides and herbicides), and illicit substances (amphetamine, methamphetamine, and cocaine) [17].

In a review, Di Monti et al. [18] describe some possibilities of multiple events and interactive mechanisms possibly responsible for alpha-synuclein alterations. These may include (i) the synergistic action of endogenous and exogenous toxins, (ii) the interactions of toxic agents with endogenous elements (e.g., the protein α-synuclein), (iii) the tissue response to an initial toxic insult, and (iv) the effects of environmental factors on the background of genetic predisposition and aging.

It's important to explain that the symptoms of Parkinson's disease sometimes can be seen outside the disease itself. In these cases, we call this clinical condition of parkinsonism, also known as "atypical Parkinson's," "secondary Parkinson's," or "Parkinson's syndrome." Parkinsonism often has an identifiable cause, such as exposure to toxins, methamphetamine, trauma, multiple strokes, other nervous system disorders, or illness. Generally, Lewy bodies are not seen in parkinsonism [14].

3. Parkinson's clinical signs, diagnosis, and rating scales

The three clinical motor cardinal signs of PD, a-/hypo-/bradykinesia, rest tremor, and rigidity, are directly related to the degeneration of dopaminergic neurons. However, other motor symptoms and signs, secondary to degeneration of nondopaminergic pathways, can be described such as loss of postural control, postural stability/balance, and gait disturbance. In addition, the most well-known nonmotor characteristic motor symptoms have also been described. There can be additional psychiatric and autonomic features found, as well as cognitive impairment, sleep disorders, olfactory dysfunction, and pain.

3.1. Clinical motor cardinal signs

1. A-/hypo-/bradykinesia: These terms are defined, collectively, as slowed voluntary movement. Separately, akinesia indicates the absence of voluntary movement, while hypokinesia

means smaller movements, and bradykinesia refers to slowness of movement. They usually determine any impairment in fine motor movements, facial expression (hypomimia), monotonic and hypophonic speech with a reduction of speed, and general motion amplitude. This can have an important impact in functional skills like arm swinging when walking, raising from a chair, handwriting, and general gesturing [14, 19].

This cardinal sign is one of the best that emerges from its origin of dysfunction, which is cited in this chapter (see **Figure 1**). It has been determined especially by a characteristic involving the movement programming of the cerebral cortex, in particular the supplementary motor area [8, 19].

It is possible to find two modulations of this cardinal sign of Parkinson's disease: freezing phenomenon and kinesia paradoxa. In the first one, the individual presents a sudden and transient motor block, mainly in the lower limbs during walking. This may include start hesitation, hesitation, or inability to move through the presence of contradictory visual cues (floors with different colors and small steps), when there is a need to change direction of gait or be still in open spaces. The second one, kinesia paradoxa, occurs under certain emotional circumstances where the patient is able to exhibit a sudden brief period of mobility (walking or even running and catching a ball). This phenomenon shows that, even though individuals with Parkinson's disease have their motor programs intact, the disease prevents them from accessing them in the correct way, requiring external stimuli for this to happen even if done poorly [19, 20].

2. *Rest tremor*: this sign is usually asymmetric, consisting of alternate contractions of agonist and antagonist muscles, including flexors, extensors, pronators, and supinators of the wrists and arms, resulting in the "pill rolling" movement of the hand. It has a medium frequency (3 to 6 Hz) and tends to disappear with action. The legs, lower jaw, or head may also be involved, resulting in an adduction-abduction movement of the lower limbs and yes-yes or no-no motion in the head [8, 21].

The pathophysiology of rest tremor is largely unknown. Clinical-pathological studies have demonstrated that patients with PD and prominent tremor have dysfunction of a subgroup of midbrain (A8) neurons and its magnitude seems to not be related to dopamine deficiency [8, 19].

3. *Rigidity*: it is a type of increase in muscle tone (also called plastic hypertonia), generally defined as an increased resistance to passive movement of a joint. Rigidity is more evident in the flexor muscles of the trunk and limbs and may be enhanced by voluntary movement. However, its presence usually determines a characteristic of stooped posture. Two types of rigidity can be described: cogwheel rigidity refers to resistance that stops and starts at the limb, the limb is moved through its range of motion, and it is the result of coexisting rigidity and tremor; lead-pipe rigidity is defined as a constant resistance to motion throughout the entire range of movement [8, 14].

It is unclear how rigidity is associated with dopamine deficiency and basal ganglia dysfunction. Nevertheless, evidence suggests that this cardinal sign has its pathogenesis in the passive mechanical properties of joints, tendons, and muscles, and spinal and supraspinal reflexes, which together determine an increased response to peripheral stimulation and an increased muscle elongation response [8].

3.2. Additional motor signs

1. *Posture disturbances*: individuals with Parkinson's disease usually develop abnormal axial postures as a result of bradykinesia, rigidity, and resting tremor. This abnormality leads to a flexed general posture, with hip and knee flexion, accompanied by shoulder and even elbow flexion. In the long term, this posture disturbance can determine severe postural deformities such as antecollis, scoliosis, camptocormia, and Pisa syndrome. Little is known about the cause of these deformities, which makes it unresponsive to most treatments [8, 19].

2. *Postural instability balance and gait disturbances*: postural instability and gait disturbances usually occur during the course of PD, generally being manifestations of the late stages of the disease. They represent a therapeutic challenge, since they show little change through traditional pharmacological treatment using dopaminergic drugs. These two impairments, especially if associated with the freezing phenomenon, are the most common cause of falls and fractures in Parkinsonians [19, 22].

One of the most important causes for these signs is the poor ability to integrate visual, vestibular, and proprioceptive inputs associated with a failure to activate central motor programs and their interaction with the mechanisms of sensitive feedback. Postural instability and gait disturbances have been associated with an akinetic-rigid syndrome, as well as an increased incidence of nonmotor features [8, 22].

3. *Other* signs *and symptoms*: in addition to the most important signs of Parkinson's disease, some other motor signs can be found, such as dysarthria, hypophonia, dysphagia, and sialorrhea. These signs occur as a result of bulbar dysfunction and as a result of orofacial-laryngeal bradykinesia and rigidity. We can still find some neuro-ophthalmological signs such as a decreased blink rate and blepharospasm, among others. Other important disturbances are linked with the respiratory system and usually contribute strongly to morbidity and mortality in PD. The obstructive or restrictive respiratory complications are probably due to the presence of the rigidity present in the trunk area [19].

3.3. Nonmotor signs and symptoms

The current literature suggests there is a prodromal or premotor stage of Parkinson's disease before the onset of motor symptoms. Nonmotor signs and symptoms of Parkinson's disease include cognitive, neuropsychiatric, sleep, autonomic, and sensory dysfunctions, which are typically not treated by the dopaminergic therapy. Patients who go on to develop Parkinson's disease commonly have experienced depression, constipation, anosmia, and rapid eye movement sleep behavior disorder in the years preceding their diagnosis. So, the presence of nonmotor features has contributed during the diagnosis process of Parkinson's disease. However, if these nonmotor signs were not evaluated well enough during the diagnostic process, they may delay the diagnosis [23, 24].

More specifically, there can be subtle cognitive deficits found affecting attentional, executive, visuospatial, and memory functions. Neuropsychiatric symptoms are also common and include depression, anxiety, apathy, and psychosis. Autonomic dysfunction can manifest as urinary frequency or urgency, constipation, orthostatic hypotension, drooling, erectile dysfunction, or

Neuropsychiatric symptoms	Depression
	Dementia
	Anxiety
	Anhedonia
	Apathy
	Psychosis (hallucination and delusion)
	Cognitive dysfunction
	Attention deficit
	Off-period–related panic attacks
	Confusion
Sleep disorders	Insomnia
	Excessive daytime sleepiness
	Nonrapid eye movement sleep-related movement disorders
	Sleep-disordered breathing
	Periodic limb movement disorder
	Rapid eye movement sleep behavior disorder
	Vivid dreaming
	Restless legs syndrome
Autonomic symptoms	Urgency
	Frequency
	Orthostatic hypotension
	Nocturia
	Erectile dysfunction
	Sweating
Gastrointestinal symptoms	Dribbling of saliva
	Ageusia
	Nausea
	Dysphagia
	Reflux and vomiting
	Constipation
	Diarrhea
	Fecal incontinence
	Unsatisfactory voiding of bowel

Sensory symptoms	Primary pain
	Secondary pain
	Fluctuation-related pain
	Paresthesia
	Olfactory disturbance
	Visual dysfunction
Other symptoms	Fatigue
	Ankle swelling
	Nonmotor fluctuations
	Blurred vision

Table 1. Nonmotor signs and symptoms of Parkinson's disease [23–25].

abnormal sweating. These clinical manifestations can have a substantial impact on the patient's quality of life [25]. We can see a long list of nonmotor signs and symptoms in **Table 1**.

Some of the most important nonmotor signs and symptoms for physiotherapists, which require special attention, are fatigue, pain, urinary bladder control, and anal sphincter control. We will discuss how physical therapy functions with these aspects of the disease later in this chapter.

3.4. Diagnosis of Parkinson's disease

During the diagnostic process of Parkinson's disease, one of the first components to be established is the presence of "parkinsonism." This clinical condition is established by the presence of the cardinal signs of the disease, of which bradykinesia is an indispensable criterion jointly with one of the other two signs [25], associated and exclusionary symptoms, atypical features in the history and on examination, and response to levodopa.

The presence of nonmotor features is important, as these may be prominent even early in the disease's course. Some diagnostic criteria have been developed by some organizations like the UK Parkinson's Disease Society Brain Bank, the National Institute of Neurological Disorders and the Stroke (NINDS), and Movement Disorder Society. All of them ask for the presence of the cardinal signs, the application of exclusion criteria and some supportive criteria [25, 26]. They can be consulted in **Table 2**.

However, the reliability and validity of them have not been clearly established. In this way, it is common to have a misdiagnosis of Parkinson's disease. The most common causes of misdiagnosis that are described in literature are Alzheimer's disease, essential tremor, and vascular parkinsonism. It should be remembered that rigidity, bradykinesia, and gait disturbance can be found during normal aging period or can be determined by other medical conditions of aging [25, 27, 28].

	United Kingdom Parkinson's Disease Society Brain Bank's	National Institute of Neurological Disorders and Stroke (NINDS)	Movement Disorder Society
Step 1		Group A features (characteristic of Parkinson's disease)	1. Diagnosis of parkinsonism
	Bradykinesia	Resting tremor	a. Bradykinesia, plus one of
	At least one of the following criteria:	Rigidity	b. Tremor
	Rigidity	Asymmetric onset	c. Rigidity
	4–6 Hz rest tremor	Group B features (suggestive of alternative diagnoses)	2. Exclusion criteria
	Postural instability not caused by primary visual, vestibular, cerebellar, or proprioceptive dysfunction	Features unusual early in the clinical course	d. Cerebellar abnormalities
Step 2		Prominent postural instability in the first 3 years after symptom onset	e. Supranuclear gaze palsy
	Exclude other causes of parkinsonism	Freezing phenomenon in the first 3 years	f. Diagnosis of behavioral variant of frontotemporal dementia or primary progressive aphasia within 5 years of disease onset
Step 3		Hallucinations unrelated to medications in the first 3 years	g. Parkinsonian features restricted to the lower limbs for more than 3 years
	At least one of the following supportive (prospective) criteria:	Dementia preceding motor symptoms or in the first year	h. Treatment with a dopamine receptor blocker or dopamine-depleting agent consistent with drug-induced parkinsonism
	Unilateral onset	Supranuclear gaze palsy (other than restriction of upward gaze) or slowing of vertical saccades	i. Absence of a response to high-dose levodopa despite at least moderate disease severity
	Rest tremor	Severe, symptomatic dysautonomia unrelated to medications	j. Cortical sensory loss, clear limb ideomotor apraxia, or progressive aphasia
	Progressive disorder	Documentation of condition known to produce parkinsonism and plausibly connected to the patient's symptoms (such as suitably located focal brain lesions or neuroleptic use within the past 6 months)	k. Normal function imaging of the dopaminergic system ("DAT scan")
	Persistent asymmetry primarily affecting side of onset	Criteria for definite Parkinson's disease	l. Diagnosis of alternative condition causing parkinsonism that could be causing the symptoms
	Excellent response (70–100%) to levodopa	All criteria for probable Parkinson's are met and	3. Supportive criteria

(Continued)

United Kingdom Parkinson's Disease Society Brain Bank's	National Institute of Neurological Disorders and Stroke (NINDS)	Movement Disorder Society
Severe levodopa-induced chorea (dyskinesia)	Histopathological confirmation of the diagnosis is obtained at autopsy	m. Clear beneficial response to dopaminergic therapy
Levodopa response for 5 years or more	Criteria for probable PD	n. Presence of levodopa-induced dyskinesia
Clinical course of 10 years or more	At least three of the four features in group A are present and	o. Rest tremor of a limb
	None of the features in group B is present (note: symptom duration ≥ 3 years is necessary to meet this requirement) and	p. The presence of either olfactory loss or cardiac sympathetic denervation on MIBG scintigraphy (although the latter is rarely done in current practice)
	Substantial and sustained response to levodopa or a dopamine agonist has been documented	4. Red flags
	Criteria for possible Parkinson's disease	q. Rapid progression of gait impairment leading to wheelchair use within 5 years
	At least two of the four features in group A are present; at least one of these is tremor or bradykinesia and	r. Absence of progression of motor symptoms over 5 years, unless related to treatment
	Either none of the features in group B is present or symptoms have been present ≤ 3 years and none of the features in group B is present and	s. Early bulbar dysfunction
	Either substantial and sustained response to levodopa or a dopamine agonist has been documented or the patient has not had an adequate trial of levodopa or a dopamine agonist	t. Inspiratory respiratory dysfunction
		u. Severe autonomic failure within the first 5 years of disease
		v. Recurrent falls because of impaired balance within 3 years of onset
		w. Disproportionate anterocollis or contractures within 10 years of disease onset
		x. Absence of any of the common nonmotor features despite 5 years of disease
		y. Unexplained pyramidal signs
		z. Bilateral symmetrical parkinsonism
		For the diagnosis of clinically established Parkinson's disease

United Kingdom Parkinson's Disease Society Brain Bank's	National Institute of Neurological Disorders and Stroke (NINDS)	Movement Disorder Society
		27. Parkinsonism
		28. Absence of exclusion criteria
		29. At least 2 supportive criteria
		For the diagnosis of clinically probable Parkinson's disease
		30. Parkinsonism
		31. Absence of exclusion criteria
		32. Balanced numbers of supportive criteria and red flags

Table 2. Options of diagnostic criteria for Parkinson's disease.

3.5. Rating scales for Parkinson's disease

A rating scale is a means of providing information on a particular feature by assigning a value to it. Parkinson's rating scales are a means of assessing the symptoms of the condition. They provide information on the course of the condition and/or assess quality of life. They may also help to evaluate treatment and management strategies, which can be useful to researchers, medical doctors, physiotherapists, and other healthcare professionals, as well as to people with Parkinson's and their caregivers [29].

In Parkinson's disease, there are a number of rating scales used. Often, more than one scale is used to give a broader picture of symptoms. The most important and used rating scale for this disease is the Unified Parkinson's Disease Rating Scale (UPDRS). The scale has three sections that evaluate key areas of disability, together with a fourth section that evaluates any complications of treatment, as shown below:

Part 1: Nonmotor experiences of daily living

Part 2: Motor experiences of daily living

Part 3: Motor examination

Part 4: Motor complications

The UPDRS features sections that require independent completion by people affected by Parkinson's and their caregivers, and sections to be completed by the clinician. The UPDRS is often used with two other Parkinson's rating scales: The Hoehn and Yahr, and the Schwab and England Activities of Daily Living (ADL) scales [20, 30].

In **Table 3**, there is a list of rating scales available and recommended by the European Parkinson's Disease Association and by the International Parkinson and Movement Disorder Society [29, 30].

MDS-owned rating scales	The European Parkinson's Disease Association (EPDA)
Global assessment scale for Wilson's disease	Unified Parkinson's disease rating scale (UPDRS)
Global dystonia scale	Hoehn and Yahr scale
MDS-unified Parkinson's disease rating scale (MDS-UPDRS)	Schwab and England activities of daily living (ADL) scale
Modified bradykinesia rating scale	PDQ-39
Nonmotor symptoms scale (NMSS)	PD NMS questionnaire
Nonmotor symptoms questionnaire (NMSQ)	NMS survey
PKAN disease rating scale (PKAN-DRS)	Parkinson's disease composite scale
Quality of life essential tremor questionnaire	King's PD pain scale
Rating scale for psychogenic movement disorders	Parkinson's disease sleep scale-PDSS-2
Rush dyskinesia rating scale	Lindop Parkinson's assessment scale
Rush video-based tic rating scale	Short-form 36 (SF-36)
UFMG Sydenham's Chorea Rating Scale (USCRS)	Sickness impact profile (SIP)
Unified dyskinesia rating scale (UDysRS)	Mini-mental state examination (MMSE)
Unified dystonia rating scale (UDRS)	Montreal cognitive assessment scale (MoCa)
Unified multiple system atrophy rating scale (UMSARS)	Caregiver strain index (CSI)

Note: Based on the European Parkinson's Disease Association [29] and International Parkinson and Movement Disorder Society [30] websites.

Table 3. Recommended rating scales for Parkinson's disease.

It is important to note that many of these scales and questionnaires are owned and licensed by some organization. Hence, it is necessary to require a rating scales permission request form before working with them.

In a nonclinical way, Braak and coworkers [31] proposed staging procedures of the pathology of Parkinson's disease, based on central nervous system involvement. Their proposal has six stages:

Stage 1: Premotor period in which typical pathological changes, Lewy neurites, and Lewy bodies spread from the olfactory bulb and vagus nerve to lower brainstem regions (medulla oblongata and pontine tegmentum).

Stage 2: Additional lesions in the raphe nuclei and gigantocellular reticular nucleus of the medulla oblongata, locus coeruleus in the pontine tegmentum.

Stage 3: The symptomatic period when pathological changes involve the midbrain including substantia nigra pars compacta, basal nuclei of Meynert. Structures affected in stages 1 and 2 develop more Lewy bodies.

Stage 4: Severe dopaminergic cell destruction in the pars compacta with additional mesocortex and allocortex involvement, especially seen in amygdala and subnuclei of the thalamus.

Stage 5: There are initial changes in neocortex (cortical lobes). Cellular death can be seen in the substantia nigra, the dorsal motor nucleus of the vagus nerve, the gigantocellular reticular nucleus, and the locus coeruleus.

Stage 6: Neocortex entirely affected (motor and sensory areas).

This kind of rate is totally based on histological development of the disease. It is important to remember that, historically, the definitive diagnosis of Parkinson's disease is closed in a postmortem autopsy [32].

4. Parkinson's disease treatment

Drug treatment: traditionally, the drugs that have shown good effects on the motor signs and symptoms of Parkinson's disease are the dopaminergic drugs.

Among them, the most used in clinical practice is levodopa or levodopa plus dopa-decarboxylase inhibitors (DDC-I), designed to replace the dopamine in the depleted striatum, undoubtedly, the most efficient medication for Parkinson's disease [33]. They improve motor functions in a cyclic way during the day period. When they reduce the motor impairment, the period is called "on time." When the motor signs and symptoms start to return, the period is called "off time" or "wearing-off period." However, during the "wearing-off period," symptoms may not be related only to movement. It is also usual for patients to report increased anxiety, fatigue, mood changes, difficulty thinking, restlessness, and sweating [29].

Initially, levodopa offers a stable alleviation of PD symptoms so it is usual for it to be offered in low doses, being well-tolerated by patients. This period of treatment is called the "honeymoon." However, as the disease becomes more advanced, the effect of the drug usually wears off quickly, and an increased frequency of dosing is often required. This marks the end of the "honeymoon" period. After some years (4–6 years), patients begin to experience, most strikingly, its intense side effects [33, 34].

These long-term complications included many kinds of motor fluctuations. In addition to the on-off phenomenon, already described above, the patients may also experience delay on, when medication takes a longer period to take its effect; freezing phenomenon, which was already discussed during the motor signs presentation; and dyskinesia, which is determined by the presence of hyperkinetic involuntary movements, including twitches, jerking, twisting, or simple restlessness but no tremor, occurring when the drug is at its peak dose, during the wearing-off period or even during off-periods of the medication [29, 34]. Several new formulations of levodopa have been developed to provide a more stable levodopa plasma concentration, reducing some of the side effects, including dyskinesia. Among them, as aforementioned is a levodopa/carbidopa combination [33].

Other drugs on treatment of motor signs are dopaminergic agonists, amantadine, dopamine receptor agonists, catechol-O-methyltransferase (COMT), and monoaminoxidase (MAO) inhibitors. Recently, new pharmacological treatment has been studied such as the use of cannabis (to reduce mainly the three cardinal signs) and the angiotensin IV ligand-based compound, which influences motor and nonmotor signs (memory) [33].

Since Parkinson's disease is not considered a pure movement disorder anymore, the treatment of nonmotor signs and symptoms is justified. However, the treatment of nonmotor symptoms is still an unsatisfactory field for patients and their families [35]. A cholinesterase inhibitor has been used for dementia treatment, while noradrenergic medications (like tricyclic antidepressants) have shown some effect in depression and serotoninergic agonists (like clozapine) in psychosis. Amantadine is used with some success in the management of levodopa-induced dyskinesia. For autonomic dysfunction, there are many options such as mineralocorticoid, fludrocortisone and adrenergic agents, the noradrenaline precursor for orthostatic hypotension, antimuscarinics for urinary urgency or incontinence, and prokinetic drugs to treat constipation [35].

Surgical treatment: lesioning procedures, such as pallidotomy and thalamotomy, were used to reduce the motor signs and symptoms of Parkinson's disease. For a period, these procedures were abandoned because of good results with pharmacological treatment using dopaminergic drugs. However, nowadays, the surgical procedures are reviving as a result of the complications of pharmacological therapies.

The technological advances in the area of medicine have led to the development of a new kind and nonablative surgical procedure: deep brain stimulation (DBS). It involves sending electrical impulses to certain parts of the brain by a neurostimulator device that is a brain implant known as a 'brain pacemaker.' The general procedure of this surgery is an intracranial electrode precisely implanted in the target area (see **Table 4**), followed by implantation of lead extension wires that connect the intracranial leads to a power-generating and programming source and, then finally, the implantation of an internal pulse generator (**Figure 2**). The main target areas can be seen in **Table 4** such as the signs/symptoms that are most prominently modulated by DBS [36, 38]. When PD symptoms are very severe and medications cannot moderate them, surgery and deep brain stimulation can be considered as the final options of treatment.

Subthalamic nucleus	Disabling motor symptoms
	Dyskinesia
	Motor fluctuations
Globus pallidus internus	Improvement of motor symptoms in general
Ventral intermediate thalamic nucleus	Tremor
Pedunculopontine nucleus	Gait instability
	Gait freezing phenomenon

Note: Based on Dallapiazza et al [36].

Table 4. Main target areas for deep brain stimulation (DBS) in Parkinson's disease.

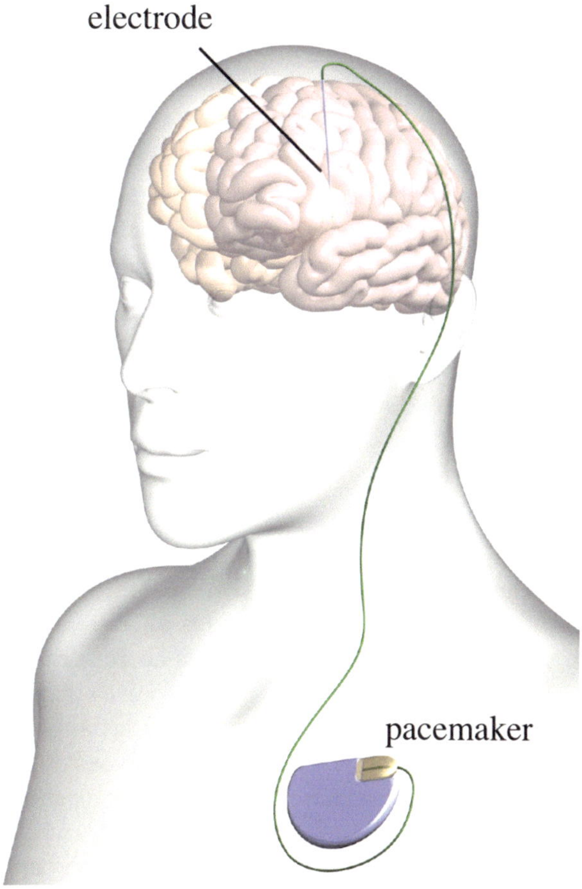

Figure 2. Typical deep brain stimulation setup. The electrode is placed in the brain and connected to a brain pacemaker permanently placed under the skin of the chest. Source: Shamir et al. [37] the use, distribution or reproduction in other forums is permitted.

Other treatments: other alternatives to Parkinson's disease management include a group of therapies other than a pharmacological approach. There is a vast variety of techniques available for this purpose, such as tai chi, yoga, massage, acupuncture, dance, traditional herbs, and molecular targeted therapies, among others.

Physical therapy shows a number of different strategies that has been frequently used in rehabilitation of Parkinson's disease patients, having the most important goal to enhance the quality of life of these individuals.

4.1. Physical therapy in Parkinson's disease treatment

Physiotherapists are members within a multiprofessional team, which has the purpose of maximizing functions and abilities and minimizing secondary complications of several diseases. They use movement rehabilitation within a context of education and support for the person as a whole. In patients with Parkinson's disease, physical therapy focuses on many functions such as transfer, posture, balance improvement and fall prevention, gait, upper limb functions, and physical capacity (including cardiorespiratory capacity) essential to carry out activities of daily life. All of these goals, worked together with cueing strategies, cognitive movement and exercises, increased independence, and safety, as a consequence, improve quality of life [10].

Some evidence presented in the literature supported that therapeutic exercises applied in individuals with Parkinson's disease were effective in improving both the motor and nonmotor impairments [39, 40]. This improvement may be linked to a number of plasticity-related physiological events including synaptogenesis, angiogenesis, and neurogenesis. This process can be mediated by use-dependent expression of endogenous neurotrophic factors. In an unedited systematic review and meta-analysis, Hirsch and his coworkers show aggregated evidence that physical exercise training increases brain-derived neurotrophic factor (BDNF) blood levels in individuals with Parkinson's disease. This BDNF increase results in concomitant reduction in motor signs and symptoms, measured by UPDRS, confirming possible effects on dopaminergic pathways [41].

Together with neuroplasticity, there is some evidence pointing to the participation of motor modules (coordinated patterns of muscle activity that combine to produce functional motor behaviors) like a physiological theory for good results of physical therapy in Parkinson's disease. For this purpose, it is proposed to consider five neuromechanical principles: motor abundance, which means that for any given task, many equivalent motor solutions are possible; motor structure, which means that motor modules reflect biomechanical task relevance; motor variability, which means that variations on motor modules are higher as much as the motor output is lower; individuality, which means that different motor repertory must be considered among different individuals; and multifunctionality, which means that muscle activity can generate a large number of different actions. It is important to emphasize that in Parkinson's disease the basal ganglia dysfunction supposedly leads to inappropriate selection of motor modules [8].

It is still important to remember that motor rehabilitation is a motor relearning practice and training where it is essential to reacquire motor skills. Although individuals with Parkinson's disease show preserved motor learning abilities, the basal ganglia dysfunction may impair the consolidation of them. Therefore, the basic rules of neural plasticity practice must be used to be successful in the rehabilitation process. It includes intensity, repetition, specificity, difficulty, and complexity of practice [8, 42].

Several rehabilitative approaches have been proposed in Parkinson's disease.

4.1.1. Resistance training and muscle strength

In the last two decades, exercise, such as resistance training, has shown to be beneficial for the improvement of both motor and nonmotor signs and symptoms. It increases low strength determined by hypokinesia and disuse, besides playing a neuroprotective effect in individuals with Parkinson's disease. Its effect is probably determined by an increase of mitochondrial respiration and of neuroplasticity mechanisms, improving the recruitment of motor unit and generating selective activation of the muscles [14, 43, 44].

However, there is no consensus about the parameters for resistance training prescription for individuals who have Parkinson's disease [43]. In a systematic review and meta-analysis, Saltychev and his coworkers [45] concluded that there is no evidence on the superiority of progressive resistance training compared with other treatments to support the use of this approach in rehabilitation procedures.

On the contrary, it is possible to find successful directions to use this therapeutic strategy in rehabilitation of individuals with Parkinson's disease from other systematic reviews, meta-analysis, and clinical research. Studies shows that low (2 times per week over 12 weeks) to moderate (2–3 times per week over 8–10 weeks) intensity resistance training appears to be effective in people with early, mild-to-moderate Parkinson's disease. They still show that this specific approach resulted in gaining muscle strength, balance, Parkinson's motor symptoms, and quality of life, with low or no improvement in gait performance, freezing phenomenon, and the number of falls [43, 44, 46, 47]. The load of the exercises can be chosen using the test of maximal strength (1-RM). The number of sets may vary between 2 and 3 during initial periods. The retest of 1-RM can provide additional information to adjust the load and sets along the rehabilitation period. The resting time between the sets can be controlled by cardiovascular parameters and can vary from 30 seconds up to 3 or 4 minutes [43, 44].

There are numerous ways to work with resistance training, and it is up to the physiotherapists to choose the most appropriate one for the individual under their care. In resistance training, the following examples of exercises can be used: bench press, lat pulldown, military press, seated row, leg 45°, barbell squat, leg curl, leg extension, calf raises, lower abdominal exercises, and manual or external (theraband, barbell, ankle-weight, and pulley system) resistance in active movement. Treadmill and bicycle intervention can be used when performing against resistance [43–45, 47]. Da Silva and her coworkers [48] suggest a long-term effect in nonmotor signs and symptoms of Parkinson's disease, especially in cognitive aspects, in individuals performing treadmill training, just as Ferreira and her coworkers [49] showed that resistance training was an effective intervention in the reduction of anxiety symptoms and improved the quality of life in this population.

4.1.2. Transcutaneous electrical stimulation to control resting tremor

Even if the treatment of Parkinson's disease tremor focuses on medication, and there is indication to deep brain stimulation for those patients with tremor recalcitrant using oral medication, electrotherapy has been shown to be beneficial to control this special cardinal sign.

Few studies have been performed to provide further evidence on the effects of electrotherapy on Parkinson's tremor reduction. The theory supporting the use of this strategy is based on evidence revealing that propriospinal neurons in the C3–4 spinal cord mediate voluntary commands from the motor cortex (in Parkinson's disease, these commands are oscillating and give rise to resting tremor) and project directly to forelimb motor neurons. This proposal assumes the importance of propriospinal neurons to interfere in tremor signal transmission, especially because there are a rich variety of afferents, including cutaneous afferents [6].

Based on this concept, Xu and coworkers [50] hypothesize that cutaneous afferents evoked by surface stimulation could produce an inhibitory effect on propriospinal neurons, which in turn could suppress tremor signals passing through the propriospinal neurons.

Additionally, evidence shows benefits of electrical stimulation, especially when applied to the superficial cutaneous radial nerve area, in reduction refractory resting tremor. This effect is possibly mediated by cutaneous reflex via premotor neuron interneurons, through a disynaptic inhibitory postsynaptic potential. Some initial research was performed to confirm this theory using transcutaneous electrical nerve stimulation (TENS), with good results [6, 52]. The position of the electrodes can be verified in **Figure 3**.

The parameters used for TENS stimulation were 200 μs pulse width at 250 Hz pulse frequency. The pulse amplitude of stimuli must be adjusted during the stimulation period. First, it is necessary to discover the radiating threshold of the patient. It occurs when the patient refers to a radiating sensation, such as a paresthesia, running from the dorsal skin to the fingers. This radiating threshold has been used as a sensory marker because it indicates that the superficial radial nerve is actually activated by electrical stimulation. After detecting the radiating threshold, the intensity of electrical stimulation must be adjusted to 1.5–1.75 times radiating threshold to produce better effects on tremor control [6].

Nowadays, researchers have been studying a way to detect the tremors and control them simultaneously and automatically by electrostimulation. They already developed and tested a closed-loop system for tremor suppression by transcutaneous electrical nerve stimulation

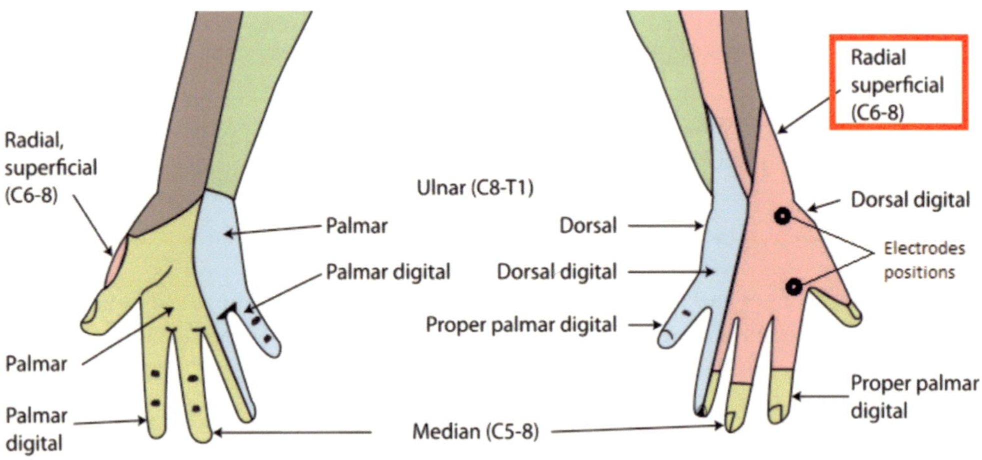

Figure 3. Use of transcutaneous electrical nerve stimulation to reduce resting tremor in Parkinson's disease. The figure brings cutaneous superficial radial nerve area and electrodes position for transcutaneous electrical nerve stimulation (TENS). Source: Modified from Gray [56]. Picture is public domain.

(TENS) using EMGs of the forearm muscles. Through this record, when a tremor is detected, a command signal triggers a stimulator to output TENS pulses to a pair of surface electrodes positioned just as described in **Figure 3**. The preliminary results showed that a closed-loop system can detect tremor properly and suppress significantly the tremor, by electrical stimulation of cutaneous afferents, in Parkinson's disease patients. Within this new concept, a tremor's glove was developed reaching also good results [50–52].

4.1.3. Aerobic training: treadmill, cycling, free walking, dance, and tai chi

It's known that aerobic exercises can reduce inflammation, suppress oxidative stress, and stabilize calcium homeostasis in the brain. So, it has been prescribed as an important activity for the elderly. The form of aerobic exercise used may be adapted to the capability of the individual. In individuals with Parkinson's disease, these exercises show important functions, once they can trigger plasticity-related changes, including synaptogenesis, enhanced glucose utilization, and neurogenesis [2, 53].

In general, aerobic training has been reported to improve both motor and nonmotor signs and symptoms of Parkinson's disease. The motor effects are extensively known and have been studied the most so far, showing the most unequivocal benefits on health across the life span. Furthermore, the neural mechanisms involving dopaminergic pathways are studied and suggest a significant preservation of nigrostriatal neuronal connections as well as striatal dopamine levels in experimental models. As a result, exercise-dependent plasticity following aerobic exercises acts on the brain in a similar manner as dopaminergic-derived treatments, using the same pathways to produce symptomatic relief [54].

In nonmotor signs and symptoms, aerobic training promotes positive and significant effects on global cognitive function, processing speed, sustained attention and mental flexibility, memory, and mood disorder aspects (anxiety and depression) in patients who are considered in a moderate stage of Parkinson's disease [49]. In sleep disorder, present in Parkinson's disease, aerobic exercise has been shown to have small-to-moderate effects. The mechanism involved in these effects evolved increased dopaminergic signaling and a wide variety of effects on nondopaminergic neurotransmitter systems, including serotonergic, noradrenergic, and GABAergic systems, which is relevant for depression, anxiety, and sleep [53, 54].

The most common and studied form of aerobic training is using a treadmill. In some systematic reviews, the majority of articles considered in analyses use treadmills for aerobic training. This approach can be used with or without a body-weight-support system, depending on the motor difficulties of the individual with Parkinson's disease. It may be related with improvement in motor signs like motor action, balance, and gait, although the evidence is not so strong [2, 48].

In the same way, free walking and Nordic walking (a total body version of walking performed with specially designed walking poles similar to ski poles) also have good effects on motor and nonmotor domains of Parkinson's disease and must be stimulated and used in physical therapy practice in rehabilitation of individuals with Parkinson's disease [55].

Similar to the aerobic training used on the treadmill, moderate intensity of interval training for cycling has shown several beneficial effects on the DA-dependent motor and nonmotor signs that compromise Parkinson's disease patients. Researchers have reported improvement on bimanual motor control, automatic interlimb coordination, executive functions, and neurological (UPDRS) symptoms [56].

An interval protocol template that can be used can be the following: from 8 to 12 weeks of training, 3 times per week, 1-hour session training with 10 minutes of warm-up, 40 minutes of aerobic training, and 10 minutes of cooldown). During the 40 minutes of aerobic training, the patient can perform 8 sets of 3 minutes of cycling or treadmill at 60–80 rpms and 2 minutes of less than 60 rpms. The heart rate also can be used as a parameter to improve effort during the training period. Hence, the physiotherapist may adjust the resistance to ensure the patient is cycling at 60–75% of his/her maximal heart rate. This effort can increase gradually during the training period [56]. A guideline with some exercise modes to be used in Parkinson's disease was provided by Meng and coworkers in a systematic review and meta-analysis [57].

Other forms of aerobic exercises have been stimulated in the rehabilitation process in Parkinson's disease. Several data have shown that dance can provide increased activation of the reward system, determining better mood aspects in people. In patients with Parkinson's disease, practicing dance has induced better responses and a substantial relevant improvement in motor symptoms (such as static and dynamic balance, freezing phenomenon, and gait) and functional mobility. This improvement determines also a better quality of life in performers. It probably occurs because rhythmic stimulation leads to time-perception compensation due to the synchronization of movement with rhythm [58, 59].

To get these effects, a dance program must include visual and auditory cues, rhythm tasks, and recreational activities that motivate socialization. Another important aspect is to reach the ideal heart rate during practice, just as discussed previously in the aerobic training protocol [58].

Oriental martial arts, such as tai chi, have been successfully used in treatment of individuals with Parkinson's disease. Tai chi combines deep breathing and slow movements and studies have provided moderate evidence that tai chi improves balance and functional mobility, reducing the number of falls, but with no significant effect in gait velocity, step length, and gait endurance improvement [33, 60, 61]. A systematic review and meta-analysis showed that tai chi, plus medication, showed greater gains than medication alone or another therapy plus medication in motor function and balance. Presumably, these gains were due to the development of new motor programs, which allow faster reactions responding to postural challenge promoting better behavioral recovery through new synaptic connections [62]. It is necessary to know and practice this technique before using it on patients.

4.1.4. Multimodal exercise program

The aim of the multimodal exercise program is to develop the patients' functional capacity, cognitive functions, posture, and locomotion. It's comprised of a variety of activities that simultaneously focus on the components of functional capacity, such as muscular resistance, motor coordination, and balance [14]. It's a 6-month program, performed 3 times per week, 1 hour per session. Each session consists of five parts (warm-up, pre-exercise stretching, the exercise session, the cooldown, and postexercise stretching). The program is divided into six phases with different uses of coordination, muscular resistance, and balance strategies [63, 64]. A description of each phase can be seen in **Table 5**.

The little data that are available in the literature point to improvement in some kinematic gait parameters of mild-to-moderate idiopathic PD patients using multimodal exercise programs [63, 64].

Phases	Capacities		
	Coordination	**Muscular resistance**	**Balance**
Phase 1	Upper and lower limb movements.	Exercises without weights.	Recreational activities that stimulated the vestibular system.
Phase 2	Trunk movements were added to upper and lower limb movements.	Light-weight equipment (hoops, ropes, and batons).	Recreational activities that stimulated the visual and vestibular systems.
Phase 3	Trunk movements were substituted by head movements.	Heavier equipment (barbells, ankle weights, and medicine balls).	Recreational activities that stimulated the visual and somatosensorial systems.
Phase 4	Head, trunk, and upper and lower limb movements.	Load was again increased with heavier equipment for resistance training (increase of intensity) or increased repetitions (increased volume).	Recreational activities integrated the vestibular, visual, and somatosensorial systems.
Phase 5	Four different movement sequences, two of which were the same for upper and lower limbs and two other sequences that alternated movements for upper and lower limbs in place and in movement.	Exercises were done with weights: leg press, pulley, seated cable rows, peck deck, and bench press. Load was adjusted according to patients' convenience (in two series of 15 repetitions).	Recreational activities included static balance, dynamic balance, half-turn, and complete turn (all with visual cues).
Phase 6	Four sequences of different movements, two sequences of alternating movement for upper and lower limbs, and two sequences of different movement for upper and lower limbs, with or without trunk movement and equipment (balloons, balls, hoops, and rope).	The same exercises with load increase. Series of 15 repetitions were added.	Recreational activities were composed of activities with tactile cues.

Note: Based on Vitório and coworkers [63].

Table 5. Multimodal exercise program in Parkinson´s disease.

4.1.5. Acupuncture

Several data show acupuncture and electroacupuncture (still performed on animal models) as beneficial strategies in Parkinson's disease treatment, used either isolated or combined with other treatments. It has been described as showing improvement in the UPDRS total score and in its subsections after an acupuncture session. So, even motor and nonmotor signs and symptoms, including pain, can be improved with the use of acupuncture [65–67]. However, the most important source of data that proves the beneficial effects of acupuncture in treatment of signs and symptoms in Parkinson's disease is provided from functional neuroimaging studies. These studies have shown huge modifications in neural functions after acupuncture sessions [68, 69].

As tai chi use was previously discussed, acupuncture requires previous academic training so that it can be used in an accurate way in the treatment of Parkinsonian individuals.

4.1.6. Hydrotherapy

Hydrotherapy has been widely used to treat individuals with Parkinson's disease. It has been proven to be effective for different gait rehabilitation programs, as well as to improve balance and quality of life, and reduce pain and falls. The warm property of water used for hydrotherapy potentially also reduces rigidity [70, 71].

In water, innumerable forms of exercises can be performed including warm-up exercises (like jumping and walking), stretching exercises, gait training, cooldown exercises, trunk mobility, balance, coordination and proprioceptive exercises, the Halliwick method, posture exercises, the Ai Chi method, aerobic exercise, the Bad Ragaz method, motor dexterity exercises, and swimming exercises, among others [71].

4.1.7. Virtual reality and exergames: integrative techniques

Virtual reality potentially optimizes motor learning in a safe environment, and by replicating real-life scenarios, it could help to improve functional activities of daily living in individuals with Parkinson's disease. However, the use of commercially available devices makes this tool contiguous to many other physical therapy instruments, leading to low evidence in the results [72]. Despite this, several studies have reported greater improvement in many signs and symptoms such as balance, gait, functional capacity, and self-confidence, improving quality of life and reducing the risk of falling [73–75].

As an example of specific virtual reality developed for Parkinson's disease rehabilitation, Gomez-Jordana and coworkers [76] developed visual cues that could be presented in an immersive, interactive virtual reality environment. With this, they created different forms of spatial and temporal information where black footprints presented at a prespecified distance apart could recreate different step lengths (spatial cues), and by controlling when the black footprints changed color to red, they could convey information about the timing of the foot placement (temporal cues). With this device, they could get significantly improved gait performance in participants.

Additionally, exercise-based video gaming (exergaming), a form of physical training that is delivered through virtual reality technology, facilitates motor learning and is efficacious in improving balance in aged populations. This approach can use commercial devices such as Nintendo Wii Fit System®, X-box 360° with Kinect®, or rehabilitation-specific software program like Jintronix® [70, 74, 77].

These devices usually combine automated game instructions as well as visual and auditory and tactile inputs to correct performance and sustain motivation levels during and following game play. Therefore, exergames employ visual and auditory feedback techniques to create a quasi-immersive environment that can facilitate motor and cognitive learning. Since individuals with Parkinson's disease are dependent on sensory cues to maintain postural stability and show difficulties with long-term consolidation of new motor skills, this sensorial integration provided by using exergames may help to upregulate neuroplasticity and facilitate motor skill acquisition and retention [77].

These resources can be used isolated or associated in a clinical approach or in a telerehabilitation program like a home-based virtual reality or home-based exergame [74].

4.1.8. Group approach

Groups are used in physical therapy to improve global health status and bring relief from typical disability symptoms of several diseases, competing with individual rehabilitation at least in short-term follow-up. Therapeutic groups have been beneficial to the health care system by decreasing the cost and time spent on rehabilitation.

Similar to other techniques, group therapy can use several kinds of exercise goals such as general mobility, using muscular strength, free movement, and relaxation exercises; trunk control, using trunk displacement and rotation during dynamic exercises performed in a sitting posture; static balance, using the same strategies for trunk control but in a standing position; dynamic balance and gait, using free gait; and gait with obstacles, stairs, ramp, uneven ground, performed in and outside the room. The use of hearing and visual cues during the procedure provides several stimulus associations for the patients. This approach was reported to improve gait, balance, and activity of daily life performance in patients with PD [78].

4.1.9. Mental imagery

Mental imagery is the cognitive process of creating visual, auditory, or kinesthetic experiences in the mind with or without overt physical execution. In many people, this procedure can help or improve motor performance. This strategy has the potential to increase the function of both the motor cortex and the spinal neurons, resulting in improved muscle function [79, 80]. Thus, it is an important technique in motor learning and control, and although it has its origin in sports science, it has been introduced into the field of neurorehabilitation.

In a few sources about mental imagery in Parkinson's disease rehabilitation, some data show a better muscle recruitment measured by electromyography or other form or neurophysiologic register. But available data are, sometimes, contradictory [80, 81].

Specifically in individuals with Parkinson's disease, this approach has shown to be beneficial to motor (measured by UPRDS-III-motor signs) and cognitive functions [79].

4.1.10. Applications (apps in cell phones or tablets): a new generation of physical therapy approach

Since smartphones became popular, numerous health-related apps have been developed for professionals, patients, and the general population. However, many of these apps are not validated, so their efficacy may be not satisfactory. Nowadays, this resource still has been used as a complementary treatment [82].

It is a well-known fact that it is important to emphasize that apps are a democratic source of information and rehabilitation, since they maintain the main principles of usability, accessibility, and equal opportunities for healthcare professionals, patients, relatives, and caregivers [82].

For Parkinson's disease, there are a few apps available, and just one with some data partially published. On the Parkinson's UK webpage, we can find a list of apps reviewed and recommended for individuals with Parkinson's disease. There are apps for sleep, volume of voice, mood, swallowing, memory (recording stories of patients), mobility, speech, and dexterity [83].

Another source from the International Parkinson's Community recommended eight extra apps. They focus on measurement and tracking the patient's symptoms, give information about Parkinson's disease, record and measure the magnitude of tremor and speech, and manage and track the individual's health condition. The only one that has some physical approach is the Parkinson's home exercise [84].

The Parkinson's Home Exercise®, promoted by the European Foundation for Health and Exercise, was easy-to-use and designed to be used by patients and physiotherapists. It provides advice and instructions for daily exercises and movements through over 50 videos and text instructions. It has a cost involved [85]. There are no references in literature about its efficacy.

Another app, developed by TEVA Pharmaceutical Industries, named Parkinsounds®, is a free app that helps patients with Parkinson's disease to find their gait rhythm using music and rhythmic beats (like a metronome). They use a predetermined music list or one that can be linked to Spotify®. Once the rhythm is chosen, Parkinsounds is able to find music that combines with the preselected rhythm adding beats in the music. The physiologic base for this strategy is centered on the synchronic activation of neurons provided by the music and the rhythmic stimulus, added to an increase of dopamine liberation [86].

Our group has been developing research using this specific app in rehabilitation of gait in Parkinson's disease. The partial data were already presented at the World Confederation of Physical Therapy Conference (research data are not still available). However, a huge acute effect could be seen in the gait of Parkinsonians using Parkinsounds, even in a long-term period of rehabilitation. We could see an improvement in width and length of gait, with a reduction of base and number of steps, which were measured in a 10 meters' route, after 10 weeks of treatment. It is important to emphasize that the walking test was performed with and without Parkinsounds® use for patients at the moment of evaluation (initial and final), and in both cases, the improvement was significant. So, it can be considered an important feature for gait rehabilitation in Parkinson's disease.

4.1.11. Whole body vibration

According to the literature data, there is no apparent consistency in the effect of whole body vibration shown on mobility, balance, and gait in individuals with Parkinson's disease [87]. However, the majority of the studies point to a favorable effect of this therapeutic strategy [87, 88].

Disregarding the differences between the various types of equipment, a lot of research has proposed some parameters that are useful in improving mobility and balance in individuals with Parkinson's disease. The majority recommend orthostatic position and 7 to 14 mm amplitude with a frequency ranging between 3 and 25 Hz, in cycles of 5 bouts of 1 minute each. Until now, there is no consensus about which frequency in better [87]. So, it is recommended that the physical therapist evaluate these functions constantly after using this resource.

The effect of whole body vibration on tremor is less prominent [87]. Moreover, it also does not appear to lead to better cardiovascular conditions reducing the feeling of fatigue when compared to treadmill training [89].

The physiological mechanism involved in the effects of whole body vibration on reducing some of the motor signs of Parkinson's disease remains elusive. Some theories suggest that whole body vibration provides tactile and proprioceptive stimulus to the whole body originated from the vertical oscillating mechanical movement or the movement along the horizontal axis, which through neuromuscular activation and metabolic mechanism may bypass dysfunctional basal ganglia, resulting in better adjustments for postural stability and gait [88, 90].

5. Conclusion

In this chapter, we can notice how profound the discussions about Parkinson's disease are, especially about treatment. Physical therapy has increased its participation in Parkinson's disease treatment. However, research is still lacking to substantiate its real effectiveness. It is imperative that further research be done to strengthen performance and the excellent results obtained with physical therapy in treating individuals with Parkinson's disease.

Acknowledgements

I would like to thank Pontifical University of Minas Gerais for funding the research cited in this chapter: PROBIC PUC Minas 95/35 {80}; Parkinsounds Project PROBIC PUC/FAPEMIG 2018/1510.

Author details

Luciana Auxiliadora de Paula Vasconcelos

Address all correspondence to: lucivasc@pucpcaldas.br

Physical Therapy Department - PUC Minas Campus, Poços de Caldas, Brazil

References

[1] Zanzoni A, Montecchi-Palazzi L, Quondam MX. A molecular interaction database. FEBS Letters. 2002;**513**:135-140. DOI: 10.1016/s0014-5793(01)03293-8

[2] Shu HF, Yang T, Yu SX, et al. Aerobic exercise for Parkinson's disease: A systematic review and meta-analysis of randomized controlled trials. PLoS One. 2014;**9**(7):e100503. DOI: 10.1371/journal.pone.0100503

[3] Alves G, Forsaa EB, Pedersen KF, Dreetz Gjerstad M, Larsen JP. Epidemiology of Parkinson's disease. Journal of Neurology. 2008;**255**(Suppl 5):18-32. DOI: 10.1007/s00415-008-5004-3

[4] Mackenzie IRA. The pathology of Parkinson's disease. British Columbia Medical Journal. 2001;**43**(3):142-147

[5] Rocca WA. The burden of Parkinson's disease: A worldwide perspective. Lancet Neurology. 2018;**17**(11):928-929. DOI: 10.1016/S1474-4422(18)30355-7

[6] Hao MZ, Xu SQ, Hu ZX, et al. Inhibition of Parkinsonian tremor with cutaneous afferent evoked by transcutaneous electrical nerve stimulation. Journal of NeuroEngineering and Rehabilitation. 2017;**14**(1):75. DOI: 10.1186/s12984-017-0286-2

[7] National Institute of Neurological Disorders and Stroke. Parkinson's Disease Information Page. 2019. Available from: https://www.ninds.nih.gov/Disorders/All-Disorders/Parkinsons-Disease-Information-Page [Accessed: June 28, 2019]

[8] Magrinelli F, Picelli A, Tocco P, et al. Pathophysiology of motor dysfunction in Parkinson's disease as the rationale for drug treatment and rehabilitation. Parkinsons Disease. 2016;**2016**:9832839. DOI: 10.1155/2016/9832839

[9] Krüger R, Klucken J, Weiss D, et al. Classification of advanced stages of Parkinson's disease: Translation into stratified treatments. Journal of Neural Transmission (Vienna). 2017;**124**(8):1015-1027. DOI: 10.1007/s00702-017-1707-x

[10] Tomlinson CL, Patel S, Meek C, et al. Physiotherapy intervention in Parkinson's disease: Systematic review and meta-analysis. BMJ. 2012;**345**:e5004, 1-14. DOI: 10.1136/bmj.e5004

[11] Stoker TB, Torsney KM, Barker RA. Emerging treatment approaches for Parkinson's disease. Frontiers in Neuroscience. 2018;**12**:693. DOI: 10.3389/fnins.2018.00693

[12] Nitrini R, Bacheschi LA. A Neurologia Que Todo Médico Deve Saber. 3rd ed. São Paulo: Atheneu; 570p. ISBN: 9788538806240

[13] Di Monte DA, Lavasani M, Manning-Bog AB. Environmental factors in Parkinson's disease. Neurotoxicology. 2002;**23**(4-5):487-502. DOI: 10.1016/S0161-813X(02)00099-2

[14] A Train Education: Continuing Education for Health Professionals. 2019. Available from: https://www.atrainceu.com/course-module/2441043-143_parkinsons-module-02 [Accessed: June 28, 2019]

[15] National Institute of Aging. What is Lewy Body Dementia?. 2019. Available from: https://www.nia.nih.gov/health/what-lewy-body-dementia [Accessed: June 28, 2019]

[16] Barcia C. Glial-mediated inflammation underlying parkinsonism. Scientifica (Cairo). 2013;**2013**:357805. DOI: 10.1155/2013/357805

[17] Ball N, Teo WP, Chandra S, Chapman J. Parkinson's disease and the environment. Frontiers in Neurology. 2019;**10**:218. DOI: 10.3389/fneur.2019.00218

[18] Dick FD, De Palma G, Ahmadi A, et al. Environmental risk factors for Parkinson's disease and parkinsonism: The Geoparkinson study. Occupational and Environmental Medicine. 2007;**64**(10):666-672. DOI: 10.1136/oem.2006.027003

[19] Thorp JE, Adamczyk PG, Ploeg HL, et al. Monitoring motor symptoms during activities of daily living in individuals with Parkinson's disease. Frontiers in Neurology. 2018;**9**:1036. DOI: 10.3389/fneur.2018.01036

[20] Banou E. Kinesia paradoxa: A challenging Parkinson's phenomenon for simulation. In: Vlamos P, Alexiou A, editors. GeNeDis 2014. Advances in Experimental Medicine and Biology. Vol. 822. Springer, Cham. DOI: 10.1007/978-3-319-08927-0_18

[21] Eshius SA, Leenders KL. Parkinson's disease: Symptoms and age dependency. In: Hof PR, Mobbs CV, editors. Functional Neurobiology of Aging. San Diego: Academic Press; 2001. pp. 675-688

[22] Kouli A, Torsney KM, Kuan W-L. Parkinson's disease: Etimology, neuropathology, and pathogenesis. In: Stoker TB, Greenland JC, editors. Parkinson's Disease: Pathology and Clinical Aspects. Brisbane (AU): Codon Publications; 2018. Available from: https://ncbi.nlm.nih.gov/books/NBK 536722/ DOI: 10.15586/codonpublications.parkinsonsdisease.2018.chl

[23] Lee HM, Koh SB. Many faces of Parkinson's disease: Non-motor symptoms of Parkinson's disease. Journal of Movement Disorders. 2015;**8**(2):92-97. DOI: 10.14802/jmd.15003

[24] Sveinbjornsdottir S. The clinical symptoms of Parkinson's disease. Journal of Neurochemistry. 2016;**139**(Suppl 1):318-324. DOI: 10.1111/jnc.13691

[25] Kouli Greenland JC, Barker RA. The differential diagnosis of Parkinson's disease. In: Stoker TB, Greenland JC, editors. The Differential Diagnosis of Parkinson's Desease. Brisbane (AU): Codon Publications; 2018. Available from: https://ncbi.nlm.nih.gov/books/NBK 536722/ DOI: 10.15586/codonpublications.parkinsonsdisease.2018.chl

[26] Jankovic J. Parkison's disease: Clinical features and diagnosis. Journal of Neurology, Neurosurgery, and Psychiatry. 2008;**79**:368-376. DOI: 10.1136/jnnp.2007.131045

[27] Postuma RB, Berg D, Stern M, et al. MDS clinical diagnostic criteria for Parkinson's disease. Movement Disorders. 2015;**30**(12):1591-1601. DOI: 10.1002/mds.26424

[28] Del Rey NL, Quiroga-Varela A, Garbayo E, et al. Advances in Parkinson's disease: 200 years later. Frontiers in Neuroanatomy. 2018;**12**:113. DOI: 10.3389/fnana.2018.00113

[29] European Parkinson's disease Association. Rating Scales. 2019. Available from: https://www.epda.eu.com/about-parkinsons/symptoms/rating-scales/ [Accessed: June 30, 2019]

[30] International Parkinson and Movement Disorder Society. 2019. Available from: https://www.parkinsons.org.uk/professionals/resources/unified-parkinsons-disease-rating-scale-updrs [Accessed: June 30, 2019]

[31] Braak H, Del Tredici K, Rüb U, et al. Staging of brain pathology related to sporadic Parkinson's disease. Neurobiology of Aging. 2003;**24**(2):197-211. DOI: 10.1016/s0197-4580(02)00065-9

[32] Cuenca L, Gil-Martinez AL, Cano-Fernandez L, et al. Parkinson's disease: A short story of 200 years. Histology and Histopathology. 2019;**34**(6):573-591. DOI: 10.14670/HH-18-073

[33] Dong J, Cui Y, Li S, Le W. Current pharmaceutical treatments and alternative therapies of Parkinson's disease. Current Neuropharmacology. 2016;**14**(4):339-355. DOI: 10.2174/1570159X14666151120123025

[34] Zahoor I, Shafi A, Haq E. Pharmacological treatment of Parkinson's disease. In: Stoker TB, Greenland JC, editors. Parkinson's Disease: Pathogenesis and Clinical Aspects. Brisbane (AU): Codon Publications; 2018. Available from: https://www.ncbi.nlm.nih.gov/books/NBK536726/ DOI: 10.15586/codonpublications.parkinsonsdisease.2018.ch7

[35] Radhakrishnan DM, Goyal V. Parkinson's disease: A review. Neurology India. 2018;**66**:26-35. DOI: 10.4103/0028-3886.226451

[36] Dallapiazza RF, De Vloo P, Fomenko A, et al. Considerations for patient and target selection in deep brain stimulation surgery for Parkinson's disease. In: Stoker TB, Greenland JC, editors. Parkinson's Disease: Pathogenesis and Clinical Aspects. Brisbane (AU): Codon Publications; 2018. Available from: https://www.ncbi.nlm.nih.gov/books/NBK536714/ DOI: 10.15586/codonpublications.parkinsonsdisease.2018.ch8

[37] Shamir R, Noecker A, McIntyre C. Deep brain stimulation. Front Young Minds. 2014;**2**:12. DOI: 10.3389/frym.2014.00012. Available from: http://kids.frontiersin.org/article/10.3389/frym.2014.00012 [Accessed: July 02, 2019]

[38] Emamzadeh FN, Surguchov A. Parkinson's disease: Biomarkers, treatment, and risk factors. Frontiers in Neuroscience. 2018;**12**:612. DOI: 10.3389/fnins.2018.00612

[39] de Dreu MJ, van der Wilk AS, Poppe E, et al. Rehabilitation, exercise therapy and music in patients with Parkinson's disease: A meta-analysis of the effects of music-based movement therapy on walking ability, balance and quality of life. Parkinsonism and Related Disorders. 2012;**18**(Suppl 1):S114-S119. DOI: 10.1016/S1353-8020(11)70036-0

[40] Goodwin VA, Richards SH, Taylor RS, et al. The effectiveness of exercise interventions for people with Parkinson's disease: A systematic review and meta-analysis. Movement Disorders. 2008;**23**(5):631-640. DOI: 10.1002/mds.21922

[41] Hirsch MA, van Wegen EEH, Newman MA, et al. Exercise-induced increase in brain-derived neurotrophic factor in human Parkinson's disease: A systematic review and meta-analysis. Translational Neurodegeneration. 2018;**7**(7). DOI: 10.1186/s40035-018-0112-1

[42] Umphred DA. Reabilitação Neurológica. 5th ed. Rio de Janeiro: Elsevier; 2009. ISBN: 9788535231250

[43] Barbalho M, Monteiro EP, Costa RR, et al. Effects of low-volume resistance training on muscle strength and functionality of people with Parkinson's disease. International Journal of Exercise Science. 2019;**12**(3):567-580

[44] Chung CLH, Thilarajah S, Tan D. Effectiveness of resistence training on muscle strength and physical function in people with Parkinson's disease: A systematic review and meta-analysis. Clinical Rehabilitation. 2016;**30**(1):11-23. DOI: 10.1177/0269215515570381

[45] Saltychev M, Bärlund E, Paltamaa J, et al. Progressive resistence training in Parkinson's disease: A systematic review and meta-analysis. BMJ Open. 2016;**6**:e008756. 1-9. DOI: 10.1136/bmjopen-2015-008756

[46] Ramazzina I, Bernazzoli B, Costantino C. Systematic review on strength training in Parkinson's disease: An unsolved question. Clinical Interventions in Aging. 2017;**12**:619-628. DOI: 10.2147/CIA.S131903

[47] Uygur M, Bellumori M, Knight CA. Effects of a low-resistance, interval bicycling intervention in Parkinson's disease. Physiotherapy Theory and Practice. 2017;**33**(12):897-904. DOI: 10.1080/09593985.2017.1359868

[48] da Silva FC, Iop RDR, de Oliveira LC, et al. Effects of physical exercise programs on cognitive function in Parkinson's disease patients: A systematic review of randomized controlled trials of the last 10 years. PLoS One. 2018;**13**(2):e0193113. DOI: 10.1371/journal.pone.0193113

[49] Ferreira RM, Alves WMGC, Lima TA, et al. The effect of resistance training on the anxiety symptoms and quality of life in elderly people with Parkinson's disease: A randomized controlled trial. Arquivos de Neuro-Psiquiatria. 2018;**76**(8):499-506. DOI: 10.1590/0004-282x20180071

[50] Xu FL, Hao MZ, Xu SQ, et al. Development of a closed-loop system for tremor suppression in patients with Parkinson's disease. In: Proceedings of the IEEE Engineering in Medicine and Biology Society; Aug 2016. pp. 1782-1785. DOI: 10.1109/EMBC.2016.7591063

[51] Gray H. Gray's Anatomy. 20th ed. Collectible Classics; 2010. ISBN: 9781435114937. Figure available from: https://pt.wikipedia.org/wiki/Nervo_cut%C3%A2neo_medial_do_bra%C3%A7o [Accessed: June 30, 2019]

[52] Jitkritsadakul O, Thanawattano C, Anan C, et al. Tremor's glove-an innovate electrical muscle stimulation therapy for intractable in Parkinson's disease: A randomized sham-controlled trial. Journal of the Neurological Sciences. 2017;**381**:331-340. DOI: 10.1016/j.jns.2017.08.3246

[53] Reynolds GO, Otto MW, Ellis TD, Cronin-Golomb A. The therapeutic potential of exercise to improve mood, cognition, and sleep in Parkinson's disease. Movement Disorders. 2016;**31**(1):23-38. DOI: 10.1002/mds.26484

[54] Duchesne C, Gheysen F, Bore A, et al. Influence of aerobic exercise training on the neural correlates of motor learning in Parkinson's disease individuals. Neuroimage: Clinical. 2016;**12**:559-569. DOI: 10.1016/j.nicl.2016.09.011

[55] Franzoni LT, Monteiro EP, Oliveira HB, et al. A 9-week Nordic and free walking improve postural balance in Parkinson's disease. Sports Medicine International Open. 2018;**2**(2):E28-E34. DOI: 10.1055/s-0043-124757

[56] Marusiak J, Fisher BE, Jaskólska A, et al. Eight weeks of aerobic interval training improves psychomotor function in patients with Parkinson's disease-randomized controlled trial. International Journal of Environmental Research and Public Health. 2019;**16**(5):880. DOI: 10.3390/ijerph16050880

[57] Ni M, Hazzard JB, Signorile JF, et al. Exercise guidelines for gait function in Parkinson's disease: A systematic review and meta-analysis. Neurorehabilitation and Neural Repair. 2018;**32**(10):872-886. DOI: 10.1177/1545968318801558

[58] Dos Santos DM, Komeroski IG, Monteiro EEP, et al. Effects of dance practice on functional mobility, motor symptoms and quality of life in people with Parkinson's disease: A systematic review and meta-analysis. Aging Clinical and Experimental Research. 2018;**30**(7):727-735. DOI: 10.1007/s40520-017-0836-2

[59] Pereira APS, Marinho V, Gupta D, et al. Music therapy and dance as gait rehabilitation in patients with Parkinson's disease: A review of evidence. Journal of Geriatric Psychiatry and Neurology. 2019;**32**(1):49-56. DOI: 10.1177/0891988718819858

[60] Liu H-H, Yeh N-C, Wu Y-F, et al. Effects of Tai Chi exercise on reducing falls and improving balance performance in Parkinson's disease: A meta-analysis. Parkinson's Disease. 2019;**2019**:9626934, 8 p. DOI: doi.org/10.1155/2019/9626934

[61] Winser SJ, Tsang WW, Krishnamurthy K, et al. Does Tai Chi improve balance and reduce falls incidence in neurological disorders? A systematic review and meta-analysis. Clinical Rehabilitation. 2018;**32**(9):1157-1168. DOI: 10.1177/0269215518773442

[62] Yang Y, Qiu WQ, Hao YL, Lv ZY, Jiao SJ, Teng JF. The efficacy of traditional Chinese medical exercise for Parkinson's disease: A systematic review and meta-analysis. PLoS One. 2015;**10**(4):e0122469. DOI: 10.1371/journal.pone.0122469

[63] Vitório R, Teixeira-Arroyo C, Lirani-Silva E, et al. Effects of 6-month, multimodal exercise program on clinical and gait parameters of patients with idiopathic Parkinson's disease: A pilot study. ISRN Neurology. 2011;**2011**:714947. DOI: 10.5402/2011/714947

[64] Orcioli-Silva D, Barbieri FA, Simieli L, et al. Effects of a multimodal exercise program on the functional capacity of Parkinson's disease patients considering disease severity and gender. Motriz. 2014;**20**(1):100-106. DOI: doi.org/10.1590/S1980-65742014000100015

[65] Jiang F, Yang T, Yin H, et al. Evidence for the use of acupuncture in treating Parkinson's disease: Update of information from the past 5 years, a mini review of the literature. Frontiers in Neurology. 2018;**9**:596. DOI: 10.3389/fneur.2018.00596

[66] Lee SH, Lim S. Clinical effectiveness of acupuncture on Parkinson disease: A PRISMA-compliant systematic review and meta-analysis. Medicine (Baltimore). 2017;**96**(3):e5836. DOI: 10.1097/MD.0000000000005836

[67] Lin JG, Chen CJ, Yang HB, Chen YH, Hung SY. Electroacupuncture promotes recovery of motor function and reduces dopaminergic neuron degeneration in rodent models of Parkinson's disease. International Journal of Molecular Sciences. 2017;**18**(9):1846. DOI: 10.3390/ijms18091846

[68] Yeo S, van den Noort M, Bosch P, Lim S. A study of the effects of 8-week acupuncture treatment on patients with Parkinson's disease. Medicine (Baltimore). 2018;**97**(50):e13434. DOI: 10.1097/MD.0000000000013434

[69] Li Z, Chen J, Cheng J, et al. Acupuncture modulates the Cerebello-Thalamo-cortical circuit and cognitive brain regions in patients of Parkinson's disease with tremor. Frontiers in Aging Neuroscience. 2018;**10**:206. DOI: 10.3389/fnagi.2018.00206

[70] Alves Da Rocha P, Mcclelland J, Morris ME. Complementary physical therapies for movement disorders in Parkinson's disease: A systematic review. European Journal of Physical and Rehabilitation Medicine. 2015;**51**(6):693-704

[71] Pinto C, Salazar AP, Marchese RR, et al. The effects of hydrotherapy on balance, functional mobility, motor status, and quality of life in patients with Parkinson disease: A systematic review and meta-analysis. PM&R: The Journal of Injury, Function, and Rehabilitation. 2019;**11**(3):278-291. DOI: 10.1016/j.pmrj.2018.09.031

[72] Dockx K, Bekkers EM, Van den Bergh V, et al. Virtual reality for rehabilitation in Parkinson's disease. Cochrane Database of Systematic Reviews. 2016;**12**(12):CD010760. DOI: 10.1002/14651858.CD010760.pub2

[73] Feng H, Li C, Liu J, et al. Virtual reality rehabilitation versus conventional physical therapy for improving balance and gait in Parkinson's disease patients: A randomized controlled trial. Medical Science Monitor. 2019;**25**:4186-4192. DOI: 10.12659/MSM.916455

[74] Gandolfi M, Geroin C, Dimitrova E, et al. Virtual reality telerehabilitation for postural instability in Parkinson's disease: A multicenter, single-blind, randomized, controlled trial. BioMed Research International. 2017;**2017**:7962826. DOI: 10.1155/2017/7962826

[75] Severiano MIR, Zeigelboim BS, Teive HAG, et al. Effect of virtual reality in Parkinson's disease: A prospective observational study. Arquivos de Neuro-Psiquiatria. 2018;**76**(2):78-84

[76] Gómez-Jordana LI, Stafford J, Peper CLE, Craig CM. Virtual footprints can improve walking performance in people with Parkinson's disease. Frontiers in Neurology. 2018;**9**:681. DOI: 10.3389/fneur.2018.00681

[77] Harris DM, Rantalainen T, Muthalib M, et al. Concurrent exergaming and transcranial direct current stimulation to improve balance in people with Parkinson's disease: Study protocol for a randomised controlled trial. Trials. 2018;**19**(1):387. DOI: 10.1186/s13063-018-2773-6

[78] Pereira DDC, Siqueira SA, Alvisi TA, Vasconcelos LAP. Group physical therapy program for patients with Parkinson's disease: Alternative rehabilitation. Fisioterapia em Movimento. 2009;**22**(2):229-237

[79] Abraham A, Hart A, Andrade I, et al. Dynamic neuro-cognitive imagery improves mental imagery ability, disease severity, and motor and cognitive functions in people with Parkinson's disease. Neural Plasticity. 2018;**2018**:6168507. DOI: 10.1155/2018/6168507

[80] Suzuki T, Bunno Y, Onigata C, et al. Excitability of spinal neural function during motor imagery in Parkinson's disease. Functional Neurology. 2014;**29**(4):263-267

[81] Kobelt M, Wirth B, Schuster-Amft C. Muscle activation during grasping with and without motor imagery in healthy volunteers and patients after stroke or with Parkinson's disease. Frontiers in Psychology. 2018;**9**:597. DOI: 10.3389/fpsyg.2018.00597

[82] Rodríguez S, Vázquez C, Casas M, et al. Neurorehabilitation and apps: A systematic review of mobile applications. Neurología. 2018;**33**(5):313-326. DOI: 10.1016/j.nrl.2015.10.005

[83] Parkinson's UK. Apps and Devices for Parkinson's. Available from: https://www.parkinsons.org.uk/information-and-support/apps-and-devices-parkinsons [Accessed: July 12, 2019]

[84] Parkinson's Life. 8 Smart Parkinson's Apps You Need to Try. Available from: https://parkinsonslife.eu/top-apps-for-the-parkinsons-community/ [Accessed: July 12, 2019]

[85] Parkinson Home Exercise. Available from: https://apps.apple.com/us/app/parkinson-home-exercises/id473641730 [Accessed: July 12, 2019]

[86] Parkinsounds. Available from: http://www.parkinsounds.com.br/ [Accessed: July 12, 2019]

[87] Dincher A, Schwarz M, Wydra G. Analysis of the effects of whole-body vibration in Parkinson disease: Systematic review and meta-analysis. PM&R. 2019;**11**(6):640-653. DOI: 10.1002/pmrj.12094

[88] Sharififar S, Coronado RA, Romero S, et al. The effect of whole body vibration on mobility and balance in Parkinson disease: A systematic review. Iranian Journal of Medical Sciences. 2014;**39**(4):318-326

[89] Corbianco S, Cavallini G, Baldereschi G, et al. Whole body vibration and treadmill training in Parkinson's disease rehabilitation effects on energy cost and recovery phases. Neurological Sciences. 2018;**39**(12):2159-2168. DOI: 10.1007/s10072-018-3566-0

[90] Madou KH, Cronin JB. The effects of whole body vibration on physical and physiological capability in special populations. Hong Kong Physiotherapy Journal. 2008;**26**:24-38

Section 4

Physical Therapy Interventions Related to Pulmonary Conditions

Chapter 7

Application of a Single-Case Research Design to Present the Effectiveness of Rehabilitation in the Clinic

Jirakrit Leelarungrayub, Yothin Pothasak,
Jynwara Kaju and Rungtiwa Kanthain

Additional information is available at the end of the chapter

http://dx.doi.org/10.5772/intechopen.90665

Abstract

Clinical benefits of rehabilitation are very difficult to present because of various factors such as very small sample sizes, no control comparison, or short period of intervention. However, clinical improvement can be presented with a single case study research design that is very interesting and challenging technique. Basic and advanced single-research designs can be performed in various patterns, for example, baseline (A) and intervention (B) phases [A-B], A-B-withdrawal (A′) phases [A-B-A′], A-B-A′- new intervention (B′) phases [A-B-A′-B], etc. In each phase, a line graph must be presented for changes using a trend line or split-middle method or mean and the standard deviation is shown. A trend or celebration line of data in the baseline period (A) should be drawn through the intervention phase (B). Then, the serial dependence or autocorrelation coefficient in each phase must be calculated by Barletta test, and the transformation of autocorrelation data should be performed when serial dependence occurs. Finally, clinically statistical improvement during intervention can be analyzed with the Bloom table, two-standard deviation band, paired t-test, binomial statistic, or C-statistical analysis. Therefore, single case study or cases of research design can be used to present the effectiveness of any intervention in the clinic.

Keywords: single-case research design, rehabilitation

1. Introduction

At present, the benefit of clinical research is very important in clinical practice. However, clinical research involving human patients or subjects has more varied bias and confounding

IntechOpen

© 2020 The Author(s). Licensee IntechOpen. This chapter is distributed under the terms of the Creative Commons Attribution License (http://creativecommons.org/licenses/by/3.0), which permits unrestricted use, distribution, and reproduction in any medium, provided the original work is properly cited.

factors than experimental research [1]. A previous report claimed that common studies in clinical research had various designs such as case–control studies, cohort study, randomized controlled trials, reviews, and meta-analyses, the same as case reports [2]. Moreover, single-subject design also is used for practice-based primary care research, due to the limitation on condition, heterogeneity, and strict criteria, but with some interesting results [3]. Previous evidence reported that clinical research can be divided broadly into two types; observational and experimental [4]. Cross-sectional, case control, cohort, and ecological study are analytical, but prevalence surveys, case series, surveillance data, and analysis of routinely collected data are a type of descriptive study. Although the best clinical research is designed with a controlled group, low bias on inclusion criteria, and good statistical analysis protocol, the limitations on various pathological conditions and inconsistency among patients are presented, whereas the value of inspiring new ideas or explaining new results from techniques during rehabilitation is of clinical concern in multiple or single cases [5–7]. Therefore, effectiveness of rehabilitation in a rare or single case can be presented with descriptive data alone, as in a previous report that presented the effect of combined thoracic and backward lifting exercise at a thoracic kyphosis angle, and intercostal muscle pain, without any graphs, tables, or statistical analysis measurement [8]. However, better results of a single-case research design can be represented by visual graphs after data collection at either baseline or intervention phases, whereas efficiency of intervention also can be evaluated with a mean level and trend changes by comparing with baseline or prior interventions [9, 10]. Finally, significant effectiveness of intervention can be analyzed simply with the Bloom Table, paired t-test, or one-way ANOVA methods, if serial dependence or autocorrelation coefficient of data is not found (**Figure 1**).

The flow chart in **Figure 1** shows a simple series procedure for performing a single-case research, (1) collecting data in both baseline and intervention phases, (2) drawing the trend line and mean level in each phase, (3) checking the series dependency of data in each phase,

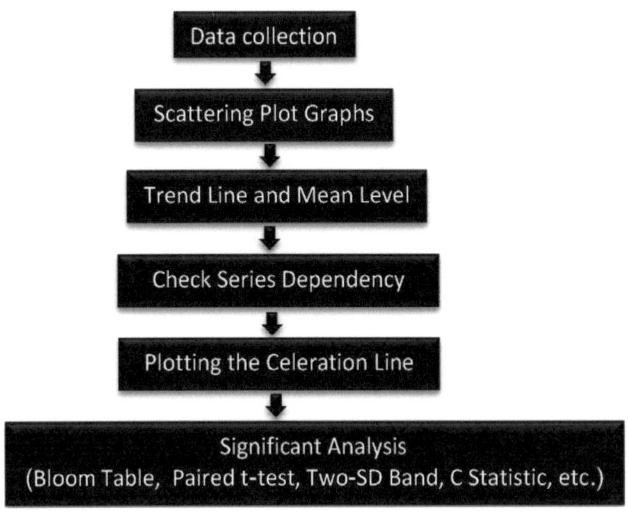

Figure 1. Flowchart of procedure on a single-case research design.

and (4) drawing the celeration line from the prior phase to the next one, and then analyzing statistically.

2. Research design

There has been a variety of single case research designs such as (1) AB, (2) reversal, (3) multiple baseline, and (4) alternating treatment [11]. The components of a single-case research design are composed of a series of interventions and frequency of assessment in multiple phases and various conditions. For instance, the effectiveness of a 7-day chest wall-stretching exercise in patients with chronic obstructive pulmonary disease (COPD) compared with 7 days in the baseline phase [12]. The same applies to 7-day pulmonary rehabilitation in patients with chronic scleroderma [13]. Therefore, various designs with a control period or baseline (A), intervention (B), withdrawn (A), or new intervention phase (B′) can be performed. Thus, a simple visual graph has been recommended with the following three designs (**Figure 2**).

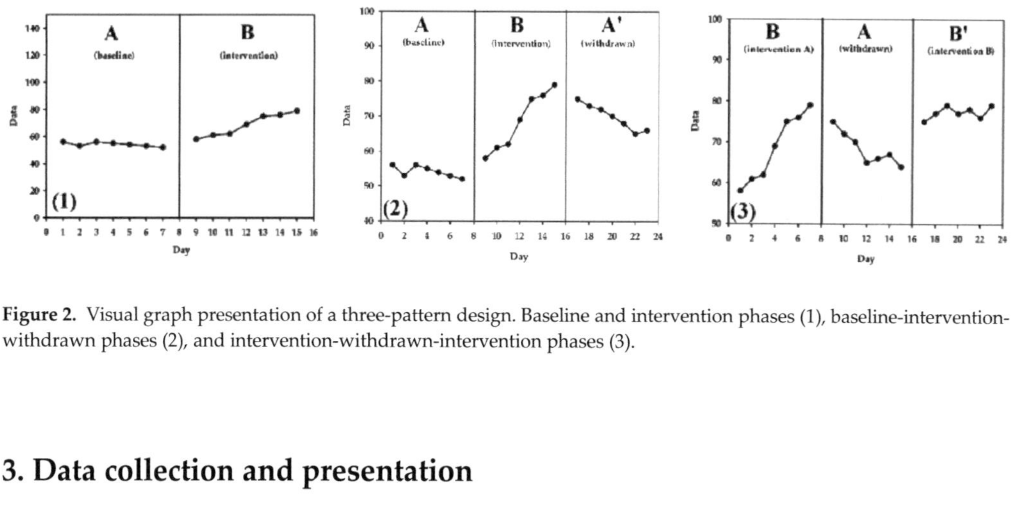

Figure 2. Visual graph presentation of a three-pattern design. Baseline and intervention phases (1), baseline-intervention-withdrawn phases (2), and intervention-withdrawn-intervention phases (3).

3. Data collection and presentation

In this design, the frequency of data collection has been suggested as at least three times or during individual periods in either the baseline or intervention phase [14], in order to present the change in trend in the baseline phase, whereas a previous report preferred an evaluation 6-8 times [15] as in **Table 1**, for example. The visual analysis involves determining the level, trend and stability of the data within in each phase, as well as immediacy of effect, consistency of data patterns, and overlap of data between baseline and intervention phases [16].

Presentation of the data or scores can be performed with scattering, plotted as a simple line graph for either single or multiple cases with a multiple baseline design, as in **Figure 3**.

Baseline phase						Intervention phase				
PImax	Day 1	Day 2	Day 3	Day 4	Day 5	Day 6	Day 7	Day 8	Day 9	Day 10
1	2	3	2	2	3	3	5	5	5	6
2	2	2	2	3	3	4	4	5	7	7
3	2	2	2	2	2	3	5	4	8	8
High value	**2**	**3**	**2**	**3**	**3**	**4**	**5**	**5**	**8**	**8**

Table 1. Chest wall excursion (cm) between baseline and intervention phases.

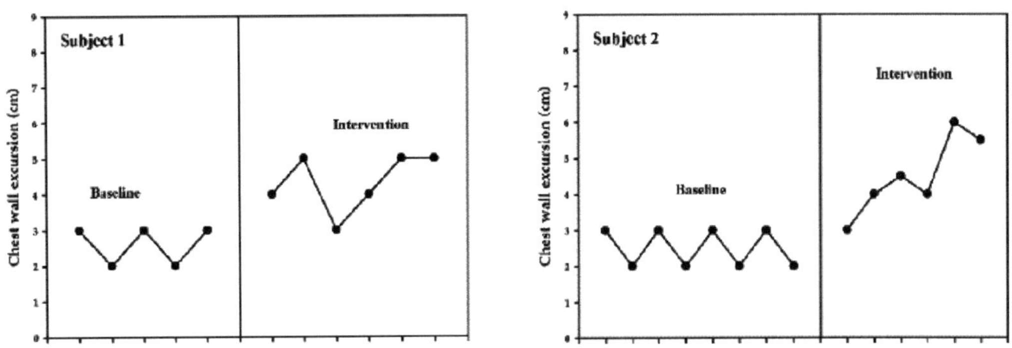

Figure 3. Line graph presentation of chest wall excursion (cm) in two cases that show the baseline and intervention phases with different scores in the baseline phase.

Presentation with a line graph has several advantages, for example, easy interpretation and understanding. Moreover, the bar graph of mean in each phase can be used.

The appropriate graphic methods can be applied to present data of changes in level, variability, trend, and slope [17] within each phase following the immediacy of effect, consistency of data patterns, and overlap of data between baseline and intervention phases [16]. For example, the mean levels of peak inspiratory pressure (PImax) between baseline (A), intervention (B), and withdrawn (A′) is shown in **Figure 4(1)** and trend lines in **Figure 4(2)**. Trend lines within a phase can demonstrate the stability of scores in the baseline phase with constant trend, as well as acceleration and deceleration trend patterns in intervention and withdrawn phases, respectively.

Interpretation of the mean and trend line in each phase presents the meaning clinically, for example, chest wall excursion (**Figure 5(1)**), dyspnea scale (**Figure 5(2)**), vital capacity, diffused capacity of lung for carbon monoxide (DLCO), etc. **Figure 5(1)** shows the constancy of chest wall excursion before treatment, which then increases with a mean level higher (3.83 cm) than that at baseline (2.19 cm). Therefore, that intervention can increase chest wall excursion in the clinic. In addition, dyspnea scale changes in **Figure 5(2)** decrease from a mean of 5.6 in the intervention phase to 4.2 in the baseline phase.

The deleterious effect of interventions can be presented, as in **Figure 5(3)**. Vital capacity reduces and decelerates tendency during given treatment; therefore, that treatment does not affect vital capacity. Finally, the last example of change in DLCO between baseline and intervention phases shows a slight increase of DLCO mean. Thus, that intervention can increase the DLCO slightly (**Figure 5(4)**).

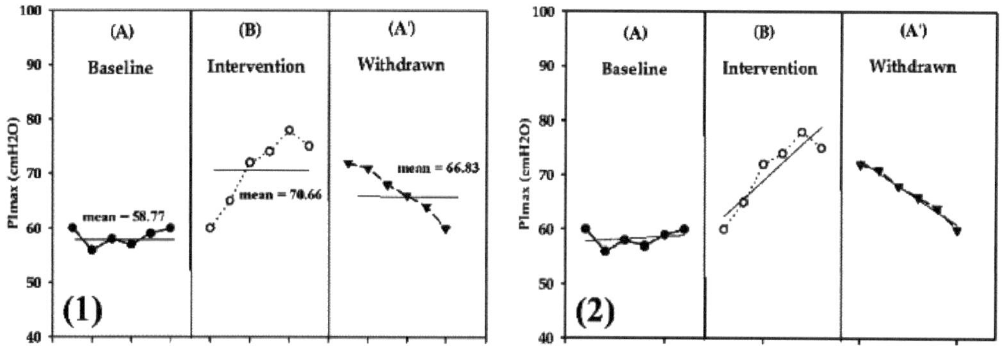

Figure 4. Demonstrated data of mean levels (1) and trend lines (2) within baseline (A), intervention (B), and withdrawn (A′) phases.

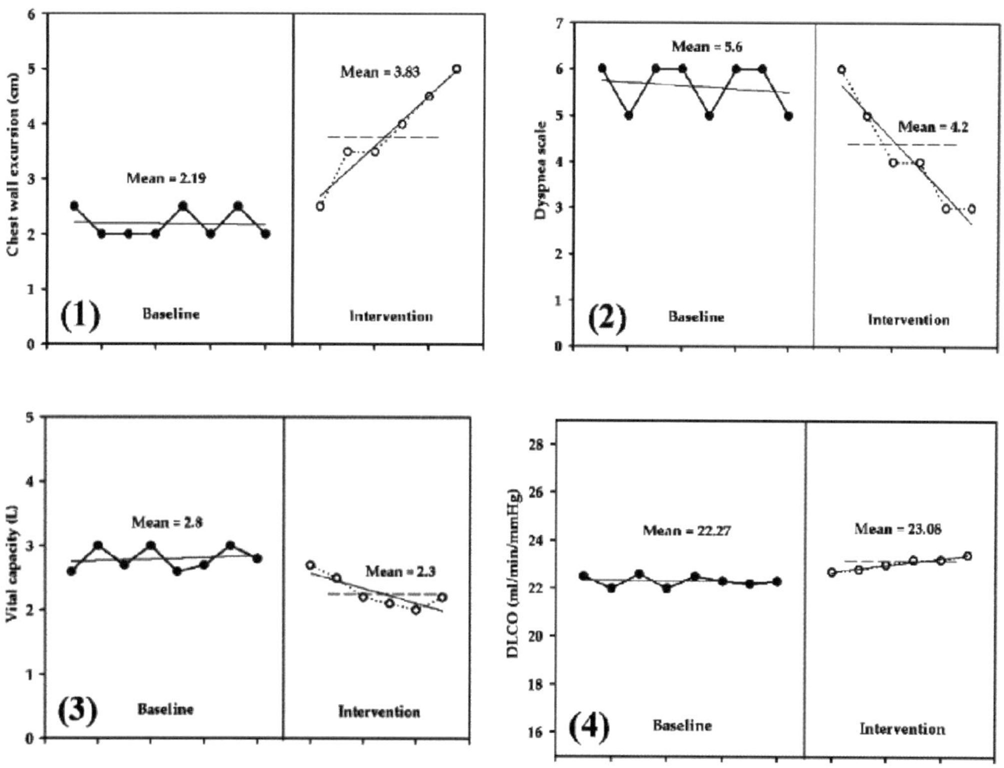

Figure 5. Graph lines of chest wall excursion (1), dyspnea scale (2), vital capacity (3), and diffusing capacity of lung for carbon monoxide (DLCO) (4) between baseline and intervention phases.

The trend line in each phase, especially between baseline and intervention phases, can show the effectiveness of rehabilitation using some techniques, for instance, the deceleration trend line of dyspnea (**Figure 5(2)**) and acceleration trend line of chest wall excursion (**Figure 5(1)**). Therefore, the effectiveness of rehabilitation in the intervention phase can be compared with the extended line from the baseline phase, which is called the **celeration line** as in **Figure 6**.

The celeration line can be found by the freehand [19], several semi-average [18], and least squares method, including computing in a specific program, such as SPSS or SigmaPlot.

The simple method of drawing the celeration line can be carried out by therapists using the semi-average [18] or "split-middle" method. For example, the data of 10 pain scores in the baseline phase; 4, 5, 4, 5, 6, 7, 6, 8, 7, and 6 have been recommended with 8–10 data in order to fit the celeration line more accurately [19, 20]. Therefore, the procedure of drawing a celeration line can be performed in the following steps:

Step 1: Plot the data (**Figure 7(1)**).

Step 2: Divide the data in half by drawing a solid vertical line and dividing each of the halves in half by drawing dashed vertical lines before plotting the median level of each half phase, so that the mean in the first half is 5 and 7 in the second half (**Figure 7(2)**).

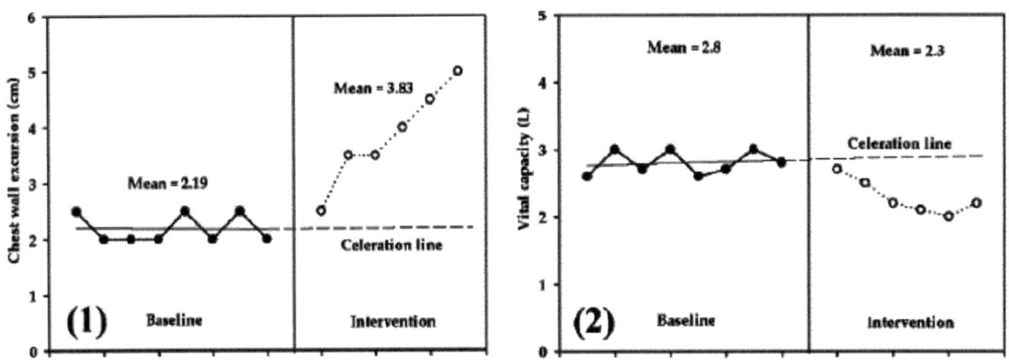

Figure 6. Line graphs showing the celeration line from the baseline phase of chest wall excursion (1) and vital capacity (2).

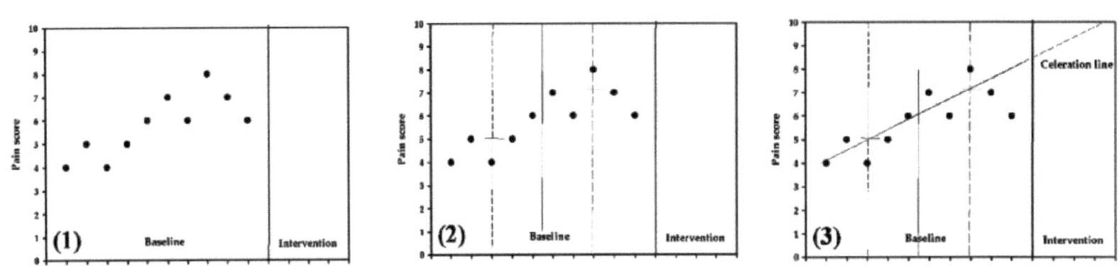

Figure 7. Plotting data in the baseline phase (1). The baseline phase is divided in half with a solid line, and each half phase is divided by dashed vertical lines with median horizontal lines (2). The celeration line is extended to the intervention phase (3).

Step 3: Finally, extend the celeration line from baseline to the intervention phase (**Figure 7(3)**).

On the other hand, the mean value of each half can be used for instant median value [18, 21].

Therefore, data presentation of the single-case research design is developed simply and understood with the mean level and trend changes in the baseline phase. In addition, the effectiveness of rehabilitation can be presented from the difference of mean level and trend line from the celeration line in the baseline phase. However, the effectiveness of rehabilitation in the intervention phase also can be compared under statistical procedure.

4. Statistical analysis

The statistical analysis must be performed as a series procedure. First of all, the data on autocorrelation or serial dependency must be evaluated so that it can violate the independence of error assumption of statistical tests [22]. Data or outcome especially should have no serial dependency on either baseline or intervention phases. Serial dependency basically means that temporally adjacent scores tend to be related to one another. For instance, the score of an individual subject for day 1 tends to predict that for day 2. A day-2 score can predict the day-3 score, etc. Previous study ranked lag 1 autocorrelation and assigned it to one of the three sets; autocorrelations ranging from 0.15 to 0.50 (low), 0.51 to 0.75 (moderate), and 0.76 to 0.94 (high) [23], which found the interaction between serial dependency and significance level. This meant that high serial dependency correlates with low significance. Therefore, the data within phase examination should have no autocorrelation (r) or serial dependency.

4.1. Serial dependency analysis

The procedure for calculating serial dependency is appraised by statistical calculation, called an autocorrelation coefficient, if the lag−1 autocorrelation for a series of performance is measured from a statistically significant evaluation ($p < 0.05$). For instance, the procedure is manual for calculating the autocorrelation coefficient in the baseline phase (**Table 1**), as in the following series:

Step 1: Calculate the mean of the scores in each phase with the sum of all data divided by total numbers.
Baseline phase: [2 + 3 + 2 + 3 + 3]/5 = 2.6

Intervention phase: [4 + 5 + 5 + 8 + 8]/5 = 6

Step 2: Find the difference values by minutes in each score (**Table 1**) with its mean.

Baseline phase	**Intervention phase**
Score-mean = difference value	**Score-mean = difference value**
2.0 − 2.6 = −0.6	4.0 − 6.0 = −2.0
3.0 − 2.6 = 0.6	5.0 − 6.0 = −1.0

Baseline phase	Intervention phase
Score-mean = difference value	Score-mean = difference value
2.0 – 2.6 = –0.6	5.0 – 6.0 = –1.0
3.0 – 2.6 = 0.6	8.0 – 6.0 = 2.0
3.0 – 2.6 = 0.6	8.0 – 6.0 = 2.0

Step 3: Calculate the sum of multiple first and second difference values from Step 2.

Baseline phase	Intervention phase
(–0.6) (0.6) = –0.36	(–2) (–1) = 2
(0.6) (–0.6) = –0.36	(–1) (–1) = 1
(–0.6) (0.6) = –0.36	(–1) (2) = –2
(0.6) (0.6) = 0.36	(2) (2) = 4
Sum = –0.72	**Sum = 5**

Step 4: Calculate the sum of the square of difference values from Step 2.

Baseline phase	Intervention phase
$(-0.6)^2 = 0.36$	$(-2)^2 = 4$
$(0.6)^2 = 0.36$	$(-1)^2 = 1$
$(-0.6)^2 = 0.36$	$(-1)^2 = 1$
$(0.6)^2 = 0.36$	$(2)^2 = 4$
$(0.6)^2 = 0.36$	$(2)^2 = 4$
Sum = 1.8	**Sum = 15**

Step 5. Calculate the autocorrelation coefficient (r) in each phase by dividing the sum value in Step 3 by the square sum of difference values in Step 4.

Baseline phase	Intervention phase
0.72/1.8 = 0.40	5/15 = 0.33

Step 6: Analyze the autocorrelation coefficient as statistically significant or not; a simple procedure called Bartlett test can be used. If the autocorrelation value (r) in Step 5 is less than $2/\sqrt{n}$ (n = number of data), the nonsignificant autocorrelation within or in the phase is confirmed. Therefore, this example = $2/\sqrt{5}$ is 0.894.

Baseline phase	Intervention phase
0.40 < 0.894	0.33 < 0.894

Final results of serial dependency calculation show that data in both phases have not demonstrated a significant degree of autocorrelation or serial dependency. Therefore, therapists may be confident in the results from disease stability in the baseline phase and intervention program. However, if the result of autocorrelation analysis shows significant serial dependency, transformation of autocorrelation should be performed again.

4.2. Transformation data

Due to significant serial dependency being presented in some phases during study, therapists cannot confirm changed results confidently from either the pathology or treatment [23]. For example, scores for dyspnea during 12 days of the baseline phase were 3, 5, 4, 5, 6, 6, 7, 8, 8, 11, 10, and 11, respectively.

Step 1: The mean score [3 + 5 + 4 + 5 + 6 + 6 + 7 + 8 + 8 + 11 + 10 + 11]/12 is 7.08.

Step 2: Difference values.

Score − mean	=	difference value
3.0 − 7.08	=	−4.08
5.0 − 7.08	=	−2.08
4.0 − 7.08	=	−3.08
5.0 − 7.08	=	−2.08
6.0 − 7.08	=	−1.08
6.0 − 7.08	=	−1.08
7.0 − 7.08	=	−0.08
8.0 − 7.08	=	0.92
8.0 − 7.08	=	0.92
11.0 − 7.08	=	3.92
10.0 − 7.08	=	2.92
11.0 − 7.08	=	4.92

Step 3: Calculate the sum of multiple first and second difference values.

(−4.08)(−2.08)	=	8.48
(−2.08)(−3.08)	=	6.41
(−3.08)(−2.08)	=	6.41

(−2.08)(−1.08)	=	2.24
(−1.08)(−1.08)	=	1.17
(−1.08)(−0.08)	=	0.08
(−0.08)(0.92)	=	−0.07
(0.92)(0.92)	=	0.85
(0.92)(3.92)	=	3.61
(3.92)(2.92)	=	11.45
(2.92)(4.92)	=	14.37
Sum	=	**54.99**

Step 4: Calculate the squared sum of difference values.

$(-4.08)^2$	=	16.65
$(-2.08)^2$	=	4.33
$(-3.08)^2$	=	9.49
$(-2.08)^2$	=	4.33
$(-1.08)^2$	=	1.17
$(-1.08)^2$	=	1.17
$(0.08)^2$	=	0.01
$(0.92)^2$	=	0.85
$(0.92)^2$	=	0.85
$(3.92)^2$	=	15.37
$(2.92)^2$	=	8.53
$(4.92)^2$	=	24.21
Sum	=	**86.92**

Step 5: Analyze the autocorrelation coefficient: 54.99/86.92 = 0.632. Analyze whether the autocorrelation coefficient is statistically significant or not, and $2/\sqrt{12}$ is 0.577 because$\sqrt{12}$ is 3.464 ($n = 12$). Therefore, these series data have significant serial dependency because 0.632 is more than 0.577. All data must be transformed by the first difference in transformation as below.

Step 6: The first score in the data is subtracted from the second, the second from the third, the third from the fourth, the fourth from the fifth, and so on, until all scores are fully completed: 3, 5, 4, 5, 6, 6, 7, 8, 8, 11, 10, and 12.

3 − 5 = −2, 5 − 4 = 1, 4 − 5 = −1, 5 − 6 = −1, 6 − 6 = 0, 6 − 7 = −1, 7 − 8 = −1, 8 − 8 = 0, 8 − 11 = −3, 11 − 10 = 1, and 10 − 11 = −1.

Thus, new data are −2, 1, −1, −1, 0, −1, −1, 0, −3, 1, and −1. When returning to calculate the serial dependency in Steps 1–5, the autocorrelation efficiency is 0. 51, which is less than 0.577. Finally, all new series data were added with a constant of any value such as 2, in order to avoid the minute value.

However, the transformation of data by the first transformation difference still failed, thus moving the average transformation to the second procedure in order to reduce the serial dependency in Step 7.

Step 7: The following moving average method reduces the serial dependency that consists of simply plotting the mean values between two adjacent data points over the entire series data.

Score			Transformed score	
3 + 5	=	8/2	=	4.0
4 + 5	=	9/2	=	4.5
6 + 6	=	12/2	=	6.0
7 + 8	=	15/2	=	7.5
8 + 11	=	19/2	=	9.5
10 + 11	=	21/2	=	10.5

Then, the new data from 12 to 6 of 4.0, 4.5, 6.0, 7.5, 9.5, and 10.5 will be returned for calculating the autocorrelation coefficient (r) in Steps 1–5. The result of the new autocorrelation coefficient calculation is 0.56, which is less than 0.82 (2/√6). Therefore, the data do not present serial dependency.

4.3. Statistical evaluation

4.3.1. Standardized statistic method

When the non-serial dependency or autocorrelation is not presented in each phases, confidential results of rehabilitation can be implied without any confounding factors from diseases or condition of auto-recovery. Finally, the procedure for identifying the statistical difference between intervention and baseline or control can be evaluated by various methods. Analysis of variance (ANOVA), F-test, and t-test between phases are widely familiar to researchers and clinicians, for example, comparing the data of expiratory tidal volume (VTE) during 10 days on a mechanical ventilator during chest physical therapy with the previous 10 days of non-treatment. The visual graphic shows the mean, autocorrelation, and trend line (**Figure 8(1)**), whereas bar graphs with a significant level calculated under the nonparametric paired t-test were presented (**Figure 8(2)**).

Before the CPT phase: 352, 350, 323, 349, 345, 350, 352, 348, 360, 354 (mean = 347.9 mL).

During the CPT phase: 364, 371, 378, 380, 410, 425, 429, 485, 501, 515 (mean = 425.8 mL).

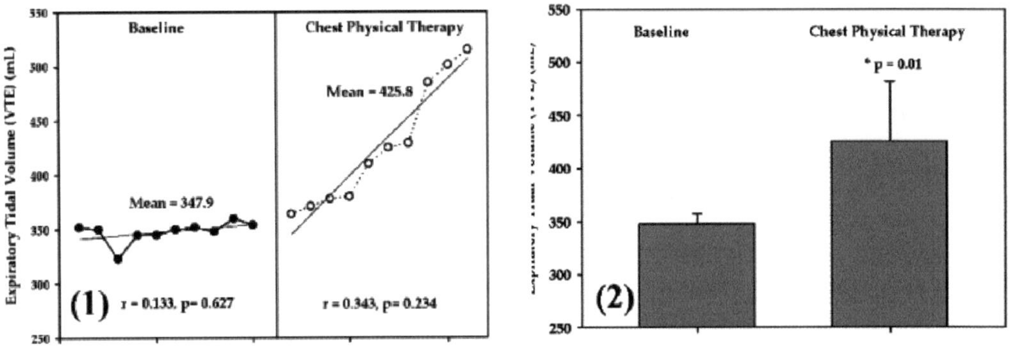

Figure 8. Line graphs of expiratory tidal volume (mL) at baseline and intervention by chest physical therapy phase (1) and t-test analysis from the Wilcoxon signed-rank test in the SPSS program (2).

4.3.2. Statistical analysis with the celeration line

When the celeration line is approached from the baseline to intervention phase, the changes should be stationary if the pathology is stable, whereas some celeration lines from baseline may decelerate muscle mass from prolonged bed rest or accelerate dyspnea from secretion obstruction. A previous report claimed that the celeration line during the intervention phase was the same as that in the baseline phase, indicating no beneficial effect from treatment [24], whereas 50% of the data points in the intervention phase fell or were below the celeration line from the baseline phase, which reflected beneficial clinical effect from treatment.

Two methods can be used to determine statistically significant changes. One method is using the probability table presented by Bloom [25] (**Table 2**), and the other is computing a simple binomial test.

	Number of treatment observations				
Proportion during baseline	**4**	**6**	**8**	**10**	**12**
0.10	3	3	3	4	4
0.15	3	3	4	4	5
0.20	3	4	5	5	6
0.25	4	4	5	6	7
0.30	4	5	6	6	7
0.35	4	5	6	7	8
0.40	4	5	6	8	9
0.45	4	6	7	8	9
0.50	4	6	7	9	10

Modified from Bloom [25], p. 203. Determined by use of the one-tailed test; $p < 0.05$.

Table 2. Number of treatment observations above the celeration line that are required to demonstrate a statistically significant effect.

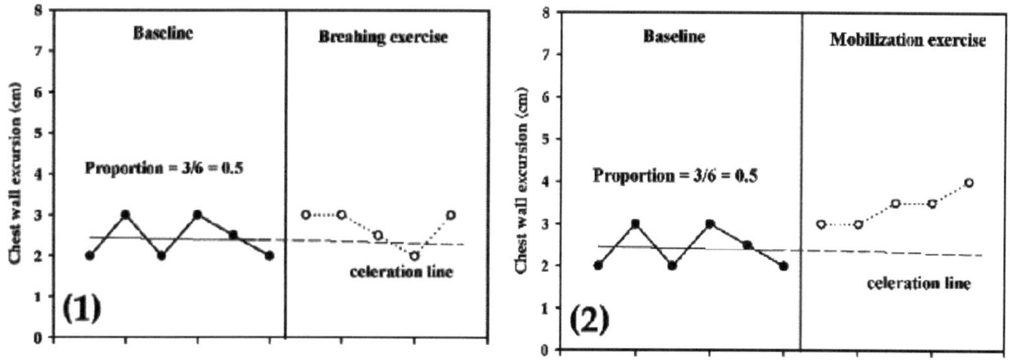

Figure 9. Comparative data of chest wall excursion (cm) between interventions: breathing exercise (1) and mobilization exercise (2).

4.3.3. Statistical analysis using the Bloom table

The method for using the Bloom Table (**Table 2**) for statistical analysis is performed in the following steps, for example, chest wall excursion with two different treatments in **Figure 9**.

Step 1: Calculate the proportion during the baseline phase, for example, in **Figure 9**. From a total of six data points, locate three points above the trend line, so the proportion is 0.6.

Step 2: Draw the extending or celeration line to the treatment phase.

Step 3: See that the first column is 0.50 in the Bloom Table and the number of treatment observations is 5. The intersection of these two values is approximately 5.

Step 4: Figure 9(1) has only four points above the trend line, whereas **Figure 9(2)** has all five points above trend line. Therefore, the mobilization exercise shows significant changes in the clinic, but the breathing exercise does not affect chest wall excursion.

4.3.4. Statistical analysis with the two-standard deviation band method

This method is a semi-statistical approach or "statistical rule of thumb" and easily performed. A previous report indicated that at least two data points fall outside the two-standard deviation band during the intervention phase, which presents a statistically significant change in intervention [26]. Nowadays, there are many computing programs that can calculate the mean and standard deviation, for instance, Microsoft Excel, SigmaPlot, etc. Therefore, a simple and quick calculation on these data can be performed, for example, calculating the data of systolic blood pressure (mmHg) between the baseline phase and exercise period.

Baseline phase: 120, 123, 121, 122, 125, 122, 123, 122, 121, 122 (mean = 122.21, SD = 1.45)

Exercise period: 120, 119, 116, 115, 117, 114, 100, 101, 100, 102 (mean = 110.4, SD = 8.45)

Thus, two-standard deviation (SD) values in the baseline phase can be calculated with two times of SD ($1.45 \times 2 = 2.9$). The upper band above the mean is a sum of 122.1 and 2.9

(122.1 + 2.9), and the lower band below the mean is 122.1 minutes 2.9 (122.1 − 2.9). Therefore, final levels of the 2-SD band are 125 and 119.2, which are drawn in **Figure 10(1)** and **(2)**.

4.3.5. Statistical analysis with the binomial test

This method was demonstrated by Kazdin [15] and White [20]. The formula for computing was based on the binomial test $\binom{x}{n}$ p^n, where n is the number of data points in the intervention phase, x is the number of data points above (or below) the celeration lines, and p is the probability of obtaining × data points above or below the projected celeration line [27]. Therefore, the binomial test from **Figure 11** can be computed by n = 5, X = 4, and p = 0.5, with results in statistical probability of $p < 0.05$.

Null hypothesis (Ho) = data points in the intervention phase being more than 5 in 10.

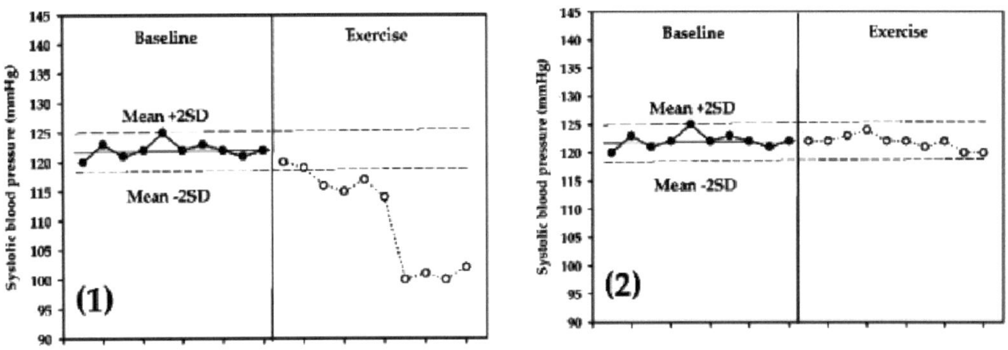

Figure 10. Line graph depicting the 2-SD band method for identifying the statistical significance between two subjects. Different results of exercise occurred in the two subjects, with the first subject showing most of the points (8 in 10 points) below the 2-SD band; thus, it can be concluded that the exercise reduces systolic blood pressure significantly (1), whereas 10 points are located within the 2-SD band in the second subject, which involves nonsignificant change when exercise is implicated (2).

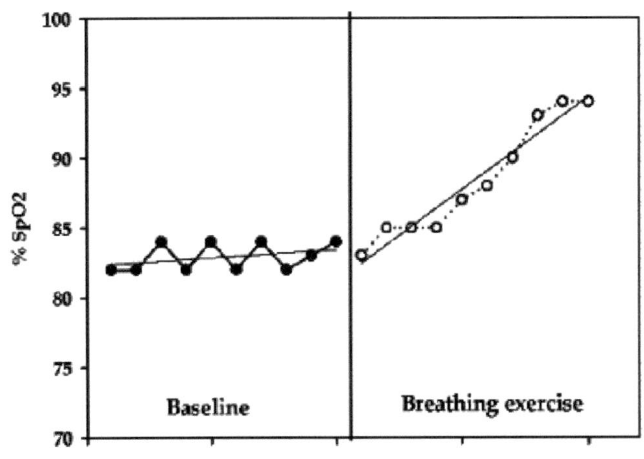

Figure 11. Line graph showing the data in baseline and breathing exercise phases.

	Category	N	Observed Prop.	Test Prop.	Aym.	Sig (1-tailed)
Data	Group 1	1.00	4	0.8	0.50	0.375
	Group 2	0.00	1	0.20		
			5	1.00		

Note: Group 1 is the number of data points above the celeration line, whereas Group 2 is the number of data points below the celeration line from the baseline phase.

Table 3. Result of the binomial test from SPSS analysis.

Alternative hypothesis (H1) = data points in the intervention phase being less than 5 in 10.

The result of the binomial test in **Table 3** shows an asymmetrically significant value (0.375) of more than 0.05, which means acceptance on the null hypothesis.

4.3.6. Statistical analysis with C statistic

The C statistic method was proposed by Bloom and Fisher (1975) [21] and Tryon (1982) [28] as a single-case research design and also reported by Caetano et al (2018) [29]. There are seven steps in using C statistic with example data shown below.

Example: data of % oxygen saturation (%SpO_2) in a postoperative cardiac patient:

Baseline phase: 82, 82, 84, 82, 84, 82, 84, 82, 83, 84

Breathing exercise: 83, 85, 85, 85, 87, 88, 90, 93, 94, 94

Step 1: Each data point in the baseline phase is subtracted from its adjacent successor data, for example, the first from second, second from third, etc. until all of the scores in the baseline phase are used.

Step 2: Each value from Step 1 is squared and the sum repeated.

Step 1			Step 2		
82 − 82	=	0	$(0)^2$	=	0
84 − 82	=	2	$(2)^2$	=	4
84 − 82	=	2	$(2)^2$	=	4
84 − 82	=	2	$(2)^2$	=	4
83 − 84	=	−1	$(-1)^2$	=	1
			Sum	=	**13**

Step 3: The mean value of the baseline points is calculated.

82 + 82 + 84 + 82 + 84 + 82 + 84 + 82 + 83 + 84 = 829/10 = 82.9

Step 4: The value of mean-difference for each set of data is calculated by subtracting each raw score from the mean value of squared results before summing up the squared mean difference.

82	–	82.9	=	−0.9	$(-0.9)^2$	=	0.81
82	–	82.9	=	−0.9	$(-0.9)^2$	=	0.81
84	–	82.9	=	1.1	$(1.1)^2$	=	1.21
82	–	82.9	=	−0.9	$(-0.9)^2$	=	0.81
84	–	82.9	=	1.1	$(1.1)^2$	=	1.21
82	–	82.9	=	−0.9	$(-0.9)^2$	=	0.81
84	–	82.9	=	1.1	$(1.1)^2$	=	1.21
82	–	82.9	=	−0.9	$(-0.9)^2$	=	0.81
83	–	82.9	=	0.1	$(0.1)^2$	=	0.01
84	–	82.9	=	1.1	$(1.1)^2$	=	1.21
					Sum	=	**8.9**

Step 5: The value from Step 4 is multiplied by 2: $8.9 \times 2 = 17.8$.

Step 6: The C score is computed using the formula.

$$
\begin{aligned}
C &= 1\text{–}[\textit{value from step } 2/\textit{value from step } 5] \\
&= 1\text{–}[13/8.9] \\
&= 1\text{–}1.46 \\
&= -0.46
\end{aligned}
$$

Step 7: The standard error for the C statistic is computed using the formula.
Standard error = $\sqrt{}(n-2)/(n-1)(n+1)$, in which n = the number of data in the series data from which the C statistic is computed.

Standard error = $\sqrt{}(10-2)/(10-1)(10+1) = \sqrt{8/99} = \sqrt{0.0808} = 0.284$

Step 8: In determining whether the C statistic is significant, a Z score is computed by dividing the C statistic value from Step 6 by the standard error from Step 7.

$$
\begin{aligned}
Z &= \textit{step } 6/\textit{step } 7 \\
&= -0.46/0.284 \\
&= -1.62
\end{aligned}
$$

Step 9: Statistical analysis: for any series data with 10 data points, a Z of 1.64 or more is significant at a level of $p < 0.05$. The results of Z calculation in the baseline phase shows −1.62, which is less than the required 1.64, indicating that the trend does not exist.

Step 10: Data in the intervention phase are included with the baseline phase and completed as in Step 2.

82 − 82 = 0	$(0)^2 = 0$
84 − 82 = 2	$(2)^2 = 4$
84 − 82 = 2	$(2)^2 = 4$
84 − 82 = 2	$(2)^2 = 4$
83 − 84 = −1	$(-1)^2 = 1$
83 − 85 = −2	$(-2)^2 = 4$
85 − 85 = 0	$(0)^2 = 0$
87 − 88 = −1	$(-1)^2 = 1$
90 − 93 = −3	$(-3)^2 = 9$
94 − 94 = 0	$(0)^2 = 0$
	Sum = **27**

Step 11: The mean value for the baseline points is calculated: 82 + 82 + 84 + 82 + 84 + 82 + 84 + 82 + 83 + 84 + 83 + 85 + 85 + 85 + 87 + 88 + 90 + 93 + 94 + 94 = 1713/20 = 85.65.

Step 12: The value of the mean-difference for each set of data is calculated by subtracting each raw score from the mean value of squared results before summing up the squared mean difference.

82	−	85.65	=	−3.65	$(-3.65)^2$	=	13.32
82	−	85.65	=	−3.65	$(-3.65)^2$	=	13.32
84	−	85.65	=	−1.65	$(1.65)^2$	=	2.72
82	−	85.65	=	−3.65	$(-3.65)^2$	=	13.32
84	−	85.65	=	−1.65	$(1.65)^2$	=	2.72
82	−	85.65	=	−3.65	$(-3.65)^2$	=	13.32
84	−	85.65	=	−1.65	$(1.65)^2$	=	2.72
82	−	85.65	=	−3.65	$(-3.65)^2$	=	13.32
83	−	85.65	=	−2.65	$(-2.65)^2$	=	7.02
84	−	85.65	=	−1.65	$(1.65)^2$	=	2.72
83	−	85.65	=	− 2.65	$(-2.65)^2$	=	7.02
85	−	85.65	=	−0.65	$(-0.65)^2$	=	0.42
85	−	85.65	=	−0.65	$(-0.65)^2$	=	0.42
85	−	85.65	=	−0.65	$(-0.65)^2$	=	0.42
87	−	85.65	=	1.35	$(1.35)^2$	=	1.82
88	−	85.65	=	2.35	$(2.35)^2$	=	5.52
90	−	85.65	=	4.35	$(4.35)^2$	=	18.92
93	−	85.65	=	7.35	$(7.35)^2$	=	54.02

94	–	85.65	=	8.35	$(8.35)^2$	=	69.72
94	–	85.65	=	8.35	$(8.35)^2$	=	69.72
					Sum	=	**312.55**

Step 13: The value from Step 12 is multiplied by 2: $312.55 \times 2 = 625.1$.

Step 14. The C score is computed using the formula.

$$C = 1 - [\textit{value from step } 10/\textit{value from step } 13]$$
$$= 1 - [27/625.1]$$
$$= 1 - 0.043$$
$$= 0.957$$

Step 15: The standard error for the C statistic is computed using the formula.
Standard error = $\sqrt{}(n-2)/(n-1)(n+1)$, in which n = the number of data in the series data from which the C statistic is computed.

Standard error = $\sqrt{}(20-2)/(20-1)(20+1) = \sqrt{18/399} = \sqrt{0.045} = 0.212$

Step 16: In determining whether the C statistic is significant, a Z score is computed by dividing the C statistic value from Step 14 by the standard error from Step 15.

$$Z = \textit{step } 6/\textit{step } 7$$
$$= 0.957/0.212$$
$$= 4.514$$

Step 17: Statistical analysis: for any series data with 20 data points, a Z of 1.64 or more is significant at a level of $p < 0.05$. The results of Z calculation in the baseline and intervention phases show 4.514, which is more than the required 1.64. This presents a statistically significant trend across the baseline and intervention phases, or the breathing exercise in this case affects oxygen saturation in the clinic when compared to the baseline phase.

5. Discussion and critical point for a single-case research study

All details and data on examples show the procedure for presenting a single-case research study, due to the limitation on conditions, rare cases, and interesting treatment [3]. A basic procedure of a single-case design, with visual graphs of 6–8 data points in each phase [15], including mean level and cerelation line in baseline phase, can be presented [8]. When the data in each period at either baseline or intervention have no series dependency, a clinically significant difference of the treatment can be evaluated by comparing the baseline or pre-treatment using the Bloom Table, C statistic, or paired t-test [22, 25, 28, 29]. Moreover, the different types of single-case experimental designs as alternating treatment, introduction/withdrawal designs, or multiple baseline designs are very interesting in physical and rehabilitation medicine [30]. However, an update on evidence in using a single-case design reported that it risks a bias tool (SCD RoB) based on current conceptualizations of biases, as well as the Cochrane risk of bias criteria. Therefore, contemporary single-case design quality should be applied for demonstrating and providing initial validation in research using such a design [31]. In order to demonstrate a single-case research study, the clinical details or characteristics of a subject must be presented as in previous study; such as illness history, medical diagnosis, laboratory results, and prior medical treatments during 7 days of pre-treatment, during treatment and/or posttreatment with an ABA study design. It is important that the condition of a patient, its stability or constancy, is reported for at least 7 days in COPD patients [12]. Their arterial blood gas (ABG), complete blood count (CBC), blood chemistry, liver function test, chest X-ray, and sputum culture also are reported. The results presented the autocorrelation values in each phase, which was less than $2/\sqrt{7}$ or 0.756. Therefore, it can be assumed that the results have no autocorrelation within the data, so changes in the data did not reflect the time dependence or pathological condition [22]. In addition, a previous study on a scleroderma patient having short-term chest physical therapy (CPT) for 7 days compared pre-treatment with an A-B design and showed that CPT significantly reduced the dyspnea score and respiratory rate and increased chest expansion and maximal inspiratory mount pressure (PImax) by using Bloom Table analysis [13]. Therefore, both previous studies present the effectiveness or benefits of rehabilitation in specific patients. Thus, in order to present the effectiveness of therapy or rehabilitation, all details of treatment also should be cleared and more details given such as techniques, frequency, intensity, and timing. When specific treatment is performed, the outcomes should be recorded daily before statistical analysis. For good data presentation, graph lines with scattered plotting, mean level, and autocorrelation must be presented in each phase. Finally, the clinical effectiveness of treatment must be shown by using the statistical protocol, such as the celeration line from the baseline to treatment phase and Bloom Table analysis. In addition, the statistic nonparametrical paired t-test or one-way ANOVA or C statistic can be used for confirmation as same as in a previous review meta-analysis suggestion [32].

6. Conclusion

The effectiveness of rehabilitation can be seen under a single-case research design as well as in practice of psychology research [33]. Firstly, data collection should be performed at least 5 days before starting intervention or treatment in order to obtain higher stability for the condition of the patient. Secondly, scattering the data from baseline and intervention with visual graph lines must be carried out. Thirdly, trend lines and the mean values in each phase should be calculated and plotted. Fourthly, series dependency or autocorrelation coefficient must be calculated and indicated on the graph. Finally, statistical analysis of the effectiveness of treatment can be performed by comparing with the celeration line, which has been drawn manually using the spilt-middle method or fit curve from baseline phase, and underlining the Bloom Table. Moreover, the nonparametrical paired t-test or binomial test can be used. Although there are some limitations in this method, due to the small data collection and series dependency of data within each phase, it has easy-to-understand visuals and shows the trend. Therefore, a single-case research design is one of the many statistical protocols that can be applied for clinical scientists or therapists in order for them to represent the effectiveness of treatment in rare cases and present interesting results. Furthermore, the results of a good research design can be developed into a standardized statistical model, with a larger sample size, control subjects, and parametric statistical protocol in the future.

Conflict of interest

All authors claim no conflict of interest.

Author details

Jirakrit Leelarungrayub*, Yothin Pothasak, Jynwara Kaju and Rungtiwa Kanthain

*Address all correspondence to: donrawee.leela@cmu.ac.th

Department of Physical Therapy, Faculty of Associated Medical Sciences, Chiang Mai University, Chiang Mai, Thailand

References

[1] Hartung DM, Touchette D. Overview of clinical research design. American Journal of Health-System Pharmacy. 2009;**66**(4):398-408. DOI: 10.2146/ajhp080300

[2] Callas PW. Searching the biomedical literature: Research study designs and critical appraisal. Clinical Laboratory Science. 2008;**21**(1):42-48

[3] Janosky JE. Use of the single subject design for practice based primary care research. Postgraduate Medicine. 2005;**81**(959):549-551

[4] Parab S, Bhalerao S. Study designs. International Journal of Ayurveda Research. 2010;**1**(2): 128-131. DOI: 10.4103/0974-7788.64406

[5] Gonnella C. Single-subject experimental paradigm as a clinical decision tool. Physical Therapy. 1989;**69**:601-609

[6] Siggelkow N. What's in a name? The Academy of Management Journal. 2007;**50**(1):30-34

[7] Thomas G. A typology for the case study in social science following a review of definition, discourse, and structure. Qualitative Inquiry. 2011;**17**(6):511-521. DOI: 10.1177/1077800411409884

[8] Yoo WG. Effect of a combined thoracic and backward lifting exercise on the thoracic kyphosis angle and intercostal muscle pain. Journal of Physical Therapy Science. 2017; **29**(8):1481-1482. DOI: 10.1589/jpts.29.1481

[9] Portney LG, Watkins MP. Foundations of Clinical Research: Applications to Practice. Philadelphia, PA: F.A. Davis Company; 2015

[10] Horner RH, Swminathan H, Sugai G, Smolkowski K. Considerations for the systematic analysis and use of single-case research. Education & Treatment of Children. 2012;**35**(2): 269-290

[11] Lobo MA, Moeyaert M, Baraldi Cunha A, Babik I. Single-case design, analysis, and quality assessment for intervention research. Journal of Neurologic Physical Therapy. 2017;**41**(3): 187-197. DOI: 10.1097/NPT.0000000000000187

[12] Leelarungrayb D, Pothongsunun P, Yankai A, Pratanaphon S. Acute clinical benefits of chest wall-stretching exercise on expired tidal volume, dyspnea and chest expansion in a patient with chronic obstructive pulmonary disease: A single case study. Journal of Bodywork and Movement Therapies. 2009;**13**(4):338-343. DOI: 10.1016/j.jbmit.2008.11.0004

[13] Leelarungrayub J, Pinkaew D, Wonglangka K, Eungpinichpong W, Klaphajone J. Short-term pulmonary rehabilitation for a female patient with chronic scleroderma under a single-case research design. Clinical Medicine Insights: Circulatory, Respiratory and Pulmonary Medicine. 2016;**10**:11-17 eCollection 2016

[14] Barlow DH, Hersen M. Single-case experimental designs. Uses in applied clinical research. Archives of General Psychiatry. 1973;**29**(3):319-325

[15] Kazdin AE. Single Case Research Designs: Methods for Clinical and Applied Setting. New York: Oxford University Press; 1982

[16] Busse RT, Kratochwill TR, Elliott SN. Meta-analysis for single-case consultation outcomes: Applications to research and practice. J School Psychol. 1995;**33**(4):269-285. DOI: 10.1016/0022-4405(95)00014-D

[17] Wolery M, Harris SR. Interpreting results of single-subject research designs. Physical Therapy. 1982;**62**(4):445-452

[18] White OR, Haring NG. Exceptional Teaching. 2nd ed. Columbus, OH: Charles; 1980

[19] Kazdin AE. Unobtrusive measures in behavioral assessment. Journal of Applied Behavior Analysis. 1979;**12**(4):713-724

[20] White OR. Data-based instruction: Evaluating educational progress. In: Cone JD, Hawkins RP, editors. Behavioral Assessments: New Directions in Clinical Psychology. New York: Brunner/Mazel; 1977

[21] Bloom M, Fischer J. Evaluating Practice: Guidelines for the Accountable Professional. Englewood Cliffs, NJ: Prentice-Hall; 1982

[22] Matyas TA, Greenwood KM. Serial dependency in single-case time series. In: Franklin RD, Allison DB, Gorman BS, editors. Design and Analysis of Single-Case Research. Mahwah, NJ: Lawrence Erlbaum Associates; 1997. pp. 215-243

[23] Jones RR, Weinrott MR, Vaught RS. Effects of serial dependency on the agreement between visual and statistical inference. Journal of Applied Behavior Analysis. 1978; **11**(2):277-283

[24] Ottenbacher KJ. Evaluating Clinical Change.: Strategies for Occupational and Physical Therapist. Sydney: Williams & Wilkins; 1986

[25] Bloom M. The Paradox of Helping: Introduction in the Philosophy of Scientific Practice. New York: Macmillan Publishing; 1975

[26] Gottman JM, Leiblum SR. How to Do Psychotherapy and how to Evaluate it. New York: Holt, Rinehart & Winston; 1974

[27] Siegel S. Nonparametric Statistics. New York: McGraw-Hill; 1956

[28] Tryon WW. A simplified time-series analysis for evaluating treatment inter-ventions. Journal of Applied Behavior Analysis. 1982;**15**(3):423-429

[29] Caetano SJ, Sonpavde G, Pond GR. C-statistic: A brief explanation of its construction, interpretation and limitations. European Journal of Cancer. 2018;**90**:130-132. DOI: 10.1016/j.ejca.2017.10.027 Epub 2017 Dec 5

[30] Krasny-Pacini A, Evans J. Single-case experimental designs to assess intervention effectiveness in rehabilitation: A practical guide. Annals of Physical and Rehabilitation Medicine. 2018;**61**(3):164-179. DOI: 10.1016/j.rehab.2017.12.002 Epub 2017 Dec 15

[31] Reichow B, Barton EE, Maggin DM. Development and applications of the single-case design risk of bias tool for evaluating single-case design research study reports. Research in Developmental Disabilities. 2018;**79**:53-64. DOI: 10.1016/j.ridd.2018.05.008 Epub 2018 Jun 27

[32] Tincani M, De Mers M. Meta-analysis of single-case research design studies on instructional pacing. Behavior Modification. 2016;**40**(6):799-824 Epub 2016 Apr 11

[33] Sexton-Radek K. Single case designs in psychology practice. Health Psychology Research. 2014;**2**(3):1551. DOI: 10.4081/hpr.2014.1551.eCollection 2014 Nov 6

Chapter 8

Targeting Limb Muscle Dysfunction in COPD

Andre Nyberg and Erik Frykholm

Additional information is available at the end of the chapter

http://dx.doi.org/10.5772/intechopen.90815

Abstract

Chronic obstructive pulmonary disease (COPD), is today one of the world's most common chronic diseases, estimated by the World Health Organization to be the third leading cause of death worldwide by the year 2030. An often neglected aspect of COPD is that the course of the disease is linked to extrapulmonary manifestations that are currently not dealt with optimally, but that has a direct and substantial impact on the condition. Limb muscle dysfunction, at the functional level defined as the reduction of either strength or endurance (or both) properties of the muscle, is highly prevalent in COPD, closely linked to critical clinical and prognostic outcomes including functional status, quality of life, and even mortality. If the goal is to improve limb muscle function among people with COPD is exercise training recommended before other treatment modalities, highly prioritized in international guidelines. In this chapter, why and how to assess and manage limb muscle dysfunction among people with COPD will be targeted, highlighting the vital role of physical therapy and the physiotherapist.

Keywords: chronic obstructive pulmonary disease, limb muscle dysfunction, muscle strength, muscle endurance, dynamic measurements, static measurements, exercise training, resistance training

1. Introduction

Chronic obstructive pulmonary disease (COPD) is one of our most common chronic diseases and accounted for 2.6% of the entire global burden of disease 2015 with 63.9 million disability-adjusted life years. From 1990 to 2015, the prevalence of COPD increased by 44.2% and is now estimated to 174.5 million people worldwide [1]. COPD is by the World Health Organization anticipated to be the third leading cause of death worldwide by the year 2030.

Although COPD is primarily a disease of the respiratory system, with structural and functional impairments of the lungs [2], the disease is often accompanied by manifestations outside

IntechOpen

© 2020 The Author(s). Licensee IntechOpen. This chapter is distributed under the terms of the Creative Commons Attribution License (http://creativecommons.org/licenses/by/3.0), which permits unrestricted use, distribution, and reproduction in any medium, provided the original work is properly cited.

the lungs. One of the most common extrapulmonary manifestations in COPD is limb muscle dysfunction, defined as a pathological change of muscle proprieties with a variety of structural and morphological abnormalities that compromise the muscle function. The latter evidenced by a reduction in the strength and/or endurance capacity of the limb muscles [3], with or without a loss of muscle mass [4]. Limb muscle dysfunction is evident in up to a third of all people with COPD and closely linked to the prognosis of the disease. For example, individual factors such as reduced mid-thigh cross-sectional area [5], fat-free mass [6], lower quadriceps strength [7], and vastus lateralis fiber type shift [8] are all predictors of mortality in COPD. Additionally, limb muscle dysfunction is also associated with other important clinical outcomes including reduced quality of life [9], reduced exercise tolerance [10–12], and higher healthcare use [13].

Thus, the clinical and prognostic importance of limb muscle dysfunction in COPD stress the importance of assessing the limb muscle and develop therapies aiming at stopping or slowing down the progression of limb muscle dysfunction, for which the physiotherapist has a crucial role. In this chapter, the etiology and pathophysiology of limb muscle dysfunction in people with COPD will be briefly overviewed; the main objective is to highlight why and how to assess and manage limb muscle dysfunction in people with COPD within the clinical context.

2. Features and importance of limb muscle dysfunction in COPD

Limb muscle dysfunction includes a variety of structural and morphological abnormalities within the muscle resulting in muscle atrophy, weakness, and reduced endurance [4, 14]. Most studied is the quadriceps muscle, this since the quadriceps muscle is an essential muscle for everyday activities such as standing up and walking.

Aspects of limb muscle dysfunction in COPD include larger amounts of intramuscular fat [15] effectively reducing the contractile mass within the muscle; mitochondrial dysfunction including a reduced absolute and relative number of mitochondria but also a changed oxidative capacity of the mitochondria [16]; and a shift from muscle fiber type I toward fiber type IIx which is inconsistent with healthy aging and displays the muscle's poor ability for aerobic work [17].

The structural changes affect functional capacity with impairments such as reduced oxidative capacity and a greater reliance on anaerobic work [18], as well as reduced muscle strength or endurance [3, 19]. It should be noted that the structural changes mentioned here apply to the quadriceps muscle, and other muscle groups, especially upper limb muscle are not affected to the same extent [20]; thus, limb muscle dysfunction is a heterogenic rather than homogenous process. Furthermore, physiological responses to activities can be different across limb muscles and depending on the type of exercise performed [21–27].

2.1. Etiology and pathophysiology of limb muscle dysfunction

People with COPD are inactive [28], and deconditioning due to disuse seems to play a vital role in limb muscle dysfunction. There is, however, evidence to suggest that the limb muscle dysfunction is linked to COPD or at least share the same contributing risk factors. Thus, limb muscle dysfunction is not as simple as a direct consequence of inactivity and disuse (**Figure 1**).

http://dx.doi.org/10.5772/intechopen.90815

First, when people with COPD are compared to people without COPD but matched with equally low physical activity levels, differences in structure and function remain [29]. Second, quadriceps weakness occurs already in the early stages of COPD [30] when the reduced respiratory capacity should be of minor importance. And third, the training response seems blunted on a structural level for people with COPD [31]. Additional systemic factors, including tobacco smoking, systemic inflammation, exacerbations, nutrition, gas exchange abnormalities, and drugs, can also influence the function of both respiratory and peripheral muscles, by inducing changes in their local microenvironment. Under all these circumstances may, protein metabolism imbalance, oxidative stress, inflammatory events, as well as muscle injury occur, determining the final structure and modulating the function of different muscle groups. For thorough reviews of the pathophysiology, we refer to other sources [4, 32]. Last, the heterogeneity of limb muscle dysfunction in COPD emphasizes a need for specificity, which is equally true for assessment of the limb muscles as well as concerning therapies. We, therefore, present aspects of limb muscle dysfunction separate and do not have a one solution fits all.

2.2. Muscle mass

Muscle mass refers to the amount of muscle available for contractile work and can be reported on a whole-body level, a segmental level, the individual muscles, or on a muscle fiber level depending on the assessment method. Reduction or loss of muscle mass is the leading cause of weight loss within the COPD population [33] and has been demonstrated to be a better predictor of health-related quality of life [9] and survival [5] than, for example, body weight or Body Mass Index (BMI) [34]. Reduced limb muscle mass over time can be defined as muscle wasting and is part of sarcopenia (that is, changes in muscle proprieties due to aging) and cachexia (defined as a complex metabolic syndrome associated with underlying illness and characterized by loss of muscle with or without loss of fat mass) [35].

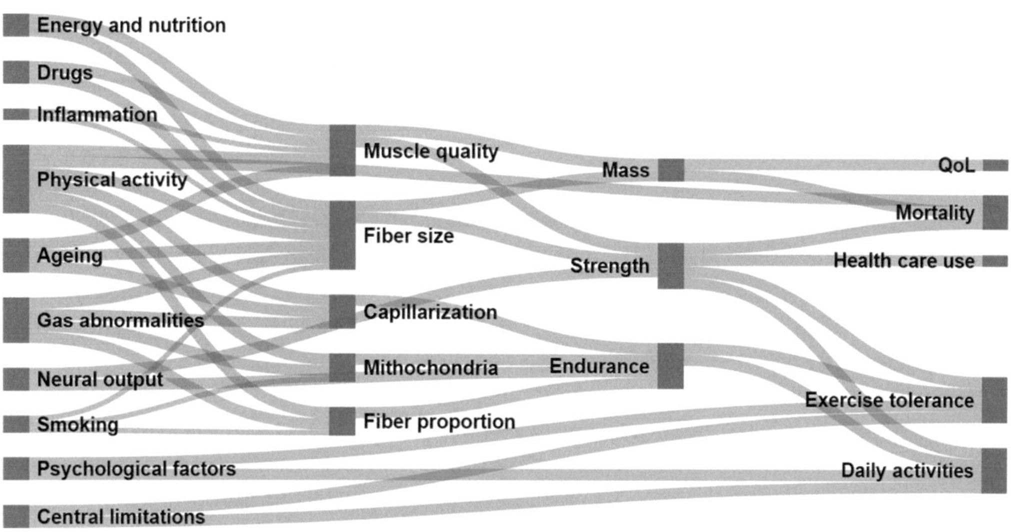

Figure 1. Illustration of the complex interplay of factors and outcomes were limb muscle dysfunction playing a role for people with COPD, some have been thoroughly studied whereas others have not.

Fat-free mass is frequently used as a proxy for muscle mass on a whole-body level and is usually reported as a fat-free mass index by dividing the fat-free mass by the individual's length in meters squared (fat-free mass/m^2). Several criteria have been suggested to define low muscle mass, but irrespective of the criteria used, low muscle mass is common in COPD [4]. Moreover, a low-fat free mass index has been reported in 26% of patients with COPD with a normal BMI [36]. Irrespective of BMI, a low-fat free mass index is a strong predictor of mortality [6], and mid-thigh cross-sectional area is a better predictor of mortality than body mass index [5]. A fat-free mass index <16 kg/m^2 (male) or <15 kg/m^2 (female) is linked with approximately a twofold increase in mortality among people with COPD [6, 37, 38]. A low-fat free mass is also associated to reduced quality of life [9]. Another important notion is that the lower limb muscles are particularly vulnerable to the muscle wasting process in COPD [39, 40], and the loss of thigh muscle mass is relatively more significant than that of whole-body weight, indicating a preferential loss of muscle mass in the legs of people with COPD [41].

2.3. Muscle strength

Reduced muscle strength or muscle weakness, defined as the force generated by a specific muscle or group of muscles in a single contraction [42], has been found in one-third of people with COPD attending hospital respiratory outpatient services [43]. However, when quadriceps strength is normalized by thigh muscle cross-sectional area or by muscle mass, the difference may no longer be significant [41, 44]. Therefore, the reduced quadriceps strength could mostly be a reflection of the loss in muscle mass [40]. This finding is not universal, and the weakness is sometimes disproportional to the reduction in muscle mass [43]. A disproportional reduction in quadriceps weakness may occur in individuals with a high dose of oral corticosteroids [41]. This may however only apply to individuals treated with a high dose of oral corticosteroids over long periods, as no further decrease in quadriceps strength was reported in short-term corticosteroid-treated people with COPD compared with untreated people with COPD [45]. Reduced limb muscle strength is associated with reduced exercise tolerance [10, 11], mortality [7], and higher healthcare use [13].

2.4. Muscle endurance

Quadriceps muscle strength and quadriceps muscle endurance are both reduced in people with COPD. However, quadriceps muscle endurance, defined as the ability to maintain or repeat a contraction over time [42], might be more reduced than quadriceps strength. For example, quadriceps muscle endurance has been reported to be reduced with up to 82% among men and up to 76% among women compared to matched people without COPD, while quadriceps muscle strength was decreased with 29 and 19% among men and women, respectively [3]. Furthermore, using a non-volitional approach with a magnetic nerve stimulator strapped around the quadriceps muscle, people with COPD had approximately 45% of the muscle endurance capacity of people without COPD [46]. However, the variability between studies is vast, and it is probably due to differences in test procedures since quadriceps muscle endurance has been assessed in numerous ways [19]. Limb muscle endurance is essential for work tolerance over time, and it has been shown that people with COPD rate leg fatigue higher than dyspnea in exercise tests [47]. Quadriceps endurance also seems to be closer related to functional tests such as the 6-minute walk test than the quadriceps strength [48–50], implicating importance for performing daily activities. Contradictory to quadriceps strength, quadriceps endurance to muscle mass ratio is lower in people with COPD compared to people without COPD [51], and people with COPD, regardless of fat-free mass, have a higher degree of fatigue during endurance tests compared to people without COPD [52]. Most studies have been conducted in a population of severe COPD, but the reduced quadriceps muscle endurance is also evident in people with mild to moderate COPD [53].

2.5. In summary

Limb muscle dysfunction encompasses several manifestations including, muscle atrophy and weakness, reduced endurance, and susceptibility to muscle fatigue, which reflects both structural and morphological muscle adaptations that are seen in limb muscles among people with COPD.

Limb muscle dysfunction is evident in up to a third of all individuals with COPD and has a direct and substantial impact on the condition. For example, limb muscle dysfunction is intimately linked to relevant clinical outcomes, including physical activity, exercise tolerance, quality of life, healthcare use, and even survival.

Thus, limb muscle dysfunction is an essential area for physical therapy and should be prioritized among physiotherapists.

3. How to assess limb muscles in clinical practice

Assessment of limb muscle mass and function should always be a priority within clinical praxis of COPD management, due to its clinical and prognostic relevance [4, 54, 55].

Considering the complexity of limb muscle dysfunction in COPD, no single test could be used to assess and monitor all aspects of the limb muscles within the COPD population, resulting in a wide range of available tests and measurement techniques [14, 54–56].

When deciding on how to assess limb muscles in clinical practice, several factors should be considered and will influence the choice of technique and strategy used. **Table 1** highlights some factors that physiotherapists need to take into account when making this decision [55].

For example, among people with COPD, assessment of limb muscle mass and function should always include the quadriceps muscle due to its clinical and prognostic value [4, 7]; however, as all assessments are muscle group-specific, other limb muscles may also be assessed to provide valuable information [4].

Furthermore, the availability of measurement equipment will likely vary between clinical settings and contexts, thus impacting the choice of the assessment strategy. The physiotherapist needs to acknowledge that measurement equipment and assessment strategies are not interchangeable and may provide different information even if the goal of the assessment would be the same [55, 57].

Different assessment strategies might also vary concerning important quality aspects, including but not limited to validity, reliability, and responsiveness. For example, test–retest reliability is of importance to consider when performing assessments before and after exercise

- What is the aim of the measurement?

For example, diagnostic purposes? Evaluation purposes?

- Which muscle(s) should we target?

For example, upper extremity/lower extremity, unilateral/bilateral, one/several muscle(s).

- Which aspect(s)?

For example, muscle mass, strength, endurance, fatigue, power, etc.

- Which type(s) of muscle contraction?

For example, static/dynamic concentric/eccentric, volitional/non-volitional.

- Which equipment?

For example, weight-machines/free-weights, elastic/functional, availability.

- Measurements quality.

For example, validity, reliability, accessibility, feasibility, responsiveness.

Table 1. Factors to consider when deciding on how to assess limb muscles [53].

interventions to interpret findings [57–61], while validity, for example, could be an issue when using simple field tests to provide information on aspects of limb muscle function [62–65].

Irrespective of the goal of the measurement technique used, standardization plays a crucial role to increase the measurement quality when assessing limb muscles in COPD, including standardization of preparation guidelines (e.g., guidelines for medications, caffeine, activities, etc. before an assessment), equipment (e.g., free weight/weight-machines/dynamometers), instructions (e.g., written/oral/visual), familiarization (to minimize learning effect), warm-up (e.g., general vs. specific warm-up of targeted muscles), positioning, the range-of-motion (e.g., start and end positions), velocity (e.g., seconds in concentric/eccentric phase of movement), and rest (between contractions/sets, etc.). For further details on what to consider to standardize assessments, we refer to previously published work [42, 54, 55].

Nevertheless, irrespective of all factors to consider when deciding on how to assess limb muscles in clinical practice, the take-home message is that the limb muscles should be evaluated. Despite the prognostic and clinical relevance of limb muscle dysfunction in people with COPD, and even though assessment of limb muscles is recommended in international guidelines [4], it remains to be an integrated part of the routine evaluation and management of COPD.

3.1. Muscle mass

Assessing only BMI is inadequate to quantify the impact of COPD on different muscle compartments or to provide valid information on muscle mass [36] since BMI does not give any information on body composition or fat distribution [54]. Instead, fat-free mass could be targeted and is frequently used as a proxy for muscle mass on a whole-body level among people with COPD [4].

The gold standard and reference method in COPD for assessing fat-free mass is through determining total body water by deuterium dilution [66]; however, this technique is invasive, and use of the method is likely limited to research centers [56]. Fat-free mass could also be assessed using simple techniques such as skinfold anthropometry. However, this technique generally overestimates the fat-free mass when compared to other techniques, especially if measured on more obese individuals [67, 68].

Two techniques that are realistic to be used in the clinical environment to monitor and provide accurate assessments of fat-free mass in COPD are bioelectrical impedance (BIA) and dual-energy X-ray absorption (DEXA). Both techniques are noninvasive and have shown to provide valid and reliable information on the distribution of fat-free mass among people with COPD [7, 67, 69–71]. BIA has the advantage of being less expensive and often more easily accessible than DEXA in clinical settings [69]. When estimating fat-free mass from BIA, it is vital to use equations that have been validated within the COPD population and to be cautious with built-in equations provided by manufacturers [72, 73]. Also of importance is that since BIA is influenced by total body water, fluid balance and time of day need to be controlled, primarily when a longitudinal assessment is performed. For example, if used as an outcome measure after an exercise training period [54]. About the latter, it should be noted that even though BIA (and DEXA) assessments could provide information for body compartments (e.g., left/right arm, trunk, left/right leg), these techniques might be less sensitive to change than if direct assessments of regional muscle mass using more advanced techniques such as computed tomography, magnetic resonance, or ultrasound imaging are performed [27, 74]. Furthermore, the correlation between local and whole-body muscle mass is weak in COPD, thus suggesting that direct assessment of regional muscle mass indeed has additional value [74]. Nevertheless, as availability of different measurement equipment likely varies between clinical settings, it is important to note that, except BMI measurements, all techniques listed above theoretically could be used to assess muscle mass in people with COPD. However, the physiotherapist needs to acknowledge and take into account the advantages and disadvantages of each technique when performing the assessment.

3.2. Muscle strength

Assessment of limb muscle strength could be done in numerous ways using both volitional (effort dependent) and non-volitional (independent from the patient's motivation and effort) techniques. Both techniques provide valid and reliable results independent of disease severity [58, 59, 65, 75]. Even though non-volitional assessments of muscle strength could be performed through electrical or magnetic stimulation of the muscle or its motor nerve [76], these non-volitional techniques are in a similar way as assessing total body water by deuterium dilution (to determine muscle mass), mainly limited to research centers and clinical research [14]. Non-volitional assessments are also rarely used within COPD research to assess the effect of exercise interventions over time [26]. Thus, voluntary, effort dependent maneuvers, is the most clinically feasible way of measuring limb muscle strength in people with COPD [77].

Limb muscle strength measurements could be performed using various devices and techniques, including strain gauges, handheld or fixed portable dynamometers, weight machines, or manual muscle testing techniques as well as more complex systems such as computerized dynamometers [78, 79]. Furthermore, such assessments could be performed using static (isometric), or by using dynamic (isotonic [fixed external loading] or isokinetic [fixed speed of movement]) techniques (**Table 2**).

To date, static measurements of quadriceps muscle strength have been put forward and recommended, as they provide essential prognostic information [7]. Static measurements of grip strength have also been used among people with COPD; however, current research is contradictory, and grip strength does not appear to be associated with disease severity or to be decreased more than among the general older population [80], even though this is not a universal finding [81]. Even though static measurements of quadriceps muscle strength is recommended, recent literature suggests that dynamic measures of limb muscle strength should not be neglected as the dynamic capacity of the muscle seems to be more closely related to factors associated with functional tasks, such as walking or standing up from a chair, than isometric (static) measurements [49, 79].

Thus, the decision on how to assess muscle strength should be dependent on the clinical question we would like to answer.

3.3. Muscle endurance and fatigue

Assessment of limb muscle endurance could in a similar way as limb muscle strength measurements were performed using both volitional and non-volitional techniques, with the former being the most clinically feasible. In COPD, direct measures of limb muscle endurance have primarily targeted the quadriceps muscle using sustained (isometric) or repeated (isokinetic/isotonic) contractions [19], providing reliable results [57].

However, as the endurance capacity of the limb muscles reflect the ability to perform tasks requiring a low number of contractions such as climbing a set of stairs as well as tasks requiring a high number of contractions such as bicycling or walking over a long distance, it is apparent that the same method cannot be used to evaluate muscle performance in both situations and that no single test can evaluate all aspects of limb muscle endurance [19].

	Isometric*	Isokinetic†	Isotonic†
Strength	Performing 3–5 MVC held for ~5 s, spaced with 30–60s rest periods at a fixed position.	Performing a minimum of 3–5 maximal contractions at an angular velocity of 60°–90°s	Performing a 1 RM test following ACMS guidelines with the addition of standardized range-of-motion and speed of contraction
Endurance	Sustained contraction at an intensity equal to 20–60% of isometric MVC until failure using visual feedback	Total work obtained from (typically 30) maximal contractions at an angular velocity of 60°–90°s	A maximum number of repetitions performed using external loads corresponding to 10% up to 50% of the individual 1 RM until failure.

MVC, maximal voluntary contraction; ACSM, American college of sports medicine; RM, repetition maximum.
*Normally 60°–90° flexion.
†Normally 90° flexion to full extension.

Table 2. Commonly used procedures for assessment of quadriceps muscle strength and endurance among people with COPD [19, 55, 58, 61, 79, 82].

Thus, to date, there is no specific recommendation on how to assess limb muscle endurance among people with COPD, and a vast variation of techniques and strategies have been used, including both static and dynamic measurements [19]. Similarly, as for limb muscle strength assessments, dynamic measurements of quadriceps endurance seem to be more closely related functional tasks than isometric measurements [49].

Furthermore, in comparison to limb muscle strength, the endurance capacity of the limb muscles does also seem to be more closely associated with both upper and lower limb functional capacity among people with COPD [50], highlighting one reason for why the endurance capacity of should not be neglected when assessing the limb muscles. For an example of commonly used procedures for quadriceps muscle testing see **Table 2**.

3.4. Functional testing

In the assessment of limb muscles in people with COPD, the use of functional tests is quickly becoming more and more popular. One key advantage of using functional tests is that they are often cheap, time-efficient, and require minimal equipment and usually a limited amount of space. Furthermore, as there is more to limb muscle function in COPD other than strictly the ability to exert a specific torque over a particular period of time [55], functional tests may provide valuable information that cannot be obtained from direct measurements of limb muscle function or mass.

Several different functional tests have been used in people with COPD, with field walking tests and different versions of the sit to stand test, being the most common in recent years [62, 83].

Similarly, as for direct measurements of limb muscle mass and function, different functional tests provide various information depending on which test is used, and the physiotherapist is required to use different tests depending on the objective of the assessment.

Furthermore, the physiotherapist should keep in mind that functional tests and limb muscle function assessments evaluate different constructs (as evident by low to moderate associations between limb muscle function assessments and functional tests), and thus cannot replace another [49, 79, 84]. Therefore, when deciding on how to assess the limb muscles in COPD, the objective should always be the driving factor.

3.5. In summary

Assessment of limb muscle mass and function should be part of the routine management of people with COPD. One aspect that sometimes is overlooked is the complexity, a wide variety of assessment methods could be used for this purpose.

Examples from this chapter include muscle mass assessed on whole-body level [6] or by a thin slice of the thigh [5], quadriceps strength, and endurance that could be measured static [43] or dynamic [40], resulting in somewhat different conclusions dependent on the type of assessment performed. As such, several factors need to be taken into account by the physiotherapist when deciding on how to assess limb muscle mass and function in COPD (see **Table 1** for further details).

Nevertheless, standardization of testing procedures is of utmost importance to provide accurate and reliable assessments, irrespective of measurement technique used.

4. How to improve limb muscles among people with COPD?

Strategies aiming at stopping or slowing down the progression of limb muscle dysfunction are highly warranted, and interventions focusing on exercise training, nutritional supplementation, and medication alone, or in combination, have all been shown to improve various aspects of limb muscle function and mass in people with COPD [4]. The focus in this section will be on the use of exercise training, this since exercise training is recommended before all other available modalities or combination of modalities [4].

4.1. Exercise training

In one sense, exercise training interventions for people with COPD are no different than for other populations; the same general exercise principles (specificity, progression, reversibility, periodization, etc.) and acute program variables (choice of exercise, order of exercise order, intensity [duration], number of sets, rest period lengths, type of muscle action, speed of movement, volume, frequency, etc.) apply [85–87]. However, for people with COPD, some of these variables might need to be altered to maximize benefits [88].

Considering the complexity of limb muscle dysfunction in COPD, no single exercise regimen could be used to target all aspects of the decreased function and altered structure of limb muscles [4, 26]. In a recent review, the effects of different modalities including aerobic or resistance training, high-intensity interval training, electric or magnetic muscle stimulation, whole-body vibration, and water-based exercise modalities to improve limb muscle function and mass among people with COPD were summarized. Overall, limb muscle strength was increased in 78%, limb muscle endurance in 92%, and muscle mass in 88% of the cases where that specific aspect of the limb muscle was measured [26] using these different modalities. On average, this corresponded to a mean increase in limb muscle strength of 15–34%, limb muscle endurance of 8.7–96.6%, and limb muscle mass of 4.2–12.1% and was highly dependent on which type of assessment strategy used. For limb muscle strength and endurance, isotonic assessment strategies seemed to be most responsive while for muscle mass, direct measurements using ultrasound demonstrated the most substantial adaptations, independent of exercise modality used [26]. However, there is considerable heterogeneity in the type of exercise modalities used, and it is currently unknown which type of exercise modality that is most effective in different subgroups of people with COPD. To date, several different exercise modalities are available for people with COPD including but not limited to resistance training (strength or endurance targeted), aerobic training (continuous or interval), whole body vibration training, neuromuscular electrical stimulation, active mind body therapies (e.g., Tai Chi, Qigong, etc.), as well as using different strategies to structure (e.g., nonlinear periodization) or to perform (e.g., single limb) exercises [21–25, 89]. Nevertheless, the most commonly used approaches are aerobic and resistance exercises, and in the design of both modalities for people with COPD, the American College of Sports Medicine frameworks [85, 86] has been recommended [88]. However, even though both continuous and interval training have shown positive effects of limb muscle function and mass in people with COPD, if the aim is to increase these aspects of the limb muscles in COPD, resistance training may be a more effective modality than aerobic exercises [90–93].

More significant effects on muscle strength have been observed after resistance training in comparison to aerobic training alone or when resistance training is added to an aerobic training protocol [88, 91, 93]. This fits with the specificity principle of exercise, that is, that exercise adaptation is specific to the type of activity and the volume and intensity of the activity performed [86, 94]. However, this also means that different kinds of resistance training protocols are necessary to target various aspects of limb muscle dysfunction. For example, if the goal is to improve limb muscle strength and mass, high-load/low-repetition programs are favorable [92, 95, 96], while if the goal is to enhance limb muscle endurance, low-load/high-repetition programs should be used [86, 96, 97]. In addition to decreased limb muscle mass and function, limb muscle dysfunction in COPD is also characterized by altered intramuscular characteristic, that is, structural and muscle metabolic alterations on the functional level result in the decreased function of limb muscles in COPD [4, 31]. Thus, of importance is that exercise-based training interventions also result in both structural and metabolic changes within the limb muscles [31], including, but not limited to, changes in fiber type proportion, fiber size, capillary to fiber ratio, muscle protein turnover regulation, and mitochondrial enzyme activity, while markers of oxidative and nitrosative stress and inflammation does not seem to be affected [31]. However, in a similar way as for effects on muscle mass and function, exercise responses are heterogeneous, dependent on the type and intensity of the activity performed. Alterations in fiber proportion, fiber size, and capillary to fiber ratio tend to increase more after combined aerobic and resistance training, but predominantly with excellent results after higher intensity interval training [31]. Thus suggesting that the intensity of the activity performed is of importance to achieve intramuscular adaptations, even though this needs to be confirmed in future studies.

4.2. In summary

Exercise training, and resistance training in particular, is the most efficacious approach to ameliorate limb muscle dysfunction among people with COPD, with the latter resulting in the most substantial improvements in limb muscle mass and function. However, COPD limb muscle is characterized by a large heterogeneity of muscle phenotypes and muscle dysfunction, stressing the importance of identifying those specific factors that should be considered in the development of individualized resistance training programs among people with COPD. Thus, no single intervention is sufficient to target all aspects of limb muscle dysfunction in the disease. To achieve intramuscular adaptations, exercise intensity seems to be an important factor, and high intensity interval training seems to be the most promising approach. Lastly, irrespective of exercise training modality, general exercise principles and acute program variables should always be incorporated when designing the exercise program.

5. Conclusions

Limb muscle dysfunction is a highly prevalent and clinically relevant manifestation of COPD, closely linked to important clinical outcomes, including exercise tolerance, quality of life, and survival. Limb muscle dysfunction seems to be heterogeneous, with the lower limbs, and the quadriceps muscle in particular, mostly affected.

Assessment of limb muscle mass and function should be routinely performed in clinical practice, and simple valid and reliable tools are available for the physiotherapist to use.

Independent of measurement strategy, standardization of measurement properties are crucial and several different factors such as type of contraction, choice of exercise or equipment need to be acknowledged by the physiotherapist when deciding on how to assess the limb muscles among people with COPD.

Lastly, to improve limb muscle mass and function, exercise training, and resistance training in particular is recommended before other available modalities, and general exercise principles and acute program variables should always be incorporated into the design of the exercise program.

Conflict of interest

The authors report no conflict of interest.

Author details

Andre Nyberg* and Erik Frykholm

*Address all correspondence to: andre.nyberg@umu.se

Department of Community Medicine and Rehabilitation, Section of Physiotherapy, Umeå University, Umeå, Sweden

References

[1] Soriano JB, Abajoir AA, Abate KH, Abera SF, Agrawal A, Ahmed MB, et al. Global, regional, and national deaths, prevalence, disability-adjusted life years, and years lived with disability for chronic obstructive pulmonary disease and asthma, 1990-2015: A systematic analysis for the Global Burden of Disease Study 2015. The Lancet Respiratory Medicine. 2017;**5**(9):691-706

[2] Beaver WL, Wasserman K, Whipp BJ. A new method for detecting anaerobic threshold by gas exchange. Journal of Applied Physiology. 1986;**60**(6):2020-2027

[3] van't Hul A, Harlaar J, Gosselink R, Hollander P, Postmus P, Kwakkel G. Quadriceps muscle endurance in patients with chronic obstructive pulmonary disease. Muscle and Nerve. 2004;**29**(2):267-274

[4] Maltais F, Decramer M, Casaburi R, Barreiro E, Burelle Y, Debigare R, et al. An official American Thoracic Society/European Respiratory Society statement: Update on limb muscle dysfunction in chronic obstructive pulmonary disease. American Journal of Respiratory and Critical Care Medicine. 2014;**189**(9):e15-e62

[5] Marquis K, Debigare R, Lacasse Y, LeBlanc P, Jobin J, Carrier G, et al. Midthigh muscle cross-sectional area is a better predictor of mortality than body mass index in patients

with chronic obstructive pulmonary disease. American Journal of Respiratory and Critical Care Medicine. 2002;**166**(6):809-813

[6] Schols AM, Broekhuizen R, Weling-Scheepers CA, Wouters EF. Body composition and mortality in chronic obstructive pulmonary disease. The American Journal of Clinical Nutrition. 2005;**82**(1):53-59

[7] Swallow EB, Reyes D, Hopkinson NS, Man WD, Porcher R, Cetti EJ, et al. Quadriceps strength predicts mortality in patients with moderate to severe chronic obstructive pulmonary disease. Thorax. 2007;**62**(2):115-120

[8] Patel MS, Natanek SA, Stratakos G, Pascual S, Martinez-Llorens J, Disano L, et al. Vastus lateralis fiber shift is an independent predictor of mortality in chronic obstructive pulmonary disease. American Journal of Respiratory and Critical Care Medicine. 2014;**190**(3):350-352

[9] Mostert R, Goris A, Weling-Scheepers C, Wouters EF, Schols AM. Tissue depletion and health related quality of life in patients with chronic obstructive pulmonary disease. Respiratory Medicine. 2000;**94**(9):859-867

[10] Gosselink R, Troosters T, Decramer M. Peripheral muscle weakness contributes to exercise limitation in COPD. American Journal of Respiratory and Critical Care Medicine. 1996;**153**(3):976-980

[11] Hamilton AL, Killian KJ, Summers E, Jones NL. Muscle strength, symptom intensity, and exercise capacity in patients with cardiorespiratory disorders. American Journal of Respiratory and Critical Care Medicine. 1995;**152**(6 Pt 1):2021-2031

[12] Coronell C, Orozco-Levi M, Mendez R, Ramirez-Sarmiento A, Galdiz JB, Gea J. Relevance of assessing quadriceps endurance in patients with COPD. The European Respiratory Journal. 2004;**24**(1):129-136

[13] Decramer M, Gosselink R, Troosters T, Verschueren M, Evers G. Muscle weakness is related to utilization of health care resources in COPD patients. The European Respiratory Journal. 1997;**10**(2):417-423

[14] Bui KL, Nyberg A, Rabinovich R, Saey D, Maltais F. The relevance of limb muscle dysfunction in chronic obstructive pulmonary disease: A review for clinicians. Clinics in Chest Medicine. 2019;**40**(2):367-383

[15] Shrikrishna D, Patel M, Tanner RJ, Seymour JM, Connolly BA, Puthucheary ZA, et al. Quadriceps wasting and physical inactivity in patients with COPD. The European Respiratory Journal. 2012;**40**(5):1115-1122

[16] Rabinovich RA, Bastos R, Ardite E, Llinas L, Orozco-Levi M, Gea J, et al. Mitochondrial dysfunction in COPD patients with low body mass index. The European Respiratory Journal. 2007;**29**(4):643-650

[17] Vogiatzis I, Terzis G, Stratakos G, Cherouveim E, Athanasopoulos D, Spetsioti S, et al. Effect of pulmonary rehabilitation on peripheral muscle fiber remodeling in patients with COPD in GOLD stages II to IV. Chest. 2011;**140**(3):744-752

[18] Allaire J, Maltais F, Doyon JF, Noel M, LeBlanc P, Carrier G, et al. Peripheral muscle endurance and the oxidative profile of the quadriceps in patients with COPD. Thorax. 2004;**59**(8):673-678

[19] Evans RA, Kaplovitch E, Beauchamp MK, Dolmage TE, Goldstein RS, Gillies CL, et al. Is quadriceps endurance reduced in COPD? A systematic review. Chest. 2015;**147**(3):673-684

[20] Gosselink R, Troosters T, Decramer M. Distribution of muscle weakness in patients with stable chronic obstructive pulmonary disease. Journal of Cardiac and Pulmonary Rehabilitation. 2000;**20**:353-360

[21] Nolan CM, Rochester CL. Exercise training modalities for people with chronic obstructive pulmonary disease. COPD. 2019;**16**(5-6):378-389

[22] Zhou J, Pang L, Chen N, Wang Z, Wang C, Hai Y, et al. Whole-body vibration training - better care for COPD patients: A systematic review and meta-analysis. International Journal of Chronic Obstructive Pulmonary Disease. 2018;**13**:3243-3254

[23] Neves CDC, Lacerda ACR, Lage VKS, Soares AA, Chaves MGA, Lima LP, et al. Whole body vibration training increases physical measures and quality of life without altering inflammatory-oxidative biomarkers in patients with moderate COPD. Journal of Applied Physiology. 2018;**125**(2):520-528

[24] Dolmage TE, Goldstein RS. Effects of one-legged exercise training of patients with COPD. Chest. 2008;**133**(2):370-376

[25] Klijn P, van Keimpema A, Legemaat M, Gosselink R, van Stel H. Nonlinear exercise training in advanced chronic obstructive pulmonary disease is superior to traditional exercise training. A randomized trial. American Journal of Respiratory and Critical Care Medicine. 2013;**188**(2):193-200

[26] De Brandt J, Spruit MA, Hansen D, Franssen FM, Derave W, Sillen MJ, et al. Changes in lower limb muscle function and muscle mass following exercise-based interventions in patients with chronic obstructive pulmonary disease: A review of the English-language literature. Chronic Respiratory Disease. 2018;**15**(2):182-219

[27] Jones S, Man WD, Gao W, Higginson IJ, Wilcock A, Maddocks M. Neuromuscular electrical stimulation for muscle weakness in adults with advanced disease. Cochrane Database of Systematic Reviews. 2016;**10**:CD009419

[28] Vorrink SN, Kort HS, Troosters T, Lammers JW. Level of daily physical activity in individuals with COPD compared with healthy controls. Respiratory Research. 2011;**12**:33

[29] Couillard A, Prefaut C. From muscle disuse to myopathy in COPD: Potential contribution of oxidative stress. The European Respiratory Journal. 2005;**26**(4):703-719

[30] Polkey MI, Moxham J. Attacking the disease spiral in chronic obstructive pulmonary disease: An update. Clinical Medicine (London, England). 2011;**11**(5):461-464

[31] De Brandt J, Spruit MA, Derave W, Hansen D, Vanfleteren LE, Burtin C. Changes in structural and metabolic muscle characteristics following exercise-based interventions

in patients with COPD: A systematic review. Expert Review of Respiratory Medicine. 2016;**10**(5):521-545

[32] Gea J, Agusti A, Roca J. Pathophysiology of muscle dysfunction in COPD. Journal of Applied Physiology. 2013;**114**(9):1222-1234

[33] Schols AM, Soeters PB, Dingemans AM, Mostert R, Frantzen PJ, Wouters EF. Prevalence and characteristics of nutritional depletion in patients with stable COPD eligible for pulmonary rehabilitation. The American Review of Respiratory Disease. 1993;**147**(5):1151-1156

[34] Baarends EM, Schols AM, Mostert R, Wouters EF. Peak exercise response in relation to tissue depletion in patients with chronic obstructive pulmonary disease. The European Respiratory Journal. 1997;**10**(12):2807-2813

[35] Muscaritoli M, Anker SD, Argiles J, Aversa Z, Bauer JM, Biolo G, et al. Consensus definition of sarcopenia, cachexia and pre-cachexia: Joint document elaborated by special interest groups (SIG) "cachexia-anorexia in chronic wasting diseases" and "nutrition in geriatrics". Clinical Nutrition. 2010;**29**(2):154-159

[36] Vestbo J, Prescott E, Almdal T, Dahl M, Nordestgaard BG, Andersen T, et al. Body mass, fat-free body mass, and prognosis in patients with chronic obstructive pulmonary disease from a random population sample: Findings from the Copenhagen City heart study. American Journal of Respiratory and Critical Care Medicine. 2006;**173**(1):79-83

[37] Collins PF, Elia M, Stratton RJ. Nutritional support and functional capacity in chronic obstructive pulmonary disease: A systematic review and meta-analysis. Respirology. 2013;**18**(4):616-629

[38] van Wetering CR, Hoogendoorn M, Broekhuizen R, Geraerts-Keeris GJ, De Munck DR, Rutten-van Molken MP, et al. Efficacy and costs of nutritional rehabilitation in muscle-wasted patients with chronic obstructive pulmonary disease in a community-based setting: A prespecified subgroup analysis of the INTERCOM trial. Journal of the American Medical Directors Association. 2010;**11**(3):179-187

[39] Hopkinson NS, Tennant RC, Dayer MJ, Swallow EB, Hansel TT, Moxham J, et al. A prospective study of decline in fat free mass and skeletal muscle strength in chronic obstructive pulmonary disease. Respiratory Research. 2007;**8**:25

[40] Engelen MP, Schols AM, Does JD, Wouters EF. Skeletal muscle weakness is associated with wasting of extremity fat-free mass but not with airflow obstruction in patients with chronic obstructive pulmonary disease. The American Journal of Clinical Nutrition. 2000;**71**(3):733-738

[41] Bernard S, LeBlanc P, Whittom F, Carrier G, Jobin J, Belleau R, et al. Peripheral muscle weakness in patients with chronic obstructive pulmonary disease. American Journal of Respiratory and Critical Care Medicine. 1998;**158**(2):629-634

[42] Thompson WRG, Pescatello NF, Linda S, et al. ACSM's Guidelines for Exercise Testing and Prescription. 8th ed. Philadelphia: Wolters Kluwer/Lippincott Williams & Wilkins; 2010

[43] Seymour JM, Spruit MA, Hopkinson NS, Natanek SA, Man WD, Jackson A, et al. The prevalence of quadriceps weakness in COPD and the relationship with disease severity. The European Respiratory Journal. 2010;**36**(1):81-88

[44] Couillard A, Maltais F, Saey D, Debigare R, Michaud A, Koechlin C, et al. Exercise-induced quadriceps oxidative stress and peripheral muscle dysfunction in patients with chronic obstructive pulmonary disease. American Journal of Respiratory and Critical Care Medicine. 2003;**167**(12):1664-1669

[45] Hopkinson NS, Man WD, Dayer MJ, Ross ET, Nickol AH, Hart N, et al. Acute effect of oral steroids on muscle function in chronic obstructive pulmonary disease. The European Respiratory Journal. 2004;**24**(1):137-142

[46] Swallow EB, Gosker HR, Ward KA, Moore AJ, Dayer MJ, Hopkinson NS, et al. A novel technique for nonvolitional assessment of quadriceps muscle endurance in humans. Journal of Applied Physiology. 2007;**103**(3):739-746

[47] Killian KJ, Leblanc P, Martin DH, Summers E, Jones NL, Campbell EJ. Exercise capacity and ventilatory, circulatory, and symptom limitation in patients with chronic airflow limitation. The American Review of Respiratory Disease. 1992;**146**(4):935-940

[48] McNamara RJ, Houben-Wilke S, Franssen FME, Smid DE, Vanfleteren L, Groenen MTJ, et al. Determinants of functional, peak and endurance exercise capacity in people with chronic obstructive pulmonary disease. Respiratory Medicine. 2018;**138**:81-87

[49] Géphine S, Frykholm E, Nyberg A, Bui K-L, Maltais F, Saey D. Relationship between functional capacity, dynamic and static muscle function assessments in people with chronic obstructive pulmonary disease (COPD). European Respiratory Journal. 2018;**52**(suppl 62):PA4154

[50] Nyberg A, Tornberg A, Wadell K. Correlation between limb muscle endurance, strength, and functional capacity in people with chronic obstructive pulmonary disease. Physiotherapy Canada. 2016;**68**(1):46-53

[51] Vilaro J, Rabinovich R, Gonzalez-deSuso JM, Troosters T, Rodriguez D, Barbera JA, et al. Clinical assessment of peripheral muscle function in patients with chronic obstructive pulmonary disease. American Journal of Physical Medicine and Rehabilitation. 2009;**88**(1):39-46

[52] Franssen FM, Broekhuizen R, Janssen PP, Wouters EF, Schols AM. Limb muscle dysfunction in COPD: Effects of muscle wasting and exercise training. Medicine and Science in Sports and Exercise. 2005;**37**(1):2-9

[53] van den Borst B, Slot IG, Hellwig VA, Vosse BA, Kelders MC, Barreiro E, et al. Loss of quadriceps muscle oxidative phenotype and decreased endurance in patients with mild-to-moderate COPD. Journal of Applied Physiology. 2013;**114**(9):1319-1328

[54] Nyberg A, Saey D, Maltais F. Why and how limb muscle mass and function should Be measured in patients with chronic obstructive pulmonary disease. Annals of the American Thoracic Society. 2015;**12**(9):1269-1277

[55] Marklund S, Bui KL, Nyberg A. Measuring and monitoring skeletal muscle function in COPD: Current perspectives. International Journal of Chronic Obstructive Pulmonary Disease. 2019;**14**:1825-1838

[56] Barreiro E, Bustamante V, Cejudo P, Galdiz JB, Gea J, de Lucas P, et al. Guidelines for the evaluation and treatment of muscle dysfunction in patients with chronic obstructive pulmonary disease. Archivos de Bronconeumología. 2015;**51**(8):384-395

[57] Frykholm E, Gephine S, Saey D, van Hees H, Lemson A, Klijn P, et al. Inter-day test-retest reliability and feasibility of isokinetic, isometric, and isotonic measurements to assess quadriceps endurance in people with chronic obstructive pulmonary disease: A multicenter study. Chronic Respiratory Disease. 2019;**16**:1479973118816497

[58] Nyberg A, Saey D, Martin M, Maltais F. Test-re-test reliability of quadriceps muscle strength measures in people with more severe chronic obstructive pulmonary disease. Journal of Rehabilitation Medicine. 2018;**50**(8):759-764

[59] Mathur S, Makrides L, Hernandez P. Test-retest reliability of isometric and isokinetic torque in patients with chronic obstructive pulmonary disease. Physiotherapy Canada. 2004;**56**:94-101

[60] Chura RL, Marciniuk DD, Clemens R, Butcher SJ. Test-retest reliability and physiological responses associated with the steep ramp anaerobic test in patients with COPD. Pulmonary Medicine. 2012;**2012**:6

[61] Fernanda Ribeiro P-AL, Garceau-Bolduc C, Coats V, François M, Saey D. Test-retest reliability of lower limb isokinetic endurance in COPD: A comparison of angular velocities. International Journal of COPD. 2015; In press

[62] Bui KL, Nyberg A, Maltais F, Saey D. Functional tests in chronic obstructive pulmonary disease part 2: Measurement properties. Annals of the American Thoracic Society. 2017;**14**(5):785-794

[63] Crook S, Busching G, Schultz K, Lehbert N, Jelusic D, Keusch S, et al. A multicentre validation of the 1-min sit-to-stand test in patients with COPD. The European Respiratory Journal. 2017;**49**(3):1601871. DOI: 10.1183/13993003.01871-2016

[64] Janaudis-Ferreira T, Beauchamp MK, Goldstein RS, Brooks D. How should we measure arm exercise capacity in patients with COPD? A systematic review. Chest. 2012;**141**(1):111-120

[65] Rodrigues FM, Demeyer H, Hornikx M, Camillo CA, Calik-Kutukcu E, Burtin C, et al. Validity and reliability of strain gauge measurement of volitional quadriceps force in patients with COPD. Chronic Respiratory Disease. 479972316687210

[66] Schols AM, Wouters EF, Soeters PB, Westerterp KR. Body composition by bioelectrical-impedance analysis compared with deuterium dilution and skinfold anthropometry in patients with chronic obstructive pulmonary disease. The American Journal of Clinical Nutrition. 1991;**53**(2):421-424

[67] Schols AM, Mostert R, Soeters PB, Wouters EF. Body composition and exercise performance in patients with chronic obstructive pulmonary disease. Thorax. 1991;**46**(10):695-699

[68] Miller A, Strauss BJ, Mol S, Kyoong A, Holmes PH, Finlay P, et al. Dual-energy X-ray absorptiometry is the method of choice to assess body composition in COPD. Respirology. 2009;**14**(3):411-418

[69] Maddocks M, Kon SS, Jones SE, Canavan JL, Nolan CM, Higginson IJ, et al. Bioelectrical impedance phase angle relates to function, disease severity and prognosis in stable chronic obstructive pulmonary disease. Clinical Nutrition. 2015;**34**(6):1245-1250

[70] Janssen I, Heymsfield SB, Baumgartner RN, Ross R. Estimation of skeletal muscle mass by bioelectrical impedance analysis. Journal of Applied Physiology. 2000;**89**(2):465-471

[71] Lerario MC, Sachs A, Lazaretti-Castro M, Saraiva LG, Jardim JR. Body composition in patients with chronic obstructive pulmonary disease: Which method to use in clinical practice? The British Journal of Nutrition. 2006;**96**(1):86-92

[72] Steiner MC, Barton RL, Singh SJ, Morgan MD. Bedside methods versus dual energy X-ray absorptiometry for body composition measurement in COPD. The European Respiratory Journal. 2002;**19**(4):626-631

[73] Rutten EP, Spruit MA, Wouters EF. Critical view on diagnosing muscle wasting by single-frequency bio-electrical impedance in COPD. Respiratory Medicine. 2010;**104**(1):91-98

[74] Seymour JM, Ward K, Sidhu PS, Puthucheary Z, Steier J, Jolley CJ, et al. Ultrasound measurement of rectus femoris cross-sectional area and the relationship with quadriceps strength in COPD. Thorax. 2009;**64**(5):418-423

[75] Bachasson D, Villiot-Danger E, Verges S, Hayot M, Perez T, Chambellan A, et al. Maximal isometric voluntary quadriceps strength assessment in COPD. Revue des Maladies Respiratoires. 2014;**31**(8):765-770

[76] Man WD, Moxham J, Polkey MI. Magnetic stimulation for the measurement of respiratory and skeletal muscle function. The European Respiratory Journal. 2004;**24**(5):846-860

[77] Polkey MI, Kyroussis D, Hamnegard CH, Mills GH, Green M, Moxham J. Quadriceps strength and fatigue assessed by magnetic stimulation of the femoral nerve in man. Muscle and Nerve. 1996;**19**(5):549-555

[78] Robles PG, Mathur S, Janaudis-Fereira T, Dolmage TE, Goldstein RS, Brooks D. Measurement of peripheral muscle strength in individuals with chronic obstructive pulmonary disease: A systematic review. Journal of Cardiopulmonary Rehabilitation and Prevention. 2011;**31**(1):11-24

[79] Bui KL, Mathur S, Dechman G, Maltais F, Camp P, Saey D. Fixed handheld dynamometry provides reliable and valid values for quadriceps isometric strength in people with chronic obstructive pulmonary disease: A multicenter study. Physical Therapy. 2019;**99**(9):1255-1267

[80] Jeong M, Kang HK, Song P, Park HK, Jung H, Lee SS, et al. Hand grip strength in patients with chronic obstructive pulmonary disease. International Journal of Chronic Obstructive Pulmonary Disease. 2017;**12**:2385-2390

[81] Strandkvist VJ, Backman H, Roding J, Stridsman C, Lindberg A. Hand grip strength is associated with forced expiratory volume in 1 second among subjects with COPD: Report from a population-based cohort study. International Journal of Chronic Obstructive Pulmonary Disease. 2016;**11**:2527-2534

[82] Janaudis-Ferreira T, Hill K, Goldstein RS, Robles-Ribeiro P, Beauchamp MK, Dolmage TE, et al. Resistance arm training in patients with COPD: A randomized controlled trial. Chest. 2011;**139**(1):151-158

[83] Bui KL, Nyberg A, Maltais F, Saey D. Functional tests in chronic obstructive pulmonary disease part 1: Clinical relevance and links to the international classification of functioning, disability and health. Annals of the American Thoracic Society. 2017;**14**(5):778-784

[84] Rausch-Osthoff AK, Kohler M, Sievi NA, Clarenbach CF, van Gestel AJ. Association between peripheral muscle strength, exercise performance, and physical activity in daily life in patients with chronic obstructive pulmonary disease. Multidisciplinary Respiratory Medicine. 2014;**9**(1):37

[85] Garber CE, Blissmer B, Deschenes MR, Franklin BA, Lamonte MJ, Lee IM, et al. American College of Sports Medicine position stand. Quantity and quality of exercise for developing and maintaining cardiorespiratory, musculoskeletal, and neuromotor fitness in apparently healthy adults: Guidance for prescribing exercise. Medicine and Science in Sports and Exercise. 2011;**43**(7):1334-1359

[86] American College of Sports Medicine. American College of Sports Medicine position stand. Progression models in resistance training for healthy adults. Medicine and Science in Sports and Exercise. 2009;**41**(3):687-708

[87] Westra B, de Wolf S, bij de Vaate E, Legemaat M, Nyberg A, Klijn P. Quality of resistance training description in COPD trials: study protocol for a systematic review. BMJ open. 2019;**9**(1):e025030

[88] Spruit MA, Singh SJ, Garvey C, ZuWallack R, Nici L, Rochester C, et al. An official American Thoracic Society/European Respiratory Society statement: Key concepts and advances in pulmonary rehabilitation. American Journal of Respiratory and Critical Care Medicine. 2013;**188**(8):e13-e64

[89] Gendron LM, Nyberg A, Saey D, Maltais F, Lacasse Y. Active mind-body movement therapies as an adjunct to or in comparison with pulmonary rehabilitation for people with chronic obstructive pulmonary disease. The Cochrane Database of Systematic Reviews. 2018;**10**:Cd012290

[90] Ortega F, Toral J, Cejudo P, Villagomez R, Sanchez H, Castillo J, et al. Comparison of effects of strength and endurance training in patients with chronic obstructive pulmonary disease. American Journal of Respiratory and Critical Care Medicine. 2002;**166**(5):669-674

[91] Vonbank K, Strasser B, Mondrzyk J, Marzluf BA, Richter B, Losch S, et al. Strength training increases maximum working capacity in patients with COPD--randomized clinical trial comparing three training modalities. Respiratory Medicine. 2012;**106**(4):557-563

[92] Iepsen UW, Jorgensen KJ, Ringbaek T, Hansen H, Skrubbeltrang C, Lange P. A combination of resistance and endurance training increases leg muscle strength in COPD: An evidence-based recommendation based on systematic review with meta-analyses. Chronic Respiratory Disease. 2015;**12**(2):132-145

[93] Iepsen UW, Jorgensen KJ, Ringbaek T, Hansen H, Skrubbeltrang C, Lange P. A systematic review of resistance training versus endurance training in COPD. Journal of Cardiopulmonary Rehabilitation and Prevention. 2015;**35**(3):163-172

[94] Wilmore JH. Principles of exercise training. In: Kenny LW, Wilmore JH, Costill DL, editors. Physiology of Sports and Exercise. 6th ed. Champaign: Human Kinetics; 2015. pp. 224-240

[95] Kraemer WJ, Ratamess NA. Fundamentals of resistance training: Progression and exercise prescription. Medicine and Science in Sports and Exercise. 2004;**36**(4):674-688

[96] Kraemer WJFS. Optimizing Strength Training: Designing Nonlinear Periodization Workouts. Champaign, IL: Human Kinetics; 2007

[97] Nyberg A, Lindstrom B, Rickenlund A, Wadell K. Low-load/high-repetition elastic band resistance training in patients with COPD: A randomized, controlled, multicenter trial. The Clinical Respiratory Journal. 2015;**9**(3):278-288

Chapter 9

Early Mobilization on Patients with Mechanical Ventilation in the ICU

Tsung-Hsien Wang

Additional information is available at the end of the chapter

http://dx.doi.org/10.5772/intechopen.89984

Abstract

Patients in intensive care unit (ICU) usually experienced being immobile and restrained, and these can induce muscle weakness, cognitive impairments, psychological difficulties, difficult weaning, and increased length of stay (LOS) in hospital. However, early mobilization has multiple benefits including improved ventilation, perfusion, muscle strength, and functional capacity.

Keywords: early mobilization, ICU-acquired weakness, intensive care unit, mechanical ventilation, delirium, sedation

1. Introduction

Patients in the intensive care unit are often immobile and restrained, which can induce muscle weakness, cognitive impairment, psychological difficulties, and difficulty weaning from mechanical ventilation (MV) and may increase the overall length of stay (LOS) in the hospital. Long-term complications such as postintensive care syndrome, intensive care unit (ICU)-acquired weakness, physical debility, and neuropsychiatric dysfunction have become a clinical and scientific focus, as their impact on long-term quality of life is becoming increasingly obvious [1].

Early mobilization, however, has multiple benefits, including improvements in ventilation, perfusion, muscle strength, and functional capacity. Early mobilization of ICU patients, defined as mobilization within 72 h of ICU admission, remains uncommon. In critically ill medical and surgical patients, mobilization is well tolerated, even in intubated patients.

The purpose of this chapter is to provide a framework for early mobilization in critically ill patients followed by a review of recent developments in the field.

IntechOpen

© 2020 The Author(s). Licensee IntechOpen. This chapter is distributed under the terms of the Creative Commons Attribution License (http://creativecommons.org/licenses/by/3.0), which permits unrestricted use, distribution, and reproduction in any medium, provided the original work is properly cited. (cc) BY

1.1. Critical care in ICU

Once a patient is admitted to the ICU, successful management should aim at patient survival. While patient with the acute present illness, serious trauma, shock, or progression of chronic illness may require intubation with mechanical ventilation. Intubation is the passage of an artificial airway into the patient's trachea, generally through the mouth (endotracheal tube (ETT) intubation) or through the nose (nasotracheal intubation).

Over the last 50 years, mechanical ventilation has been an important tool for maintaining a patient's breathing and improving patient survival and recovery from life-threatening diseases. As a result of mechanical ventilation, the mortality rate in intensive care units has notably decreased. Recent data show that the mortality rate is 25–30% in patients with acute respiratory failure [2]; the focus now must pivot to the sequela of survivors after critical illness. The sequela still exist, even after patients are discharged from the hospital, and the symptoms include functional limitations, cognitive impairment, and mental disorders in the months or even years after a critical illness.

On the other side, many standard ICU interventions have been shown to have negative effects when used excessively: tidal volumes that are too large [3], too many blood transfusions [4], too much oxygen [5], and too much sedation [6] can all have negative effects on outcomes.

Over the past 10 years, there have been substantial decreases in mortality from such conditions as acute respiratory failure and sepsis. Recent data, however, show that many survivors are sent to rehabilitation centers. There is a high rate of mortality among survivors within the first year after ICU discharge, although it is unknown how many survivors could have returned home to stay with their family. For those who survive, the latest data show that 50–70% of ICU survivors will suffer cognitive impairment and 60–80% of survivors will suffer functional impairments or ICU-acquired weakness (ICU-AW) [7].

2. Muscle injury during mechanical ventilation

After critical illness, muscle weakness emerges not only in the peripheral muscles but also in the respiratory muscles, and it is believed to be a key factor leading to prolonged disability. Limb muscle atrophy and functional limitations persist for months after recovery from a critical illness. Muscle weakness of the diaphragm is a key risk factor for prolonged mechanical ventilation and causes long-term complications and death.

2.1. Intensive care unit-acquired weakness

Intensive care unit-acquired weakness is the most common neuromuscular impairment in critically ill patients. There are several distinguishable types of ICU-AW, including critical illness polyneuropathy, critical illness myopathy, or a combination of the two. Diagnosing ICU-AW is difficult, although most clinicians use the Medical Research Council (MRC) sum score. Handgrip is also often used to evaluate limb weakness and to determine if a patient is ventilator dependent or may have difficulty weaning from a mechanical ventilator. Regardless

http://dx.doi.org/10.5772/intechopen.89984

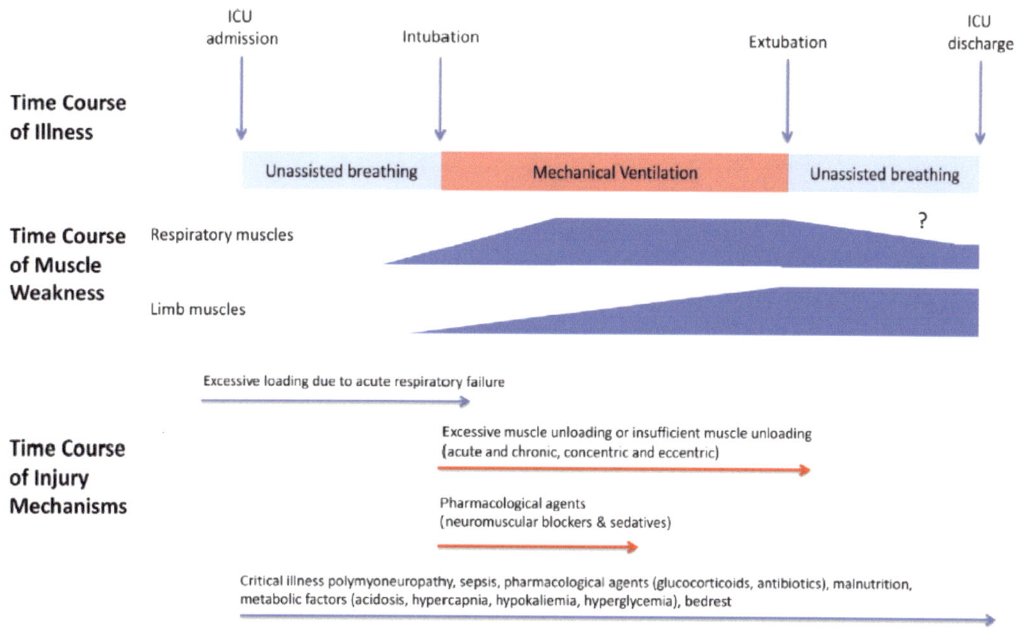

Figure 1. Time course of limb and respiratory muscle weakness during mechanical ventilation. Respiratory muscle weakness develops more rapidly than limb muscle weakness. Its influence on outcome is greater at an early stage (data from [9]).

of the type of ICU-AW, clinicians must evaluate the patient's muscle strength and assess the electrophysiological functioning of the peripheral muscles and nerves. ICU-AW is associated with difficulty in weaning from the ventilator, prolonged ICU stay, and higher hospitalization charges and increases long-term morbidity and mortality [8].

Most studies include limited cases of diagnosed ICU-AW because they usually evaluate patient weakness later in the course of disease or near hospital discharge. It is currently unknown whether peripheral muscle weakness causes prolonged ventilator use. Recently, Dres and colleagues revealed that, while limb muscle weakness noted at a patient's first spontaneous breathing trial was not correlated with prolonged mechanical ventilation, diaphragm muscle weakness did correlate. This result suggests that diaphragm muscle weakness induces prolonged mechanical ventilation, which in turn increases the risk of developing sustained limb muscle weakness and associated long-term functional impairment (**Figure 1**).

2.2. Definition

The term ICU-AW does not evaluate the time from admission to the ICU to the development of muscle weakness in a patient. In truth, it more likely describes the final resulting weakness that begins with any severe disease, regardless of the location of care. It is very important to diagnose ICU-AW after the onset of critical illness, which is a major distinguishing factor between ICU-AW and Guillain-Barre syndrome or other neuromuscular diseases that might cause acute respiratory failure after ICU admission (**Figure 2**).

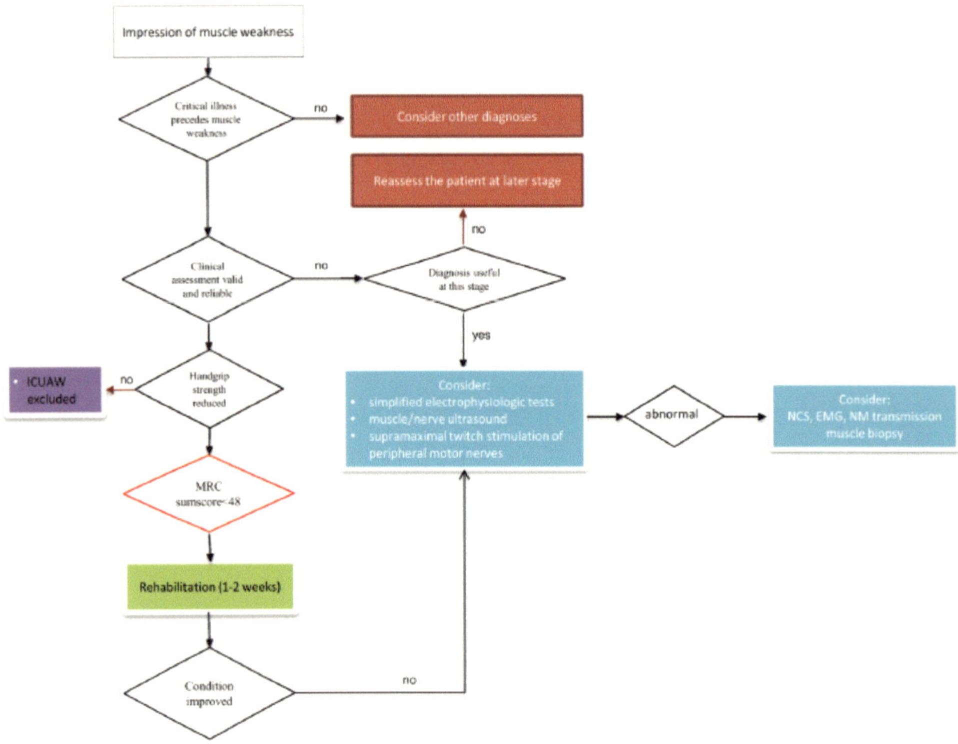

Figure 2. Diagnostic approach to patients developing intensive care unit-acquired weakness. EMG, electromyography; ICU-AW, intensive care unit-acquired weakness; MRC, Medical Research Council; NCS, nerve conduction study; NM, neuromuscular (data from [10]).

2.3. Epidemiology of ICU-acquired weakness

Neuromuscular dysfunction has long been recognized as correlating with critical illness. Sir William Osler proposed a "rapid loss of flesh" in patients with severe sepsis in 1892.

In the 1960s, Mertens reported polyneuropathy in patients in a coma state, and proof of acute myopathy was found in a patient with acute severe asthma. De Jonghe et al. reported that the incidence rate of ICU-AW used by the Medical Research Council is 25.3% of patients receiving mechanical ventilation for 7 days who had clear consciousness and could follow commands. Dhand et al. reported overall, 30–50% of critically ill patients suffer from CIP, CIM, or a combination of them.

2.4. Mechanisms

Patients with systemic inflammatory response syndrome and multiple organ dysfunction experiencing respiratory insufficiency are prone to CIP/CIM. Inflammation, apoptosis, thrombosis, and oxidant injury constitute the basis of both multiple organ failure (MOF) and peripheral neuromuscular abnormalities [11], so neuromuscular weakness because of CIP/CIM is due to neural system participation in MOF [12].

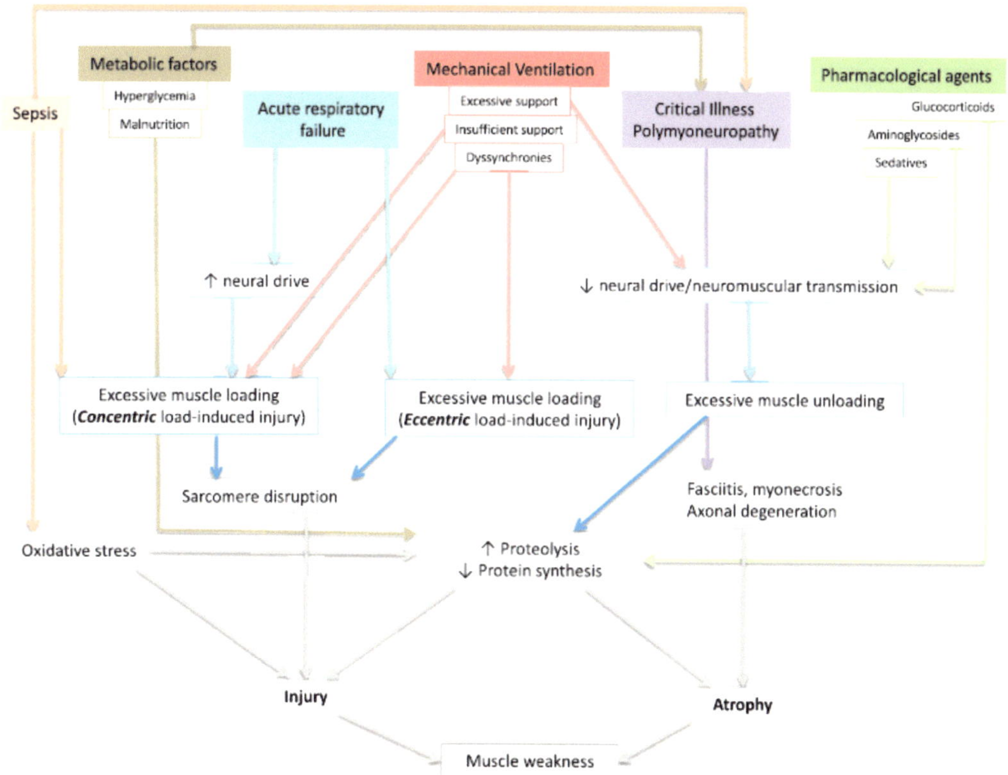

Figure 3. Mechanisms of injury to the limb and respiratory muscles during mechanical ventilation (data from [9]).

According to Bolton et al., microcirculation damage in peripheral nerves and muscles triggered by sepsis has a critical role in the CIP/CIM pathogenesis. A wide range of factors contribute to muscle injury and weakness in the context of critical illness. Schreiber et al. provide a summary of these factors, focusing especially on those mechanisms offering potential targets for intervention (**Figure 3**).

2.5. Critical illness polyneuropathy

Critical illness polyneuropathy is a sensory-motor axonal polyneuropathy. Electrophysiological studies show a reduction in the amplitudes of compound muscle action potentials (CMAPs) and sensory nerve action potentials (SNAPs), with normal or near-normal nerve conduction velocity.

2.6. Critical illness myopathy

Critical illness myopathy is an acute original myopathy and is not correlated with denervation, which differentiates the electrophysiological and morphological reports [10].

These conditions often coexist, and the combination of CIP and CIM—indicated as critical illness myopathy and neuropathy (CRIMYNE) or critical illness polyneuropathy and myopathy (CIPNM)—is the most common overlap syndrome (**Table 1**).

Condition	Definition	Diagnosis
Intensive care unit-acquired weakness	Clinically detected, diffuse, symmetric weakness involving all extremities and respiratory muscles arising after the onset of critical illness	Medical Research Council sum score of less than 48/60 or mean MRC score of 4 in all testable muscle groups Dominant-hand handgrip dynamometry scores of less than 11 kg (interquartile range (IQR) 10–40) in males and less than 7 kg (IQR 0–7.3) in females
Critical illness polyneuropathy (CIP)	An axonal, sensory-motor polyneuropathy with reduced nerve excitability and loss of axons with preserved myelin sheet	Reduced amplitude of compound muscle action potentials and sensory nerve action potentials with normal or mildly reduced nerve conduction velocity on electroneurography
Critical illness myopathy (CIM)	A primary acute myopathy with reduced muscle membrane excitability and loss of myosin filaments, fiber atrophy, and necrosis	Reduced amplitude of compound muscle action potentials and normal sensory nerve action potentials on electroneurography and reduced muscle excitability on direct muscle stimulation and myopathic motor unit potentials on needle electromyography
Combined critical illness polyneuropathy and myopathy	Combined CIP and CIM	Reduced amplitude of compound muscle action potentials and sensory nerve action potentials combined with myopathic features on needle electromyography

Data from [13].

Table 1. Definition and diagnostic criteria of intensive care unit-acquired weakness, critical illness polyneuropathy, critical illness myopathy, and combined critical illness polyneuropathy and myopathy.

2.7. Risk factors

There is an abundance of risk factors related to ICU-AW. In addition to disease severity and ICU length of stay, SIRS, sepsis, multiple organ dysfunction syndrome, female sex, severe asthma attack, electrical and ionic abnormalities, immobilization, malnutrition, central nervous system failure, renal failure, low serum albumin, and vasopressor use have all been correlated with a trend toward more severe neuromuscular dysfunction in critically ill patients.

2.8. Bed rest

Disuse of muscles causes rapid muscle weakness and atrophy. Studies show that following 2 weeks of immobilization, young healthy adults experience a loss of muscle mass of 5–9% in the quadriceps and a decrease of 20–27% in muscle strength. These impacts are often accelerated and more obvious in aging adults, with a 3–6-fold greater rate of muscle wasting [14]. In mechanically ventilated patients, skeletal muscle cross-sectional area can decrease by 12.5% over the first week in the ICU [14].

The harmful impacts of prolonged immobilization on muscle structure and function have long been known. During critical illness, the muscles are always in an unloaded condition due to disease progression, sedation, and mechanical ventilation. This unloaded condition

Skeletal muscle atrophy and weakness
Joint contractures
Thromboembolic disease
Insulin resistance
Microvascular dysfunction
Systemic inflammation
Atelectasis
Pressure ulcers
Data from [17].

Table 2. Complications of bed rest.

impacts not only the limb muscles but also the respiratory muscles, and it leads to muscle atrophy resulting from inactivity and a reduction in myofibril tension [15].

Due to the nature of critical illness, medications (e.g., sedation), and devices (e.g., continuous renal replacement therapy) used in the ICU, patients spend a great amount of time immobilized in bed [16].

However, critically ill patients frequently remain on bed rest for many days to weeks and suffer complications of bed rest (**Tables 2** and **3**). Prolonged bed rest and physical activity restraint can result in ICU-AW, pressure ulcers, lung atelectasis, aspiration pneumonia, bone mineral loss, muscle atrophy, hypotension, tachycardia, and cardiac output decreases, which result in obvious declines in physical function [19].

2.9. Sedation

Many medications used to treat critically ill patients have myopathic effects. Sedatives can exert both direct injurious effects and indirect effects by promoting rest and disuse atrophy. Heavy sedation from some medications such as benzodiazepines, propofol, fentanyl, and morphine is needed in most critical illnesses in order for patients to cooperate with a mechanical ventilator. Sustained neuromuscular blockade should be limited; it is therefore helpful to decrease the dose and duration of NMBD administration, especially in high-risk patients suffering from hepatic or kidney failure. Therapy with NMBDs and steroids for over 48 h increases the risk of acute myopathy, so the duration of their administration should be as short as possible.

Neuromuscular blocking agents and steroids should be managed carefully, and when possible, safe, and clinically sound to do so, a daily interruption of sedation should be cautiously undertaken. Heavy sedation should be adjusted following evidence-based strategies to minimize immobilization. If a patient is agitated and requires a continuous sedative infusion, short-acting titratable agents such as propofol are preferable over benzodiazepines to minimize immobility.

Musculoskeletal
• Decreased muscle protein synthesis
• Muscle atrophy and decrease in lean muscle mass
• Decreased muscle strength
• Decreased exercise capacity
• Connective tissue shortening and joint contractures
• Decreased bone density
• Pressure ulcers
Pulmonary
• Atelectasis
• Pneumonia
• Decreased maximal inspiratory pressure and forced vital capacity
Cardiovascular
• Decreased total cardiac and left ventricular size
• Decreased lower extremity venous compliance
• Orthostatic intolerance
• Decreased cardiac output, stroke volume, and peripheral vascular resistance
• Impaired microvascular function
• Decreased cardiac response to carotid sinus stimulation
Endocrine and metabolism
• Decreased insulin sensitivity
• Decreased aldosterone and plasma renin activity
• Increased atrial natriuretic peptide
Data from [18].

Table 3. Selected adverse effects of prolonged bed rest.

2.10. Sepsis

Infection is a major risk factor for the development of marked diaphragm weakness in mechanically ventilated patients [20]. In patients with sepsis, diaphragm muscle strength has been shown to decrease by an average of 50%. General muscle weakness in sepsis is mediated by cytokines, oxidative stress, and the activation of proteolytic pathways. Sepsis also weakens the body's ability to deliver oxygen and impairs its use at the cellular level, disrupting muscle metabolism and contractile function. Therefore, sepsis enhances muscle membrane fragility, increasing its sensitivity to the damaging effects of loading. The bed rest and immobilization associated with sepsis, however, may intensify the effects of the systemic infection [9].

2.11. Delirium and ICU-AW

Delirium is defined as an acute onset mental disturbance including loss of awareness and cognitive impairment that changes over time. Delirium is a major complication in critical illness as it shows a decompensation of brain function, a sudden brain failure, in response to other pathophysiologic stressors [21].

It occurs in 60–80% of critically ill patients who are receiving mechanical ventilation and in 20–50% of critically ill patients who are not receiving mechanical ventilation [22]. Prevalence rates of delirium in ICU-AW range between 20 and 40%. Hypoactive delirium in particular is correlated with progressive clinical outcomes, such as prolonged mechanical ventilation use, longer ICU and hospital length of stay, increased mortality rates, and cognitive impairment for up to 1 year after discharge [23, 24]. However there is some strategy to prevent delirium (**Table 4**).

2.12. Muscle weakness, nutrition, metabolism in ICU patients

A major concern in patients with critical illness is their inability to fulfill their own nutritional needs, especially when using mechanical ventilation. Observational data show that malnutrition is accompanied by poor outcomes in critical illness, and many providers have assumed that this means that the use of artificial nutrition in these patients improves outcomes, regardless of baseline nutritional status.

Nutritional status is associated with weakness: starvation in healthy volunteers causes loss of muscle mass, strength, and function [8].

Although the practice of providing nutrition to these patients is almost universal, the specifics vary widely from one ICU to another and even among providers.

Nutrition in the intensive care unit remains challenging; patients in the ICU are always treated using a multidisciplinary team approach, and care is determined by the patient's condition, the severity of their disease, and what they need.

However, differences in preferences among care providers increase the variations in opinions related to controversial topics, especially in nutritional support. In critically ill patients,

Components of Henderson's theory	**Bundle components**
Breathe normally	Sedation cessation
Participate in various forms of recreation	Pain management
Communicate with others in expressing emotions, needs, fears, or opinions	Sensory stimulation
Move and maintain desirable positions	Early mobility
Sleep and rest	Sleep promotion

Avoid environmental dangers and injury of others. Data from [22].

Table 4. Components of Henderson's theory that align with components of the delirium prevention bundle.

nasogastric tube feeding is often used due to its simplicity, relatively low cost, and decrease in risk of catheter-induced complications.

Insufficient nutritional support in enterally fed patients remains a global concern; however, as predicted and evaluated, energy insufficiency has been associated with poor outcomes. For the first week following admission to the ICU, most patients experience energy deficits, and these deficits are even more obvious when enteral nutrition is the only available method. Sustained nothing per os (NPO) status in the ICU and the corresponding loss of lean body mass should be at least as relevant as it is for other hospitalized patients.

Inflammation, infection, immobilization, and fatigue may result in noticeable delays in recovery, but a formal evaluation of the 1-year post-hospitalization impact in a large population of critically ill patients has not been completed, although dysfunctional status was found 5 years after an experience of acute respiratory distress syndrome. Overnutrition is more easily identified since many of its impacts are obvious and measurable, such as difficulty weaning from a ventilator, heart disease, and fatty liver disease; other effects of overnutrition, such as increased susceptibility to infection, are difficult to observe. Overnutrition has more often been achieved with parenteral nutrition rather than enteral nutrition. Additionally, overnutrition combined with bed rest has been found to lead to a greater loss of lean body mass.

A variety of metabolic derangements associated with critical illness can exacerbate muscle weakness. Respiratory acidosis, hypercapnia, and hypokalemia contribute to reversible diaphragm weakness, whereas metabolic acidosis seems to have no effect [25]. Hypercapnia can increase ventilator-induced diaphragmatic dysfunction, and hyperglycemia is a significant risk factor for muscle damage. Long-term malnutrition is likened to ICU-AW as a result of a shortage of protein in muscle tissue.

3. Early mobilization in IC

A lack of muscle loading and no contraction are a major cause of muscle damage and weakness, so patient mobilization initiated as soon as possible is necessary to prevent this damage. Patient performance of early mobilization with mechanical ventilation can be feasible and safe. The advantage of passive range of motion exercises should not be ignored, as they can lengthen the muscles when there is no active muscle contraction, leading to significant relief of muscle atrophy [26].

3.1. Safety and feasibility

Immobilization and restraint always occur during a patient's stay in the ICU, leading to the development of some complications, such as physical functional impairment, cognitive dysfunction, and neuromuscular weakness. Early mobilization has been proven to be a feasible, safe, and important preventive measure. Many studies have shown that early mobilization can be performed safely and without adverse events, even when the patient is receiving mechanical ventilation, using an extracorporeal membrane oxygenation device or receiving continuous venovenous hemofiltration [27].

http://dx.doi.org/10.5772/intechopen.89984

System	Starting criteria	Stopping criteria
Cardiovascular	Heart rate: 60–130 beats/min	Heart rate: <60 or >130 beats/min
	Systolic blood pressure, 90–180 mmHg, or mean arterial pressure, 60–100 mmHg	Systolic blood pressure, <90 or >180 mmHg, or mean arterial pressure, <60 or >100 mmHg
Respiratory	Respiratory rate: 5–40 breaths/min	Respiratory rate: <5 or >40 breaths/min
	SpO2 ≥ 88%	SpO2 < 88%
	FiO2 < 0.6	Concerns about the disconnection of the artificial airway
	PEEP <10	
	Artificial airway is properly secured	
Other	Able to open eyes to voice	Changes in consciousness
		New/symptomatic arrhythmia
		Chest pain
		Ventilator asynchrony
		Falling down
		Medical device removal
		Patient intolerance or refusal

SpO2, peripheral capillary oxygen saturation; FiO2, fraction of inspired oxygen; PEEP, positive end-expiratory pressure. Data from [31].

Table 5. Examples of safety criteria for starting and stopping rehabilitation in the intensive care unit.

Early mobilization in the ICU has been advocated as a therapeutic strategy to prevent ICU-AW, reducing the negative effects of immobility on muscles and other organ systems [28]. Mobilization in the ICU is feasible and safe provided that consensus guidelines are followed [29]. The potential incidence of adverse events is low, with a cumulative incidence of 2.6%, a rate of hemodynamic events of 3.8%, and saturation instability of 1.9 per 1000 mobilization sessions. Additionally, medical issues are rare, with one study showing a rate of 0.6% of 14,398 mobilization sessions [30]. Premobilization screening criteria to identify patients for whom rehabilitation is suitable and criteria for discontinuing mobilization should be established for each ICU (**Table 5**).

3.2. Beneficial effects of early mobilization

The current definition of mobilization is the performance of physical activity sufficient to stimulate an acute physiological impact that improves ventilation, circulation, perfusion, muscle metabolism, and alertness and decreases rates of venous stasis and deep vein thrombosis. The present definition of early mobilization refers to physical activity performed within the first 72 h of a critical illness [32].

The evidence of the impact of early mobilization in the ICU continues to increase. ICU physical therapy has also been shown to have a positive impact on patient outcomes, such as functional ability, muscle strength, and ambulation capacity at discharge.

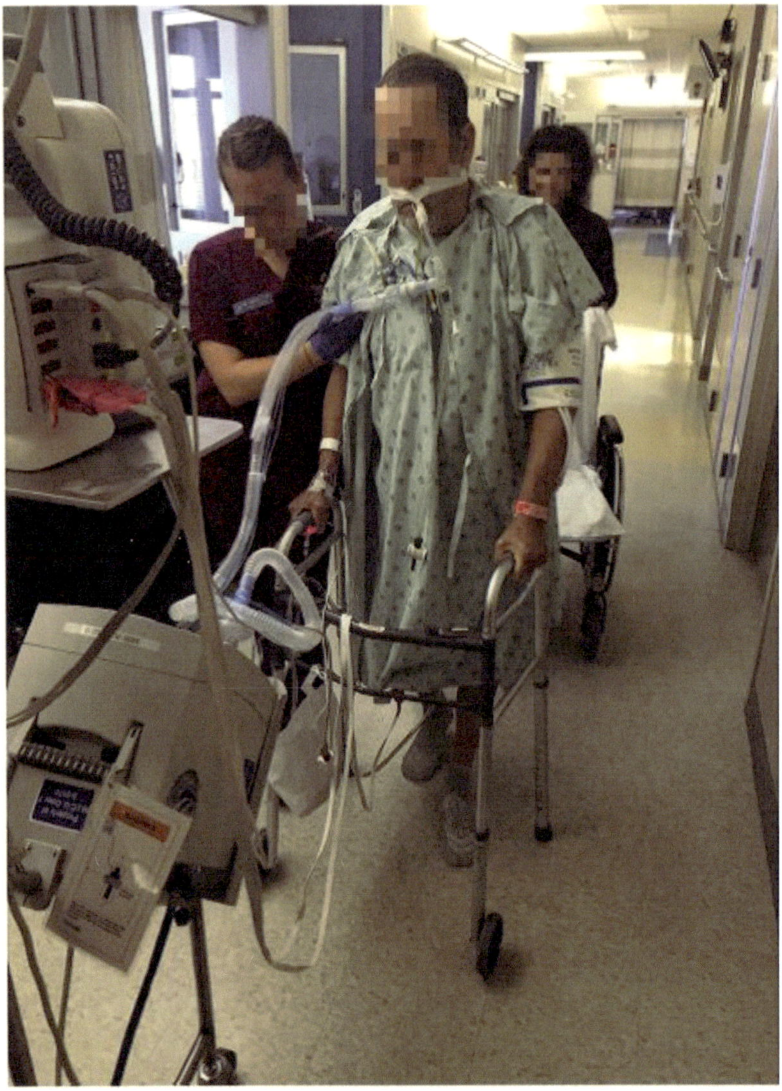

Figure 4. Photo showing a patient receiving mechanical ventilation via an endotracheal tube while ambulating in the ICU with a physical therapist. Data from [14].

Early mobilization in mechanically ventilated critically ill patients is feasible and safe [27, 33, 34] and can decrease duration of mechanical ventilation and intensive care unit length of stay. It is also associated with a shorter duration of delirium, a better functional outcome at hospital discharge, and lower 1-year mortality [35, 36]. Early mobilization has multiple benefits including improved ventilation, perfusion, muscle strength, and functional capacity. Several surveys reporting mobilization therapy practice are published worldwide, and despite all of the reported benefits, the prevalence of early mobilization in ICU patients is still low [37]. Together with other chest physiotherapy modalities, early mobilization can result in a decreased extubation failure rate and shorter durations of mechanical ventilation and ICU stay [38]. **Figure 4** illustrates a patient receiving mechanical ventilation via an ETT and ambulating with a physical therapist in the ICU.

Late initiation may reduce the efficacy of mobilization as the beneficial effects of physical therapy have been found in studies in which the treatment was started early after ICU admission [39]; however, definition of "earliness" remains undefined.

3.3. Special patient groups (ECMO)

Patients undergoing mechanical ventilation or extracorporeal circulation systems such as extracorporeal membrane oxygenation (ECMO) or hemofiltration need particular attention.

The use of ECMO for patients is increasing globally, including in patients with heart or respiratory failure awaiting organ transplantation, and there is an increasing need to assess the safety, feasibility, and functional prognosis regarding the performance of early mobilization in this patient population [40].

Early ICU physiotherapy while on ECMO for ARDS as a bridge to recovery is feasible; Munshi et al. suggest that there may be an association with improved ICU mortality. However, this needs to be further corroborated in future studies. Future research is needed to identify potential barriers, optimal timing, dosage, and safety profile.

4. Barriers and facilitators to mobilization

Although there is a growing base of evidence showing short-term benefits of early mobilization, such as shorter delirium duration, more ventilator-free days, and decreased ICU and hospital LOS, translation into clinical practice remains difficult for this complex intervention. Dubb et al. provided some common barriers that medical staff may encounter regarding early mobilization as well as possible ways to overcome them.

4.1. Cultural barriers

In many medical centers, present ICU culture is a crucial and potentially modifiable barrier to the initiation of ICU physical therapy and early mobilization. However, inadequate care coordination, timing conflicts with different medical procedures, and priorities for treatment are common barriers [41, 42]. Lastly, probably one of the most important barriers to address in implementation of early mobilization is in relation to the culture of the ICU, reported as an obstruction in almost 60% of studies [43]. This encompasses staff not viewing early mobilization as a priority for the patient and/or inadequate knowledge about the benefits of early mobilization and techniques available to implement it at the appropriate level for the patient.

Overcoming these barriers requires a structured multidisciplinary effort, with clear communication and recognition of the importance of early mobilization and rehabilitation [44].

4.2. Sedation

The widespread use of sedation in the ICU can be a major barrier to mobilizing patients who are critically ill. Implementation of early mobilization into practice was however limited, mostly due to sedation practices and clinician's safety concerns. Sedation minimization can be combined with early mobility via implementing the ABCDE bundle [45], in which all patients undergo daily coordinated spontaneous awakening trials, spontaneous breathing trials, sedation and delirium screening, and early mobility and rehabilitation.

4.3. Endotracheal tubes

The presence of an endotracheal tube is another commonly perceived barrier. To assist with overcoming this barrier, Pohlman et al. detailed the steps undertaken to start PT and OT interventions after a median of only 1.5 days of intubation in 49 patients who had undergone endotracheal intubation. There were no catheter-related adverse events [27]. Similar results were obtained in other studies [46, 47].

4.4. Costs

Increased medical staffing needs and costs correlated with early mobilization are commonly recognized barriers. Utilizing a special early mobilization team, Morris et al. did not find an increase in overall costs after accounting for additional costs related to this team, and they also found a significantly reduced risk of readmission or mortality in the year after ICU discharge.

There are multiple facets to ensuring the effective implementation of early mobilization, with interdisciplinary coordination and communication being an integral component (**Table 6**).

Patient-associated factors
• Unstable physiologic stability (cardiovascular, respiratory, neurologic)
• High sedation levels
• Presence of delirium/agitation
• Pain
• Medical limitations (procedures, orders)
Structural issues
• Low staff numbers
• Inexperienced clinical staff
• Deficiency in staff training
• Lack of defined EM programs
Process factors
• Absence of coordinated review for suitability for EM
• No EM leadership
• Poor communication
Cultural factors
• Nonexistent education regarding risks and benefits of EM
• Lack of prioritizing EM in daily care plans
• Deficient knowledge regarding EM techniques and equipment
Data from [48].

Table 6. Barriers to implementation of early mobilization in intensive care unit barrier.

5. Discussion

This chapter shows that early mobilization in the ICU demonstrated benefits on patient outcomes. The intervention improves ventilation, circulation, perfusion, muscle metabolism, and alertness and decreases rates of venous stasis and deep vein thrombosis.

Based on the findings from these reviews, no study has shown any adverse events associated with early mobilization. When safety consensus guidelines are followed and a team approach is used to ensure safety in clinical practice, early mobilization in the ICU may be an appropriate treatment strategy. It is important to recognize that not all potential safety events carry equal clinical importance (e.g., high blood pressure vs. cardiac arrest).

Patient safety is paramount in any exercise intervention. Patients with high illness severity, coma, and/or delirium are particularly vulnerable, and the utmost care must be undertaken during exercise interventions in these high-risk patients. Although many studies have shown that early mobilization is safe and feasible and one study indicated that healthcare professionals are able to identify the benefits associated with early mobilization, only 21% of physicians and 18% of nurses believe that the potential risks outweigh the benefits of early mobilization.

The optimal timing for initiation of mobilization has yet to be defined. ICU-AW can begin within the first 48 h of ICU admission; early mobilization of ICU patients, defined as mobilization within 72 h of ICU admission; and late mobilization as starting after the first 3 days of ICU admission. Other research suggests that early mobilization is currently defined as occurring within the first 2–5 days of ICU admission. Arriving at a definitive definition of early mobilization is difficult because the condition of a patient in the ICU changes daily. Further research is required to provide a conclusive definition of early mobilization.

6. Conclusion

Early mobilization and physical rehabilitation of critically ill patients appears to be safe, with a low risk of potential safety events, even when implemented as part of routine clinical practice. Early mobilization, defined as mobilization within 72 h of ICU admission, is well tolerated and feasible and should be the standard of care. However, implicating early mobilization is arduous and may need a cultural change in intensive care with an interprofessional approach.

Increases in ICU-associated neuromuscular dysfunction are resulting in both short- and long-term physical functional impairments. Bed rest and restraint play a major role in the development of neuromuscular disorders and functional ability impairments, and early mobilization and physical therapy may be able to mitigate these problems. The complete effects of early mobilization in the ICU need to be evaluated using a standardized execution protocol to determine the optimal timing, exercise dosage, and progression of mobilization, as well as determining criteria for the intensity and duration of physical therapy most likely to optimize patients' physical condition during critical illness [49].

Achieving early mobilization in practice requires a shift in unit culture and dedication from mobility champions following individualized procedures and protocols to ensure its safe application.

Author details

Tsung-Hsien Wang[1,2*]

*Address all correspondence to: wth75529@gmail.com

1 School and Graduate Institute of Physical Therapy, College of Medicine, National Taiwan University, Taipei, Taiwan

2 Department of Critical Care Medicine, Landseed International Hospital, Taoyuan, Taiwan

References

[1] Rawal G, Yadav S, Kumar R. Postintensive care syndrome: An overview. Journal of Translational Internal Medicine. 2017;**5**:90-92

[2] Esteban A, Frutos-Vivar F, Muriel A, et al. Evolution of mortality over time in patients receiving mechanical ventilation. American Journal of Respiratory and Critical Care Medicine. 2013;**188**(2):220-230

[3] The ARDS Network. Ketoconazole for early treatment of acute lung injury and acute respiratory distress syndrome: A randomized controlled trial. Journal of the American Medical Association. 2000;**283**(15):1995-2002

[4] Hebert PC, Wells G, Blajchman MA, et al. A multicenter, randomized, controlled clinical trial of transfusion requirements in critical care. Transfusion requirements in critical care investigators, Canadian critical care trials group. The New England Journal of Medicine. 1999;**340**(6):409-417

[5] Girardis M, Busani S, Damiani E, et al. Effect of conservative vs conventional oxygen therapy on mortality among patients in an intensive care unit: The oxygen-ICU randomized clinical trial. Journal of the American Medical Association. 2016;**316**(15):1583-1589

[6] Shehabi Y, Bellomo R, Kadiman S, et al. Sedation intensity in the first 48 hours of mechanical ventilation and 180-day mortality: A multinational prospective longitudinal cohort study. Critical Care Medicine. 2018;**46**(6):850-859

[7] Wischmeyer PE, San-Millan I. Winning the war against ICU-acquired weakness: New innovations in nutrition and exercise physiology. Critical Care. 2015;**19**(Suppl 3):S6

[8] Latronico N, Herridge M, Hopkins RO, et al. The ICM research agenda on intensive care unit-acquired weakness. Intensive Care Medicine. 2017;**43**(9):1270-1281

[9] Schreiber A, Bertoni M, Goligher EC. Avoiding respiratory and peripheral muscle injury during mechanical ventilation: Diaphragm-protective ventilation and early mobilization. Critical Care Clinics. 2018;**34**(3):357-381

[10] Latronico N, Bolton CF. Critical illness polyneuropathy and myopathy: A major cause of muscle weakness and paralysis. Lancet Neurology. 2011;**10**(10):931-941

[11] Pandit L, Agrawal A. Neuromuscular disorders in critical illness. Clinical Neurology and Neurosurgery. 2006;**108**:621-627

[12] De Jonghe B, Cook D, Sharshar T, Lefaucheur JP, Carlet J, Outin H. Acquired neuromuscular disorders in critically ill patients: A systematic review. Intensive Care Medicine. 1998;**24**:1242-1250

[13] Piva S, Fagoni N, Latronico N. Intensive care unit-acquired weakness: Unanswered questions and targets for future research. F1000Research. 2019:8

[14] Hashem MD, Parker AM, Needham DM. Early mobilization and rehabilitation of patients who are critically ill. Chest. 2016;**150**(3):722-731

[15] Tesch PA, Lundberg TR, Fernandez-Gonzalo R. Unilateral lower limb suspension: From subject selection to "omic" responses. Journal of Applied Physiology. 2016;**120**(10):1207-1214

[16] Castro-Avila AC, Seron P, Fan E, Gaete M, Mickan S. Effect of early rehabilitation during intensive care unit stay on functional status: Systematic review and meta-analysis. PLoS One. 2015;**10**(7):e0130722

[17] Brower RG. Consequences of bed rest. Critical Care Medicine. 2009;**37**(10 Suppl):S422-S428

[18] Truong AD, Fan E, Brower RG, Needham DM. Bench-to-bedside review: Mobilizing patients in the intensive care unit—From pathophysiology to clinical trials. Critical Care. 2009;**13**(4):216

[19] Needham DM. Mobilizing patients in the intensive care unit: Improving neuromuscular weakness and physical function. Journal of the American Medical Association. 2008;**300**(14):1685-1690

[20] Demoule A, Jung B, Prodanovic H, et al. Diaphragm dysfunction on admission to the intensive care unit. Prevalence, risk factors, and prognostic impact—A prospective study. American Journal of Respiratory and Critical Care Medicine. 2013;**188**(2):213-219

[21] Pandharipande PP, Ely EW, Arora RC, et al. The intensive care delirium research agenda: A multinational, interprofessional perspective. Intensive Care Medicine. 2017;**43**(9):1329-1339

[22] Smith CD, Grami P. Feasibility and effectiveness of a delirium prevention bundle in critically ill patients. American Journal of Critical Care. 2016;**26**(1):19-27

[23] Salluh JI, Latronico N. Does this critically ill patient with delirium require any drug treatment? Intensive Care Medicine. 2019;**45**(4):501-504

[24] Pandharipande PP, Girard TD, Jackson JC, et al. Long-term cognitive impairment after critical illness. The New England Journal of Medicine. 2013;**369**(14):1306-1316

[25] Michelet P, Carreira S, Demoule A, et al. Effects of acute respiratory and metabolic acidosis on diaphragm muscle obtained from rats. Anesthesiology. 2015;**122**(4):876-883

[26] Griffiths RD, Palmer TE, Helliwell T, MacLennan P, MacMillan RR. Effect of passive stretching on the wasting of muscle in the critically ill. Nutrition. 1995;**11**(5):428-432

[27] Damluji A, Zanni JM, Mantheiy E, Colantuoni E, Kho ME, Needham DM. Safety and feasibility of femoral catheters during physical rehabilitation in the intensive care unit. Journal of Critical Care. 2013;**28**(4):535 e539-515

[28] Denehy L, Lanphere J, Needham DM. Ten reasons why ICU patients should be mobilized early. Intensive Care Medicine. 2017;**43**(1):86-90

[29] Hodgson CL, Stiller K, Needham DM, et al. Expert consensus and recommendations on safety criteria for active mobilization of mechanically ventilated critically ill adults. Critical Care. 2014;**18**(6):658

[30] Nydahl P, Sricharoenchai T, Chandra S, et al. Safety of patient mobilization and rehabilitation in the intensive care unit. Systematic review with meta-analysis. Annals of the American Thoracic Society. 2017;**14**(5):766-777

[31] Devlin JW, Skrobik Y, Gelinas C, et al. Clinical practice guidelines for the prevention and management of pain, agitation/sedation, delirium, immobility, and sleep disruption in adult patients in the ICU. Critical Care Medicine. 2018;**46**(9):e825-e873

[32] Hodgson CL, Berney S, Harrold M, Saxena M, Bellomo R. Clinical review: Early patient mobilization in the ICU. Critical Care. 2013;**17**(1):207

[33] Pires-Neto RC, Kawaguchi YMF, Hirota AS, et al. Very early passive cycling exercise in mechanically ventilated critically ill patients: Physiological and safety aspects-a case series. PLoS One. 2013;**8**(9):e74182

[34] Sricharoenchai T, Parker AM, Zanni JM, Nelliot A, Dinglas VD, Needham DM. Safety of physical therapy interventions in critically ill patients: A single-center prospective evaluation of 1110 intensive care unit admissions. Journal of Critical Care. 2014;**29**(3):395-400

[35] Morris PE, Goad A, Thompson C, et al. Early intensive care unit mobility therapy in the treatment of acute respiratory failure. Critical Care Medicine. 2008;**36**(8):2238-2243

[36] Schweickert WD, Pohlman MC, Pohlman AS, et al. Early physical and occupational therapy in mechanically ventilated, critically ill patients: A randomised controlled trial. Lancet. 2009;**373**(9678):1874-1882

[37] Berney SC, Harrold M, Webb SA, et al. Intensive care unit mobility practices in Australia and New Zealand: A point prevalence study. Critical Care and Resuscitation. 2013;**15**(4):260-265

[38] Wang TH, Wu CP, Wang LY. Chest physiotherapy with early mobilization may improve extubation outcome in critically ill patients in the intensive care units. The Clinical Respiratory Journal. 2018;**12**(11):2613-2621

[39] Schaller S, Nydahl P, Blobner M, et al. What does the EPICC trial really tell us? Thorax. 2018;**73**(3):213-221

[40] Abrams D, Javidfar J, Farrand E, et al. Early mobilization of patients receiving extracorporeal membrane oxygenation: A retrospective cohort study. Critical Care. 2014;**18**(1):R38

[41] Bakhru RN, Wiebe DJ, McWilliams DJ, Spuhler VJ, Schweickert WD. An environmental scan for early mobilization practices in U.S. ICUs. Critical Care Medicine. 2015;**43**(11):2360-2369

[42] Leditschke IA, Green M, Irvine J, Bissett B, Mitchell IA. What are the barriers to mobilizing intensive care patients? Cardiopulmonary Physical Therapy Journal. 2012;**23**(1):26-29

[43] Dubb R, Nydahl P, Hermes C, et al. Barriers and strategies for early mobilization of patients in intensive care units. Annals of the American Thoracic Society. 2016;**13**(5):724-730

[44] Hopkins RO, Spuhler VJ, Thomsen GE. Transforming ICU culture to facilitate early mobility. Critical Care Clinics. 2007;**23**(1):81-96

[45] Morandi A, Brummel NE, Ely EW. Sedation, delirium and mechanical ventilation: The 'ABCDE' approach. Current Opinion in Critical Care. 2011;**17**(1):43-49

[46] Perme C, Lettvin C, Throckmorton TA, Mitchell K, Masud F. Early mobility and walking for patients with femoral arterial catheters in intensive care unit: A case series. Journal of Acute Care Physical Therapy. 2011;**2**(1):32-36

[47] Perme C, Nalty T, Winkelman C, Kenji Nawa R, Masud F. Safety and efficacy of mobility interventions in patients with femoral catheters in the ICU: A prospective observational study. Cardiopulmonary Physical Therapy Journal. 2013;**24**(2):12-17

[48] Paton M, Lane R, Hodgson CL. Early mobilization in the intensive care unit to improve long-term recovery. Critical Care Clinics. 2018;**34**(4):557-571

[49] Needham DM, Sepulveda KA, Dinglas VD, et al. Core outcome measures for clinical research in acute respiratory failure survivors. An international modified Delphi consensus study. American Journal of Respiratory and Critical Care Medicine. 2017;**196**(9):1122-1130

Section 5

Physical Therapy Interventions Associated with Chronic Clinical Conditions

Chapter 10

Increased Physical Activity in a Public Health Perspective

Hilde D.G. Nielsen

Additional information is available at the end of the chapter

http://dx.doi.org/10.5772/intechopen.89526

Abstract

Human beings are born to be physically active. Being physically active gives several advantages and is essential for a healthy life. Physical inactivity is to date one of the major risk factors for developing non-communicable diseases (NCD), which are responsible for nearly 70% of all deaths. It is well documented in the literature that daily physical activity reduces the risk of non-communicable diseases NCDs. The level of physical activity differs between regions of the world and between the countries. Moreover, there are age and gender differences. WHOs Global action plan on Physical Activity and Health 2018–2030 and the UN Sustainable Goal are an important document and blueprint in the work for promoting a healthier world with reduced physical inactivity. Global action plans must be translated into national needs and adapted according to local variations. Successful implementation can only be achieved with anchoring of the strategies and policies at the top and within all sectors. Prioritization of actions and cooperation are also important factors for successful implementation. Work with the aim of increasing physical activity is intersectoral. Every sector is influenced, and no sector can disclaim liability. Physical inactivity is a global, increasing public health problem, and it will not disappear by itself.

Keywords: physical activity, physical inactivity, effects of physical activity, non-communicable diseases, policies and strategies, trends globally, gender differences

1. Introduction

Non-communicable diseases (NCDs), also known as chronic diseases, are diseases of long duration and are consequences of a combination of genetic, physiological, environmental, and behavioral factors. The rise of NCDs heart disease, stroke, cancer, diabetes, and chronic

IntechOpen

© 2019 The Author(s). Licensee IntechOpen. This chapter is distributed under the terms of the Creative Commons Attribution License (http://creativecommons.org/licenses/by/3.0), which permits unrestricted use, distribution, and reproduction in any medium, provided the original work is properly cited.

lung disease has been driven primarily by four major risk factors: tobacco use, alcohol use, physical inactivity, and unhealthy diets [1].

Physical inactivity is a public health problem and is considered as one of the greatest challenges for the future [1]. The time we spend being physically active during leisure is not enough to compensate for the great reduction in everyday physical activity and the increase of sedentary activities associated with life of today. The negative consequences of inactivity are many; physical, mental, and social. For example, inactive people are more likely to be overweight, and inactivity causes many redundant deaths each year [2].

Physical activity is described as any bodily movement produced by skeletal muscles, which requires energy expenditure [3]. It is well documented that regular physical activity reduces the risk of the non-communicable diseases like hypertension [4], coronary heart disease [5], stroke [4], diabetes 2 [6], some cancer types [2], and mental illness [2]. Being physically active improves bone and functional health [7] and maintains energy balance and weight control [8].

There exist large differences in physical activity between the different geographic regions of the world. In 2016, more than a quarter of the world's adults (27%) were insufficiently physically active. In the period between 2001 and 2016, the prevalence of insufficient physical activity ranged from 16% in Oceania to 39% in Latin America and the Caribbean [9]. During the same period, the frequency of physical inactivity increased more than 5% in high-income Western countries, while southeast Asia had a decrease of physical inactivity with 5% [9]. In 2016, insufficient physical activity in high-income countries was more than double compared to the prevalence in low-income countries. The prevalence increased over time in high-income countries from 32% in 2001 to 37% in 2016, whereas it was stable in low-income countries, 6% in 2001 and 2016 [9].

In addition to difference in physical activity levels between regions, there are also differences between genders. Women were less physically active compared to men in all regions except the east and southeast Asia. The lowest levels of reported physical inactivity were observed in men from the regions Oceania, east and southeast Asia, and sub-Saharan Africa in 2016 [9].

This chapter consists of seven sections. First, a short introduction of physical activity, physical inactivity, non-communicable diseases, and some regions and gender differences related to physical activity. Second, a description of global health determinants of physical activity is given. Third, follows a section describing the importance of anchoring and cooperation of policy documents for promoting physical activity. Subsequently follows two sections, one describing the benefits of being physically active and one describing the consequences of physical inactivity. Finally, some reflections of necessary actions to increase the level of physical activity are outlined.

2. Global determinants of physical activity

Since the nineteenth century, there has been a steep increase in the knowledge of exercise and its effects on health. We have a large number of journals and books with quality research within the field. The main challenge today is the never-ending work of how to use the results of the research in line with the major changes in the society that do not inherently promote increased physical activity. We know it is important to be physically active, but we have not managed to decrease the negative trend of increased inactivity globally. The health effects of physical activity are the same all over the world, but the local society in which the activity (or no activity) is performed is continuously developing.

2.1. Increased number of older inactive persons

Older adults are more physically inactive compared to younger adults, and this is a major public health concern [10]. Not only is physical inactivity identified as the fourth leading risk factor for global mortality [11], but is it also a major contributing factor for disability and poor health outcomes [12]. Lack of physical activity is related to approximately 3 million deaths per year and to 6–10% of the occurrence of major non-communicable diseases [13]. Older adults have a more sedentary lifestyle [5]. Rates of self-reported physical inactivity in those aged 55 years and older varied from 5 to 29% across Europe [14].

2.2. Increased urbanization and decreased physical activity

Urbanization leads to more violence, traffic, low air quality, and increased pollution. Many places lack access to parks and free sports and recreation areas. It seems that increased urban living discourage physical activity. Assah et al. found that living in an urban area was associated with lower levels of energy expenditure from physical activity and a higher prevalence of metabolic syndrome compared to rural dwelling adults in Cameroon [15]. Similar differences in physical activity were found in urban versus rural dwelling minors in the United States [16] and female adolescents in Portugal [17]. Other studies [18, 19] have demonstrated no or an inverse relationship between physical activity and the degree of urbanization.

2.3. Modernization leads to less physical activity

Mechanization is the process of replacing manual labor with machinery. New technology improves task efficiency, personal safety, and mobility. On the other hand, technology decreases the physical effort required for self-transport and the performance of occupational and domestic activities. Mechanization and automatization contribute to less physical activity levels even in those cases where equivalent physical activity during the spare time place was equal [11].

2.4. Large variations in women's physical activity level globally

There are large differences in women's level of physical activity in different countries. Women in Uganda are active during domestic work or house chores, farming, tending shops or small businesses, active transport to church, markets, and gardens [11, 20]. In comparison, only 34% of the women in Norway meet the national recommendation of physical activity [21]. Women living in countries with high gender equality were more likely to be physically active compared to their counterparts living in countries with low gender equality. This phenomenon is the same for men. Some of the barriers to physical exercise that women face include family responsibilities, as well as cultural or social beliefs, economic or employment status, and level of education.

2.5. Climate change influences physical activity habits

Climate change affects physical activity habits. Extreme cold, heat, and rain lead to less physical activity [22]. On the other hand, increasing temperature in places which are affected by cold climate may over time increase the level of physical activity. The challenges with increased physical inactivity occur in locations which already experience high temperatures [22] and which already have overwhelming problems with population health. Climate change with global warming will play a growing role on physical activity levels in the future [22, 23].

3. Policy strategies for promoting physical activity

A policy consists of a set of ideas or a plan of what to do in situations that have been agreed to officially by a group of people, a government, or a political party. Today there exist several policies for promoting physical activity. A key factor for successful policy or a strategy document for promoting increased physical activity is cross-sectorial anchoring. Compared to earlier times in which the focus has been to generate as much knowledge as possible on the physiological health effects of being physical active, especially within the health sector, the focus now is how to implement the knowledge cross-sectional. The health sector is not the only sector responsible for physical activity. To increase the level of physical activity in the cities, there must be room for establishing green lounges and making bicycle roads and paths for the pedestrians (collaboration between the sectors transport, climate, and finance). Children should learn how to make the active choices and why we must be physically active at school from educated personnel (collaboration between the sectors health, knowledge, and education). Buildings must be adapted to the possibility of being active (collaboration between architecture and health). It should not be necessary to search for stairs and get the feeling that things are cumbersome, and the autowalks could, for example, keep as slow speed as possible which will lead more of us to walk. Every workplace that is affected by restructuring and mechanization should introduce the possibility of being physically active at work (collaboration between the sectors labor, health, and finance). A universal design for increased physical activity should be in focus in every sector.

In 2004, the 57th World Health Assembly (WHA) endorsed the World Health Organization's (WHO) Global Strategy on Diet, Physical Activity and Health. The strategy was developed with all concerned stakeholders in response to a request from Member States at World Health Assembly 2002 (Resolution WHA55.23). The strategy is followed up with the WHO Global action plan on Physical Activity and Health 2018–2030: more active people for a healthier world, which was launched in 2018. The global aim is to reduce physical inactivity across the globe by 10% by 2025 and 30% by 2030, setting out a plan with four objectives and 20 recommended policy actions.

UN Sustainable Goal was decided by the member countries in 2015. The Sustainable Development Goals are a call for action by all countries – low, high, and middle-income. Actions for healthy life through physical activity are to be found in Goal 3, where the aim is to ensure healthy lives and promoting the well-being at all ages.

At the national level, there is a need for a scale-up of implementations of effective policies in all countries. Implementation of national plans requires bold leadership and full engagement across sectors. The advantages with collaboration which support increased physical activity across sectors is that it generates significant returns through policies which support increased physical activity also leads to other benefits to health, local economies, community wellbeing, and environmental sustainability.

For both global and national strategies, it is difficult to keep up the efforts of increasing physical activity all the time, but in the long run, this should be part of all planning. It is time consuming and resource demanding to integrate the promotion of physical activity between various sectors, and very often one area will lose in the battle with other sectors' needs. For example, resources for in-hospital treatment or building a motor road may often be more available that for public health initiatives.

4. Why being physically active is so important

Good health and quality of life are important for the individual. The health and quality of life of the population have an impact on social development and are themselves influenced by how society changes. Good living conditions, good health, quality of life, and well-being are inter-linked.

Children who are physically active have a number of health benefits during their whole life [24]. Children who are not physical active from early age will not have these benefits and it might be difficult to catch up with it later in life. With a generally decreasing level of physical activity [25], parents or other people who are in daily contact with children are responsible for stimulating to develop positive exercise habits among children. Physical activity is crucial for children to achieve normal growth and development of muscle strength and motor skills [24] and it is of great importance to the skeleton. Weight-bearing activities, such as running, jumping, and walking, all influence the skeleton in a positive way. Physical activity strengthens the skeleton in the same way as exercise strengthens the muscles. A passive lifestyle leads to thin bones, low mineral content, and reduced strength [2]. Bone structure is completely developed when you are 20 years old. This means you can never compensate for what you did not do before turning 20.

Being in good shape results in using less energy to execute various activities. Consequently, fit persons have more excess energy and can do more things in everyday life. Adults and elderly people who are physically active and in good physical shape will also to a greater extent be self-reliant in everyday life and stay home longer. The fitness decreases with age, but the effects of cardiovascular exercise (aerobe) are the same in healthy elderly as in younger ones. The body's muscle mass decreases as you get older, and this leads to reduced muscle strength, but it is never too late to start being physically active. People who start exercising in adulthood have much to gain. Positive gains start already at very low training volumes, which mean small efforts make a big difference. Going beyond such very low training volumes, there is a clear connection between the time you spend on physical activity and the fitness.

5. Consequences of physical inactivity

A hundred years ago, the main task for the public health work was to stop the infection diseases. Today, public health work is more focused on reducing the incidence of the non-infectious lifestyle diseases. Compared to earlier times, more people are being diagnosed with cardiovascular diseases, diabetes, chronic lung diseases, and cancer as a result of multiple factors such as tobacco use, unhealthy diet, physical inactivity, and alcohol use.

NCDs kill about 41 million people each year, equivalent to 70% of all deaths globally [1]. Fifteen millions of all deaths attributed to NCDs occur between the ages of 30 and 69 years. An estimation is that over 85% of the 15 million deaths occur in low- and middle-income countries [1]. Social inequality is still a challenge.

The economic burden of physical inactivity remains unquantified at the global level, although some estimates have been made. Ding et al. reported, based on data from 142 countries, representing 93% of the population of the world, that direct health-care costs for coronary heart disease, stroke, type 2 diabetes, breast cancer, and colon cancer attributable to physical inactivity amounts to $ 53.8 billion worldwide in 2013, of which $31.2 billion was paid by the public sector, $12.9 billion by the private sector, and $9.7 billion by households. High-income countries bear a larger proportion of the economic burden (80.8% of health-care costs and 60.4% of indirect costs) [26]. Physical inactivity related deaths contribute to $13.7 billion in productivity losses worldwide [26].

6. How to increase the level of physical activity in all ages

The challenge today is that in many cases we do not need to be physically active to survive in our work and leisure. Activities that we earlier needed for surviving, for example, hunting and collecting food, are replaced with, that is, driving cars, sitting on a bus or a train or even standing still in an escalator. The ordinary daily life activities are no longer enough to keep us healthy, but the resulting inactive lifestyle leads to several health problems.

Children are more inactive compared to earlier. Eighty percent of the young population in Europe does not reach the minimum recommended amounts of physical activity [4]. Adults are more inactive compared to earlier. We get a situation with inactive children, an increasing number of adults with a less healthy lifestyle, along with an increasing number of elderly people who needs health and care services. This is a growing problem that can be difficult to handle if we do not address it actively.

Kindergarten and schools have a great opportunity to contribute developing a healthy lifestyle, but this requires focus and priority from the national government in the form of resources and financing. The education training for teachers and other personnel that work with children is also an important arena for providing the personnel with the right knowledge. Developing a healthy lifestyle is a lifelong trip. It is not enough to be physically active occasionally, and we must be physically active every day without the feeling that we are doing something extra. We must learn to choose to walk the stairs again and again rather than standing in an escalator, we must, when it is possible, choose to walk to the shop or school rather than driving a car. We must learn to take the physically active choices. And if we do not do this, the negative consequences will escalate.

The workplace is a good arena for either influencing adults to being active during a workday or giving the workers an arena for being active [27]. Examples exist in which the workplace gives room for physical activity during the work time [27, 28]. It might seem unnecessary and expensive right away, but in a long term, it is the right priority, which will be expressed through less absence at work and a more efficient workforce that creates more values for the company.

The retired population should have access to society-based actions from the government for being active, for example, open activity in parks, meeting centers for elderly, etc. Smart cities must facilitate free physical activity, which will give us a large population in good physically health and with a strong mental health.

Future society must be built on how we can be physical active. In every plan for building roads for traffic, a plan for establishing bicycling road and pavement should be included. For every area which will be used for automatized vehicles, there should be made a room for recreation and sport. This is difficult to manage in geographic areas with a large population density.

7. Methods for registering of physical activity

There are several methods for measuring level of physical activity. Each method works according to the purpose of the method, but it is difficult to compare data when comparing level of physical activity between groups, countries, regions, and between gender. For example, when comparing countries, there is a large difference in reported number of the fraction of a population that meets recommendations for physical activity. These numbers depend on how you define and operationalize the recommendations, as well as how data are collected and processed.

The most common method for registering physical activity is questionnaires [29]. Among the several hundred variants which are available, the easiest way is to ask about a person's exercise habits and grade the answers. A more demanding questionnaire contains more concrete questions about what the persons have been doing and for how long time the activity was executed. International Physical Activity Questionnaire (IPAQ) was developed in 2000 [30] and is used to classify individuals into different activity categories described in the recommendation for physical activity.

Diaries are often used when the aim is to measure how the activity is distributed through a day. Diaries give information about the persons' state and what has been done [29].

Pedometer gives a rough measure of the activity and is particularly suited in combination with activity enhancing tools. In this way, people can follow the activity development themselves by getting direct feedback.

Acceleration is a direct measure of body movement, and the higher the acceleration, the higher the intensity. In addition to the total physical activity, an accelerometer can also measure the intensity, duration, and frequency, that is, the pattern of the activity. Another advantage of an accelerometer is that it can assess inactivity and sedentary behavior. However, an accelerometer is more expensive than a pedometer, but it is preferable if high precision is needed.

There is a need for standardized methods and harmonization of data from different countries. There is also a lack of data from low- and middle-income countries, which would be very useful for making better comparisons and analyses between different types of countries.

8. Summary

Physical activity every day is essential for a long healthy life. Physical activity is an important element in the fight against non-communicable diseases. It is never too late to start being physically active. Being physically active must be integrated in our daily life from walking age to end of life. This will be beneficial for each and one of us, but also for the society as a whole.

Public health work must facilitate good health for all and contribute to less social inequalities in health. One of the hallmarks of public health work is the cross-sectoral effort and understanding of how important it is that the entire society makes an effort to influence factors that promote health and well-being. Private actors and volunteers must collaborate with public authorities. Efficient public health work entails good organization of work, a system for monitoring efforts, and developments in health status and risk factors. This applies both at national, municipal, and county level.

Public health work is demanding. It is demanding to try to make people change their lifestyle and living habits (stop smoking, being physically active, etc.), because it is hard to make the population understand that it is necessary.

Preventive public health work does not give the results right away, and it is a slow job, which needs to be prioritized by the governments. Public health work is not free, but it is cheaper compared to treat everybody who in the future will be diagnosed with a chronic disease. It is never too late to turn this negative trend.

Physical activity should be something we do without thinking that we are physically active. Many people do not like to exercise or to be physically active, and because the daily life for most people does not require physical activity, the challenge is to integrate the activity naturally in our lives. Being physically active does not demand new shoes, new clothes, or any other fancy equipment. It must be a natural part of what we are.

Teachers, health care personnel, and other personnel who are in daily contact with people should be educated in the importance of physical activity. Knowledge about the effects and how to put together an activity program must be mandatory in the relevant educations. Efforts for preventive public health work must increase, along with the social status of preventive workers. Preventive health care is not something that can be addressed with medicine or a single treatment. Preventive public health work starts with children and adolescents and lasts throughout their lives. It is a continuous work. In the long term, the work will pay off and produce results in terms of fewer diagnosed with non-communicable diseases.

There is a need for data regarding levels of physical activity, especially data from low- and middle-income countries. Obtaining data from all countries are essential for tailoring global physical activity promotion to population specific needs/trends.

Author details

Hilde D.G. Nielsen

Address all correspondence to: hildegnielsen@outlook.com

The Research Council of Norway, Norway

References

[1] WHO. Noncommunicable Diseases. 2018

[2] Booth FW, Roberts CK, Laye MJ. Lack of exercise is a major cause of chronic diseases. Comprehensive Physiology. 2012;**2**(2):1143-1211

[3] Caspersen CJ, Powell KE, Christenson GM. Physical activity, exercise, and physical fitness: Definitions and distinctions for health-related research. Public Health Reports. 1985;**100**(2):126-131

[4] Pescatello LS, Franklin BA, Fagard R, Farquhar WB, Kelley GA, Ray CA, et al. Exercise and hypertension. Medicine and Science in Sports and Exercise. 2004;**36**(3):533-553

[5] Exercise and Acute Cardiovascular Events. Placing the risks into perspective. Medicine and Science in Sports and Exercise. 2007;**39**(5):886-897

[6] Colberg SR, Fernhall B, Regensteiner JG, Blissmer BJ, Rubin RR, Chasan-Taber L, et al. Exercise and type 2 diabetes: American College of Sports Medicine and the American Diabetes Association joint position statement. Medicine and Science in Sports and Exercise. 2010;**42**(12):2282-2303

[7] Kohrt WM, Bloomfield SA, Little KD, Nelson ME, Yingling VR. Physical activity and bone health. Medicine and Science in Sports and Exercise. 2004;**36**(11):1985-1996

[8] Donnely JE, Blair SN, Jakicic JM, Manore MM, Rankin JW, Snith BK. Appropriate physical activity intervention strategies for weight loss and prevention of weight regain for adults. Medicine and Science in Sports and Exercise. 2009;**41**(2):459-471

[9] Guthold R, Stevens GA, Riley LM, Bull FC. Worldwide trends in insufficient physical activity from 2001 to 2016: A pooled analysis of 358 population-based surveys with 1.9 million participants. The Lancet Global Health. 2018;**6**(10):e1077-e1e86

[10] Tiedemann A, Hassett L, Sherrington C. A novel approach to the issue of physical inactivity in older age. Preventive Medicine Reports. 2015;**2**:595-597

[11] WHO. Global Recommendations on Physical Activity for Health. 2010

[12] Peterson MJ, Giuliani C, Morey MC, Pieper CF, Evenson KR, Mercer V, et al. Physical activity as a preventative factor for frailty: The health, aging, and body composition study. The Journals of Gerontology: Series A. 2009;**64A**(1):61-68

[13] Lim SS, Vos T, Flaxman AD, Danaei G, Shibuya K, Adair-Rohani H, et al. A comparative risk assessment of burden of disease and injury attributable to 67 risk factors and risk factor clusters in 21 regions, 1990-2010: A systematic analysis for the global burden of disease study 2010. Lancet. 2012;**380**(9859):2224-2260

[14] Gomes M, Figueiredo D, Teixeira L, Poveda V, Paúl C, Santos-Silva A, et al. Physical inactivity among older adults across Europe based on the SHARE database. Age and Ageing. 2016;**46**(1):71-77

[15] Assah FK, Ekelund U, Brage S, Mbanya JC, Wareham NJ. Urbanization, physical activity, and metabolic health in sub-Saharan Africa. Diabetes Care. 2011;**34**(2):491-496

[16] Springer AE, Hoelscher DM, Kelder SH. Prevalence of physical activity and sedentary behaviors in US high school students by metropolitan status and geographic region. Journal of Physical Activity & Health. 2006;**3**(4):365-380

[17] Machado-Rodrigues AM, Coelho ESMJ, Mota J, Padez C, Martins RA, Cumming SP, et al. Urban-rural contrasts in fitness, physical activity, and sedentary behaviour in adolescents. Health Promotion International. 2014;**29**(1):118-129

[18] Robertson MC, Song J, Taylor WC, Durand CP, Basen-Engquist KM. Urban-rural differences in aerobic physical activity, muscle strengthening exercise, and screen-time sedentary behavior. The Journal of Rural Health. 2018;**34**(4):401-410

[19] Trivedi T, Liu J, Probst J, Merchant A, Jhones S, Martin AB. Obesity and obesity-related behaviors among rural and urban adults in the USA. Rural and Remote Health. 2015;**15**(4):3267

[20] Guwatudde D, Kirunda BE, Wesonga R, Mutungi G, Kajjura R, Kasule H, et al. Physical activity levels among adults in Uganda: Findings from a countrywide cross-sectional survey. Journal of Physical Activity and Health. 2016;**13**(9):938-945

[21] Fysisk aktivitet og sedat tid blant voksne og eldre i Norge - Nasjonal kartlegging 2014-2015. Norwegian

[22] Obradovich N, Fowler JH. Climate change may alter human physical activity patterns. Nature Human Behaviour. 2017;**1**:0097

[23] Townsend M, Mahoney M, Jones JA, Ball K, Salmon J, Finch CF. Too hot to trot? Exploring potential links between climate change, physical activity and health. Journal of Science and Medicine in Sport. 2003;**6**(3):260-265

[24] American College of Sports Medicine. Physical Activity in Children and Adolescents. 2015

[25] Garber CE, Blissmer B, Deschenes MR, Franklin BA, Lamonte MJ, Lee IM, et al. American College of Sports Medicine position stand. Quantity and quality of exercise for developing and maintaining cardiorespiratory, musculoskeletal, and neuromotor fitness in apparently healthy adults: Guidance for prescribing exercise. Medicine and Science in Sports andEexercise. 2011;**43**(7):1334-1359

[26] Ding D, Lawson KD, Kolbe-Alexander TL, Finkelstein EA, Katzmarzyk PT, van Mechelen W, et al. The economic burden of physical inactivity: A global analysis of major non-communicable diseases. Lancet. 2016;**388**(10051):1311-1324

[27] Forum WHO. Preventing noncommunicable diseases in the workplace through diet and physical activity: WHO/World Economic Forum report of a joint event. Genova; 2008

[28] Abdin S, Welch RK, Byron-Daniel J, Meyrick J. The effectiveness of physical activity interventions in improving well-being across office-based workplace settings: A systematic review. Public Health. 2018;**160**:70-76

[29] Welk GJ. Physical Activity Assessments for Health-Related Research. Human Kinetics. US; 2002

[30] Bassett DR Jr. International physical activity questionnaire: 12-country reliability and validity. Medicine and Science in Sports and Exercise. 2003;**35**(8):1396

Chapter 11

Extracorporeal Shock Wave Therapy in Chronic Wound Care

Simona Maria Carmignano

Additional information is available at the end of the chapter

http://dx.doi.org/10.5772/intechopen.89592

Abstract

Chronic wounds are wounds, which failed healing and timely reparative process to produce anatomic and functional integrity over a period of 3 months. New physical therapy for chronic wounds is extracorporeal shock wave therapy (ESWT). ESWT generators can be focused, defocused, and radial. ESWT is non-invasiveness, low-associated complication rates, efficacy for indications refractory to other standards of practice, and cost-effectiveness. ESWT determines mechanotransduction that is possible as most of the cells of the body, thank to surface receptors and other transmission signals. In the specific field of ESWT, different biochemical substances are able to influence the processes of different cell lineages, besides to induce the formation of new small blood vessels. So, ESWT enhanced cell proliferation at the local wound tissue level, stimulated extracellular matrix metabolism, decreased apoptosis, and downregulated oxygen-mediated burst of leukocytes, probably stimulating homing and differentiation of stem cells with high tissue regenerating potential. From numerous experimental and clinical data, it is possible to conclude that ESWT would improve not only the wounds healing process but also the regeneration events.

Keywords: extracorporeal shock wave therapy, wound healing, chronic wound, regenerative medicine

1. Introduction

Chronic wounds are defined as wounds, which failed healing and timely reparative process to produce anatomic and functional integrity over a period of 3 months [1].

All wounds beyond their etiological origin such as venous or arterial insufficiency or diabetes can be potentially chronic. The transition from an acute to a chronic wound injury can occur at any stage of his recovery [2–4].

IntechOpen

© 2019 The Author(s). Licensee IntechOpen. This chapter is distributed under the terms of the Creative Commons Attribution License (http://creativecommons.org/licenses/by/3.0), which permits unrestricted use, distribution, and reproduction in any medium, provided the original work is properly cited. (cc) BY

Clinical treatment includes wound bed preparation with surgical and nonsurgical debridement [5], application of specialized dressings providing the wound with a moist environment [6], and medical or surgical intervention to achieve adequate vascular inflow and outflow and sufficient offloading to avoid pressure necrosis [7]. A relatively new physical therapy application for chronic wounds is represented by extracorporeal shock wave therapy (ESWT) [8]. Other approaches include hyperbaric oxygen therapy (HBOT) [9, 10], vacuum-assisted wound closure [11–13], low level laser therapy [14, 15], and electrical stimulation [16].

2. ESWT and chronic wound healing

Nowadays, in clinical practice, three different types of ESW generators are available, equipped with different types of sources, and they can also be differentiated as: focused, defocused, and radial. Focused ESWT is generated by electromagnetic, electro-hydraulic, and piezoelectric sources [17–20].

Pressure pulses rise rapidly in the range of 10–100 MegaPascal Pressure (MPa) and concentrate the acoustic energy beam with a penetration depth of approximately 12 cm. A metallic half-ellipsoid-shape reflector focused the almost spherical acoustic waves, which has been generated in the first focal point of ellipsoid directly to a second focal pit that is the therapeutic target [21, 22].

ESWT defocused produces an acoustic planar wave, generated by electromagnetic and electrohydraulic devices. These applicators use a parabolic reflector that generates a parallel wave with a diameter size of the reflector in order to apply the shock waves to a larger area [23, 24]. Radial waves (rSW) are a low-to-medium-energy shock wave (less than 0.1 mJ/mm^2) generated through the acceleration of a projectile pneumatically propelled inside a barrel in the handpiece of the device. The high kinetic energy is transferred directly to the skin, on which the applicator is directly placed, and then transmitted radially (hence the expression "radial waves") to the target zone [25], scattering and dampening by the third power of the penetration depth in the tissue while deepening up to 3.5 cm, without focusing the shock wave field in the tissue.

Compared with the conventional focused shock wave—whose focus is centered on the target site instead of on the tip of the applicator and whose wave shows a higher peak and a very short rise in pressure—the radial shock wave differs for the centering of the focus (placed on the tip of the applicator instead of on the target site) and the shape of the waves themselves (showing a lower peak pressure and a very long rise), and the propagation is limited to the most superficial (but larger) areas of the body [26].

3. ESWT and basic science: mechanotransduction and modulation of gene transcription

Therapeutic efficacy of low-energy defocused ESWT on delayed healing or chronic wounds has been demonstrated in experimental studies and clinical trials [27]. Advantages of ESWT, compared with other therapeutic interventions, include non-invasiveness, associated complication rates, efficacy of indications refractory to other standards of practice, and cost-effectiveness [28].

ESWT determines the mechanotransduction that is a complex process characterized by several steps: (1) transduction of mechanical forces in receptors detected by signals on cells, (2) conversion of mechanical signal into electrical and biochemical messages for obtaining a cellular response, cytoplasmic level, (3) transfer of a signal from the sensor to effectors molecules, in nucleus, and finally (4) biological changes determined by gene activation. It is a biological mechanism that involves numerous cells and organs [29–31]: for example, endothelial cells respond to shear stress stimulation, but also others as tenocytes, bone cells, and fibroblasts.

ESWT induces production of different biochemical substances that are able to influence the processes of different cell lineages, besides to induce the formation of new small blood vessels [32].

In fact, a lot of studies showed how ESWT is effective in stimulating several endogenous growth factors such as epidermal growth factor, insulin-like growth factor 1, vascular endothelial growth factor (VEGF), and (nitric oxide) NO production, inducing angiogenesis and promoting the healing of tendons, muscles, cartilage, bone and skin, fractures, ulcers, and complex lesions [33, 34].

Angiogenesis is one of the basic conditions for supporting healing processes in the different affected tissues. Structural mechanical stress, induced by ESWT changes in cytoskeleton and increase in NOS activity and VEGF-A expression, acts as an angiogenesis process. Furthermore in vitro, it modulates the release of anti-inflammatory cytokine (IL1, IL-6, and IL10) and transforming growth factor 1TGF1-VEGF, that promote the migration of macrophages, fibroblasts, and epithelial cells, enhancing collagen deposition into the damaged area [35–40].

Furthermore, if applied in multiple ESWT treatments, it was possible to obtain active degradation of the fibrous abnormal tissues, thanks to a synergistic modifications in pro- and anti-fibrotic proteins (TGF-β1 and matrix metalloproteinase 2, respectively), thus underlining a possible role in fibrotic tissue reabsorption/remodeling [41, 42].

ESWT influences the toll-like receptor 3 (TLR3) pathway [43], which plays a fundamental role in pathogen recognition and activation of innate immunity, so ESWT modulates the inflammatory responses related to immunology pathway [44–49].

The most recent and relevant ESWT evidence is the effect on modulation of gene expression, thus increasing the possibility of a regenerative action.

In animal models, ESWT has been shown to produce favorable molecular microenvironment in the wound tissue, suppress early pro-inflammatory cytokines and chemokines, and enhance expression of several wound healing relevant genes [46, 50, 51].

ESWT increases the Platelet-Cell Adhesion Molecule-1 (PECAM-1) production on leukocytes and on endothelial cells, which mediate a physical link between the cell surface and the nuclear envelope, and it is critically involved in the trans-endothelial migration processes at inflammatory sites, endothelial cell migration, and formation of new blood vessels. This may transmit mechanical or biochemical signals that may modulate the genetic expression of cells [50, 52]. Furthermore, PECAM-1 is not only involved in cell adhesion but also is intimately involved in signaling, for example, by binding and modulating nuclear/cytoplasmatic β catenin localization. At the membrane, β-catenin forms complexes with E-cadherin to generate cell adhesion complexes responsible for maintaining the structural integrity of many epithelial tissues. On the other hand, accumulation of β-catenin in the nucleus, in response to Wnt signaling pathways (a group of signal transduction pathways, made of proteins that pass signals into a cell through cell surface receptors), facilitates complex formation with T cell-specific (TCF) transcription factors. TCF leads to activation of a genetic program influencing a range of cellular processes, as cell growth and cell movement [53, 54] (**Figure 1**).

ESWT indirect effect on modulation of gene transcription has been found to include expression of c-Myc gene, regulation of metalloproteinase matrilysin (the smallest member of metalloproteinase enzymes), modulation of the activating protein-1 (AP-1) transcription complex, particularly cc-Jun and Fra-1 components that are essential for MMP-1 gene expression, urokinase-type plasminogen activator receptor, zonula occludens-1 (ZO-1) protein, and cyclin D1 [55].

In vivo shock wave treatment increases Ras-dependent superoxide, which in turn regulated cytosolic extracellular regulated kinase (ERK) phosphorylation and hypoxia-inducible factor-1a transactivation, which is considered as the master transcriptional regulator of cellular and developmental response to hypoxia [56].

ESWT treatment upregulates expression of cell nuclear antigen (PCNA), which is important for both DNA synthesis and repair; furthermore, it increases TGF genes (mRNA) [57].

TGF α is predominantly expressed in keratinocytes and has a profound autocrine mitogenic effect on keratinocytes, augments angiogenesis in wound healing, and it is upregulated in keratinocytes after skin injuries; TGFβ 1 mRNA shows higher values in ESW-treated fibroblasts, relating to increased expression of VEGF and endothelial NOS (eNOS), also known as constitutive NOS (cNOS), as well as genes encoding collagens types I and III [58, 59].

Shock wave treatment is capable of inducing an increase of activated fibroblasts, CD34-positive fibrocytes, and fXIIIa-positive dendritic cells; this process is thought to lead to the deposition of new collagen, characterized by thinner collagen fascicles and parallel orientation to the dermoepidermal junction. Additionally, ESWT may play a significant role in the increase in CD31-positive vessel density in the dermis allowing an improved tissue metabolism [60]. In animal models, ESWT modulates expression of angiogenesis pathway-specific genes such as those encoding for ELR motif (glutamic acid-leucine-arginine sequence) positive (ELR + -CXC) chemokines, CC-chemokines, and cytokines [51].

In addition, shock wave exposure induces strong expression of stromal cell-derived mRNA factor 1, which influences medium induced chemo-attraction of CD34+ cells, hematopoietic stem cells, and the effect on bone marrow-derived mononuclear cells facilitating cell differentiation to endothelial phenotype [61].

So, ESWT-enhanced cell proliferation at the local wound tissue level stimulated extracellular matrix metabolism, decreased apoptosis, and downregulated oxygen-mediated burst of leukocytes, probably stimulating homing and differentiation of stem cells with high tissue regenerating potential.

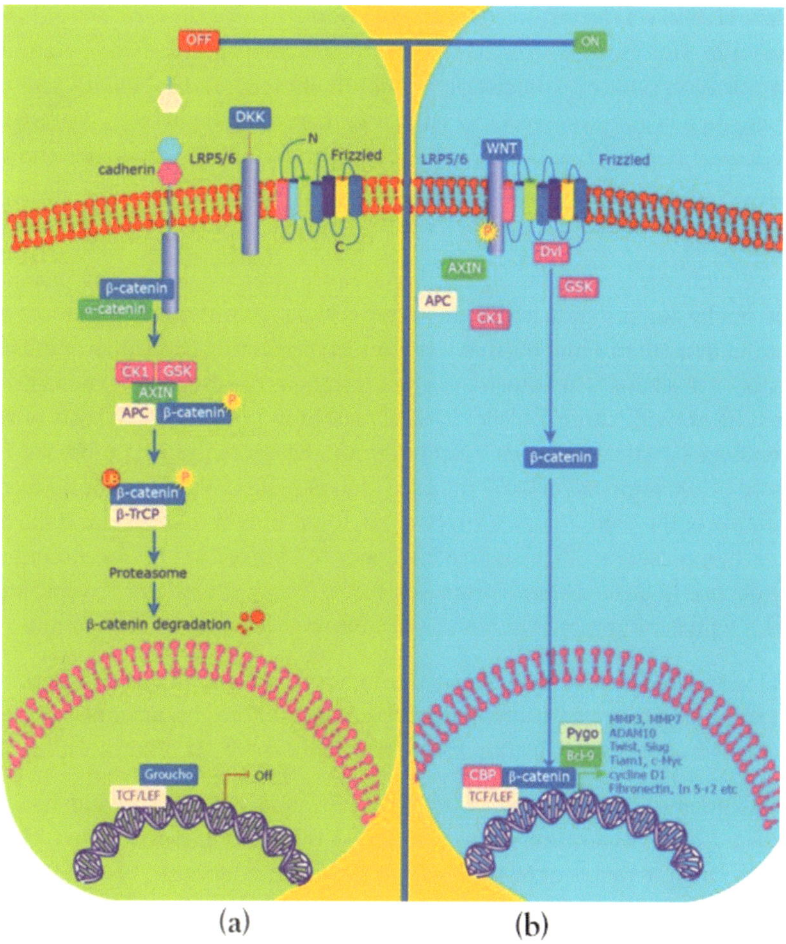

Figure 1. (a) Wnt signaling—"Off" In the absence of Wnt, β-catenin is phosphorylated, so transcriptional process is stopped (b) Wnt signaling—"On" In the presence of Wnt ligands, a signaling cascade is initiated. β-catenin accumulates in the cytoplasm and is free to translocate into the nucleus where it acts as transcriptional coactivator of transcriptional factors of the TCF/LEF family. Modified from: https://www.sigmaaldrich.com/technical-documents/articles/biology/wnt-b-catenin.html.

4. ESWT in chronic wound: clinical studies

In the published literature, there are hypothesis-generating experimental data as well as clinical observations that suggest a heretofore unproven systemic effect of ESWT.

Schaden et al. in 2007 [62] demonstrated safety and potential efficacy of electrohydraulic unfocused shock waves applied to acute and chronic wounds (33.3% acute and 66.7% chronic wounds) of various etiologies (post-traumatic, venous, pressure, and arterial wounds). A total of 208 patients were included in the study and treated with the unfocused electrohydraulic device (DermaGold). Each treatment was placed onto wound dressing applied: from 100 to 1000 pulses were applied according to wound size (100 pulses/cm^2) initially, weekly, and then biweekly. The study describes the complete reepithelialization of wounds in 75% patients:

significant association was found between complete epithelialization and wound size (wounds <10 cm^2 healed in 81.0 vs. 61.8% for wounds >10 cm^2) as well as between complete healing and wound duration (wounds persisting >1 month showed 57.1% healing rate vs. wounds <1 month that had a healing rate of 83%). With regard to wound etiology, venous stasis ulcers showed the lowest healing rates (36%), whereas all other wound etiologies showed at least a healing rate of 66% (arterial insufficiency ulcer—66.7%, decubital ulcer—71.4%, disturbed healing wounds—75.6%, posttraumatic tissue necrosis—86.6%, and burn wounds—100%).

Application of high energy unfocused shock waves for difficult wounds was confirmed by a work carried out by Saggini et al. [63]. In this study, 30 patients affected by chronic ulcers in the lower limb from more than 3 months that were unresponsive to conservative or advanced dressing treatments or mechanical debridement were included. A group of 10 consecutive patients, randomly recruited, with chronic ulcers in the lower limb treated on the basis of regular conservative dressings have been used as a control group. Electrohydraulic unfocused ESWT treatment consisted of 100 impulses at 0.037 mJ/mm^2 each per cm^2 of the row wound area (Evotron). The focal volume of the hand handled probes was 10–15 mm in diameter, and the total energy applied for each impulse was 3.5 mJ, with a frequency of 4 Hz or 240 impulses/minute. At the end of the study period, 16 ulcers healed completely (50%). Every patient underwent single sessions every 2 weeks, with a minimum of four and a maximum of 10 sessions for a complete treatment.

The wounds were classified on the basis of the location, width (cm), length (cm), row surface area (cm^2), percentage of granulation tissue, percentage of fibrin tissue or necrotic tissue, presence of exudates, bacterial colonization (positive culture swabs or tissue scrapings), and pain.

Presence of exudates was determined as: none, minimal, moderate, and heavy, adapted from the wound bed preparation score developed by Falanga [64]. Complete healing was documented within the first four to six sessions. In all of the wounds, the amount of exudates decreased considerably, and the increasing percentage of granulation tissue compared with the fibrin/necrotic tissue was statistically significant. At the end of the study period, in the non-healed ulcers, a considerable improvement in the wound bed blood supply was documented. Improvement of all these parameters was noted within the first four to six sessions.

Wang et al. [65] included 74 patients with diabetic skin ulcers of the foot for comparing ESWT and hyperbaric oxygen therapy (HBOT). They were randomly divided into two groups (38 subjects in each group). ESWT, electrohydraulic focused, protocol provides two sessions for 6 weeks (300 + 100 pulses/cm^2 at an energy flux density of 0.11 mJ/mm^2). The HBOT was performed five times a week for a total of 20 treatments using a sealed multiplace chamber at a pressure of 2.5 atmospheres for 90 minutes total (25-minute sessions with 5-minute breaks). Post-treatment wound care was the same in both groups. Outcome variables included clinical assessment of the ulcers with photo documentation, blood flow perfusion scan, bacteriological examination, histological study, and immune-histochemical analysis. In ESWT group, results showed a significant increase of eNOS, VEFG, and proliferation cell nuclear antigen (PCNA) and a decrease of terminal deoxynucleotidyl transferase-mediated UTP nick end labeling (TUNEL) with reduction of apoptotic phenomena. It reported significant improvement in local blood perfusion in the participants that had DFU and treated with ESWT (0.61, $P < 0.002$) compared with those treated with HBOT (0.50). Complete ulcer healing was found in 31% of the ESWT group compared with 22% of the HBOT group. Furthermore, in more than 50% was observed a reduction of wound surface and was observed in 89% of shock wave-treated ulcers compared with 72% of HBOT-treated ulcers. They concluded that ESWT of chronic diabetic foot ulcer is superior to HBOT, and it appears that ESWT results in increased angiogenesis and cellular events consistent with decreased cell apoptosis.

Other scientific literature, Wang et al. [66], confirmed that ESWT appeared to be more effective than HBOT for treatment of chronic wound, in a prospective open-label, randomized, but not blinded study. Patients were randomly divided into two groups: the ESWT, group consisted of 39 patients with total of 44 chronic diabetic foot ulcers, while the HBOT group consisted of 38 patients and 40 foot ulcers. ESWT treatment was carried out with an electrohydraulic-unfocused device, derma PACE device, and the dosage was ulcer size dependent with the numbers of impulses equal to the treatment area in $cm^2 \times 8$, with a minimum of 500 impulses at energy setting E2 (equivalent to 0.23 mJ/mm^2 energy flux density) at a rate of 4 shocks per second twice per week for a total of six treatments. The HBOT group received hyperbaric was performed with patients in a sealed multi-place chamber at a pressure of 2.5 atmospheres absolute daily for a total of 20 treatments. The assessment, at 3 and 6 weeks, then once every 3 months, was carried out by local blood flow perfusion scan and histopathological examination after biopsy specimens. Clinical assessment of the ulcer status was performed by physical examination including visual observation and photo-documentation.

Clinical results showed completely healed ulcers in 57 and 25% ($P = 0.003$); ≥50% improved ulcers in 32 and 15% ($P = 0.071$); unchanged ulcers in 11 and 60% ($P < 0.001$), and none worsened for the ESWT and the HBOT group, respectively. Another interesting observation was that even though prior to study-based treatment levels of oxygenation were comparable, oxygenation levels were significantly higher after shockwave therapy than after HBOT ($P = 0.002$). In histopathological examination, the ESWT group showed considerable increases in cell proliferation, cell concentration, and cell activity and a decrease in cell apoptosis as compared to the HBOT group.

Moretti et al. [67] evaluate the effect of ESWT in 30 patients affected by neuropathic diabetic foot ulcers. One group was treated with standard care and ESWT with an focused electromagnetic device, three sessions (every 72 hours), with 100 pulses per 1 cm^2 of wound delivered at each session at a flux density of 0.03 mJ/mm^2; while the control group was treated with only standard care. The wound area and its following reductions were measured with the Rhinoceros program running and the reepithelialization was measured as the time to complete ulcer healing was measured as the number of days from the start of treatment to the date in which each patient achieved complete wound healing. If the healing did not occur within the 20 weeks of the study, the patient was considered to be non-healing. The proportions of ulcers that healed in 20 weeks in the A and B groups were 53.33 and 33.33%, respectively. For the ulcers that healed during the 20-week period, the healing times were 60.8 ± 4.7 days (mean ± DS) in group A and 82.2 ± 4.7 days (mean ± DS) in group B patients ($P < 0.001$). A significant difference was observed in the index of the re-epithelization between the two groups, with values of 2.97 ± 0.34 mm^2/die (mean ± DS) in the ESWT group and 1.30 ± 0.26 mm^2/die (mean ± DS) in the control group ($P < 0.001$). Both the healing rate and the healing time were increased in the ESWT group, and the differences were statistically significant.

Larking et al. [68] investigated the response to ESWT of pressure ulcers in a randomized, placebo-controlled crossover study. All patients included in the study were patients with disabilities, presenting pressure ulcers for more than 3 months in different anatomical sites. The protocol consisted of a 3-week baseline observation period to confirm stable wound conditions, and subsequently, ulcers were allocated randomly to ESWT or placebo group and followed-up for 4 weeks receiving treatment each week. After this 4-week period and a 2-week washout period, study crossover to the other treatment ensued. Interestingly, regardless of which group they belonged to (initial treatment group or cross-over treatment group), all nine ulcers showed significant improvement (average of three measurements of ulceration was recorded) at 6–8 weeks after the initial shockwave treatment. This phenomenon was discussed as follows that shock waves may first determine debridement of the wounds receiving proper wound bed, which is then conditioned for healing.

Ottomann et al. in 2012 [69] performed a prospective randomized phase II trial of accelerated reepithelialization of superficial second-degree burn wounds using extracorporeal shock wave therapy. A total of 100 patients were included and then randomly assigned in two groups: control group received a standard treatment debridement of devitalized skin (epidermis) and topical antiseptic therapy and the experimental group received the standard treatment and a single application of defocused ESWT (100 impulses/cm at 0.1 mJ/mm) applied once to the study burn, after debridement. Patients receiving shock wave therapy showed significantly reduced mean time to complete (>95%) second-degree burn wound epithelialization (9.6 ± 1.7 vs. 12.5 ± 2.2 days). The study concludes that application of a single defocused shock wave treatment to the superficial second-degree burn wound after debridement/topical antiseptic therapy significantly was able to accelerate healing.

Saggini et al. in 2013 [70] by a randomized, controlled trial, with blind assessment, assessed the efficacy of unfocused shock wave treatment in patients with diabetic ulcers, pressure ulcers, traumatic ulcers, and vascular ulcers, through the analysis of the percentage of wound healing (calculated as the reduction in wound area divided for the initial area percent), the antibacterial effect, through the evaluation of specific buffers and searching for possible occurrence of infection during therapy. A total of 124 patients with ulcers at least from 3 to 24 months were treated with a frequency of 1 session every 7 days for 7 weeks. A total of 62 subjects were included in Group A and treated with ESWT unfocused probe with Dermagold electrohydraulic system; the mean energy applied for each pulse in Group A was equal to 0.10 mJ/mm^2 per cm^2 (0.09/0.11 mJ/mm2) with a total energy density equal to 1250 J. A total of 62 subjects were included in Group B but 22 withdrawn, so 40 were treated with ESWT electrohydraulic unfocused device (Evotron); the mean energy applied in Group B was equal to 0.037 mJ/mm^2 per cm^2 with a total energy density equal to 462 J. In both Groups A and B were administered 300–600 impulses per session relating to the wound area at a frequency of 4 Hz or 240 pulses per minute. Results showed a reduction of 80% of mean area of wound in Group A: particularly, the 23 diabetic wounds in this group achieved a 85% mean decrease of the row surface area from a mean surface area of 1.45 cm^2 to a final average surface area of 0.2 cm^2; the 10 pressure wounds demonstrated a 68% mean decrease of the row surface area rising from a mean surface area equal to 9.8 cm^2 to a final surface area of 3.1 cm^2. The 10 traumatic wounds obtained an 85% decrease of the row surface area rising from a mean surface area of 1 cm^2

to a mean surface area of 0.15 cm^2. Nineteen vascular wounds demonstrated a 76% decrease of the row surface area rising from a mean surface area of 2.75 cm^2 to a mean surface area of 0.65 cm^2. At the end of protocol (7 weeks), 44 patients achieved complete wound healing, while the remaining 18 obtained a partial recovery. As for the pain, there was a 79% mean visual analogical scale (VAS) reduction. The mean surface area in Group B, equal to 3.4 cm^2 at the beginning, decreased by 67%: diabetic wounds in this group achieved a 60% mean decrease of the row surface area rising from a mean surface area of 1.2 cm^2 to a final average surface area of 0.48 cm^2; traumatic wounds obtained an 85% decrease of the row surface area rising from a mean surface area of 1.2 cm^2 to a mean surface area of 0.18 cm^2; pressure wounds demonstrated a 72% mean decrease of the row surface area rising from a mean surface area equal to 8.8 cm^2 to a final surface area of 2.5 cm^2; vascular wounds demonstrated a 61% decrease of the row surface area rising from a mean surface area of 3.5 cm^2 to a mean surface area of 1.37 cm^2; as for wounds in patients with cryoglobulinemia was found a 33% decrease of the row surface area. At the end of therapy, 40% of patients had reached a completed healing, 37.5% a partially healed, and 22.5% unchanged. As for pain, in Group B, there was a 48% mean VAS reduction (2.7 reduction points compared to the initial value) with a final mean value equal to 3 (range 1–6). No wound in Group B developed infection during therapy; such evidence may confirm and correlate to bactericidal effect of this system because of dejection of *Staphylococcus aureus* in culture swabs. Authors concluded that the greater improvement in Group A is linked to the higher total flux density of energy transferred from the probe, as regards the application time, a significant reduction in wound areas was observed after 7 weeks and a peak of increase of the results, in terms of wound size reduction, between the third and the fourth week of treatment, so therefore the time required to obtain the regenerative effects would be at least 7 days between one.

Omar et al. [71] in a single blinded randomized controlled study included 35 patients with chronic diabetic foot ulcer. They assessed the efficacy of ESWT on the healing rate, wound surface area, and wound bed preparation. In experimental group (19 patients/24 ulcers), patients received ESWT with a pneumatic unfocused device, twice a week at a frequency of 100 pulse/cm^2 and energy flux density of 0.11 mJ/cm^2; all patients received standardized wound care consisting of debridement, blood-glucose control agents, and footwear modification for pressure reduction.

Clinical outcome measures focused on wound surface area (WSA), the percentage of reduction in the WSA, rate of healing and wound bed preparation at baseline, after the end of the interventions (W8), and at 20-week follow-up (W20).

Results showed completely healed ulcers in 33.3 and 54% in ESWT-groups and 14.28 and 28.5% in the control group after intervention (W8), and at follow-up (W20), respectively. The average healing time was significantly lower (64.5 ± 8.06 days vs. 81.17 ± 4.35 days, $P < 0.05$) in the ESWT-group compared with the control group. The authors concluded that ESWT-treated ulcers had a significant reduction in wound size and median time required for ulcer healing.

Nossair et al. [72] evaluated the effectiveness of shock wave therapy in enhancing diabetic wound healing. Forty patients with lower limb ulcerations were included in this study and divided randomly into two groups: one treated with shock wave therapy (pneumatic unfocused device) beside medications and traditional wound care methods (Group A), while the other treated with medical treatment and traditional wound care (Group B). The protocol consists of a course of three sessions (a session every 1 week for 12 weeks), with 500 pulses per 1 cm^2 of wound delivered at each session at a flux density of 0.1 mJ/mm^2; three sessions, one session every week.

The control group performed the essentials of foot ulcer care, namely debridement, adequate pressure relief, and treatment of infection. Assessments were made at baseline and after 12 weeks as reducing wound surface area and epithelialization rate. After 12 weeks, there was significant decrease in the surface area of both group, and they become (1.92 ± 3.28) and (4.65 ± 3.43) for shock wave and control group, respectively. A significant difference was observed in the wound surface area and in the rate of epithelialization between both groups after 12 weeks. The rate of epithelialization for shock wave and control group were (83.26 ± ±27.43)% and (48.66 ± 31.68)%, respectively, ($P < 0.001$). The results of this study revealed that there was a significant difference in wound surface area only after 12 weeks (post-treatment) of the treatment between in shock wave group and the control group ($P = 0.0001$).

Another scientific work [73] describes the safety and efficacy of ESWT in patients with non-healing diabetic foot ulcer of various etiologies such as peripheral arterial disease and neuropathy. Five patients received electromagnetic unfocused ESWT in 6–8 weekly sessions, delivered as 500 shocks at wound margin and 1000 shocks distal to the wound (lower leg), spread over the entire muscle area at a flux density of 0.25 mJ/mm^2, using the Cactor hand piece of the Duolith SD1 device.

Clinical assessment was carried out 2 weeks after the final session of treatment. Wound area was measured using digital photography, pressure sensitivity was evaluated by the monofilament test, and calculation of the ankle brachial index (ABI) was done at each visit.

After 6–8 weekly sessions of ESWT, a significant reduction in ulcer surface area was observed in four patients with a mean post-treatment ulcer size of 6.33 cm^2 ± 5.00 (mean reduction: 1.21 ± 0.82 cm^2, $P = 0.03$).

All patients showed improvement in the ABI and monofilament test after treatment (mean ABI and monofilament test score of 0.9 ± 0.12, p value: 0.00 and 4/10 after treatment, respectively). It is interesting that the increase of ABI in all patients after treatment confirms the strong angiogenic effect of ESWT leading to enhanced limb perfusion. The majority of clinical trials investigate the effectiveness of short-term ESWT, instead Wang et al. [74] evaluate the long-term effects of ESWT in chronic foot with 5-year follow-up; they included 38 patients with 40 ulcers in the diabetes mellitus (DM) group and 29 patients with 32 ulcers in the non-diabetes mellitus (non-DM) group. All patients received unfocused ESWT with a derma PACE device, and dosage is ulcer size dependent. The number of pulses was calculated as follows: ¼ of the treatment area ($cm^2 \times 8$); but it had reach to 500 shocks (4Hz-equivalent to 0.11 mJ/mm^2 energy flow density) twice/week for six treatments.

The follow-up examinations were performed in 1, 3, 6, and 12 months and then once a year. The evaluations included clinical assessment of the ulcer status, including the size, shape, and depth with photo documentation, local blood flow perfusion scan, and the mortality and morbidity including the rates of amputation in 1 and 5 years after ESWT. Tissue viability was evaluated by local blood flow perfusion scan preoperatively and at 6 weeks, 1 year, and 5 years postoperatively.

After ESWT, the blood flow perfusion rates significantly improved in both DM (P ¼ 0.011) and non-DM (P ¼ 0.033) groups. The improvements of blood flow perfusion rate began at 6 weeks and lasted for up to 1 year after ESWT. The blood perfusion rates significantly decreased in both groups from 1 to 5 years compared with the data before treatment, at 6 weeks (P ¼ 0.006) and 1 year ($P < 0.001$). The blood flow perfusion rate of the non-DM group is significantly better than that of the DM group from 1 to 5 years after ESWT (P ¼ 0.04).

The clinical outcomes, mortality, and morbidity were compared with a control data of 149 patients with diabetic foot ulcers previously treated by the author. The experimental group shown a better overall clinical outcomes of healed and improved ulcers at 1 year (73 vs. 64.4%) compared with the historical controls, although the differences did not reach statistical significance (P ¼ 0.338). The mortality rate was 9.4% in the historical controls and 0% at 1 year (P ¼ 0.044) and 24% at 5 years (P ¼ 0.017) in the experimental ESWT patients. The historical controls showed significantly higher amputation rates compared with the ESWT group at 1 year ($P < 0.001$) and 5 years ($P < 0.001$) and more operations other than amputation than ESWT group the at 1 year (P ¼ 0.003) and at 5 years (P ¼ 0.010), respectively. At the conclusion of this study, Wang et al. concluded that ESWT appears effective in the treatment of chronic diabetic and non-diabetic foot ulcers. However, the effects of ESWT significantly decreased from 1 to 5 years after treatment.

5. Discussion

The importance to describe current perspectives of management of soft tissue wounds is linked to the serious medical and social problem for which it stands, and the purpose of this narrative review is to evaluate evidence of effectiveness of ESWT on chronic wound and indicate an application guideline in relation to our experience [75, 76]. The primary goal in the treatment of soft tissue wounds is to produce beneficial stimuli in the tissue, which stimulate and support tissue repair and regeneration.

Modern wound bed preparation strategies are to applied immediate [77–79] and after the rational use of advanced wound care therapies when wounds do not respond sufficiently to good standard care after 4 weeks or sooner as circumstances dictate: negative pressure wound therapy, HBOT, biophysical electrical stimulation, diathermy, pulsed electromagnetic fields, pulsed radiofrequency energy, and low-frequency non-contact ultrasound—MIST and ESWT [80]. The described ESWT studies revealed a lack of uniformity classification of ulcers (etiology, grade, and size) and a variety of types and parameters of treatment and the duration of ulcers varied across identified studies (1–24 months) or the initial ulcer size (1 cm^2 up to 10 cm^2); therefore, it is appropriated to group them based on measuring the therapeutic effect of ESWT. In this chapter review, the relevant clinical outcomes were focused on wound healing and reepithelialization time. However, the methods used to define them are varied. The evidences have shown clinical efficacy as regards speed of healing highlighting the size of the wound. Furthermore, ESWT is a safe mode and associated with a low rate of complications during its application both short-term and medium-term periods of follow-up. All included studies provided sufficient details to allow the repetition of the intervention protocol. However, we can highlight differences in frequency, dosage, duration and the generator type, the duration of the protocols, and the device used. This heterogeneity of parameters can make difficult comparisons between studies with aim to standardize the application of ESWT in chronic ulcers. In many cited studies, the number of pulses in a single ESWT session ranged from 10 to 500 pulses/cm^2 (206.4 ± 172.3 pulses/cm^2), but the most frequent value was 100 pulses/cm^2 of wound area. Not all studies did describe frequency parameters which instead can be considered important in order to evaluate the application and effects of ESWT. According to the review of clinical research studies, in the case of chronic wounds, ESWT sessions were typically once or twice per week, as well as once every 2 weeks. The total number of treatment sessions ranged between three and six. The average time of a single ESWT session was 1–3 minutes, depending on the size of the wound.

So, ESWT represents a new application of translational medicine and a current border not only as an advanced physical therapy but also as a regenerative application [81]. This regenerative potential is linked to mechanotransduction, thanks to cytoplasmic cellular and extracellular cascade [82], that generates a gene expression modulation. This complex biological phenomenon determines a change in the key factors of regenerative skin process.

In fact, ESWT can reduce expression of several metalloproteinases and interleukins (MMPs and ILs) [83]; it stimulates proliferation and collagen synthesis, mediated by early up-regulation of proliferating cell nuclear antigen (PCNA) and TGF-beta1 gene expression, endogenous NO release and synthesis and TGFbeta1 protein and then collagen synthesis [84]; in vitro it improves functional activities of ruptured tendon-derived tenocytes (proliferation and migration), which could probably contribute to tendon healing in vivo [85]; it can enhance osteogenic differentiation of mesenchymal stem cells, through superoxide-mediated signal transduction [86]; furthermore, the ESWT facilitates the regeneration process of the soft tissues by early expression of angiogenesis-related growth factors [87–90].

In addition, shock wave exposure induces strong expression of stromal cell-derived mRNA factor 1, which influences medium induced chemoattraction of CD34+ cells and hematopoietic stem cells, and the effect on bone marrow-derived mononuclear cells facilitates cell differentiation to endothelial phenotype. These molecular effects and gene expression are reflected in positive clinic results [8]. All this reduces the health and social costs.

Considering all this evidences, I could recommend for treatment chronic ulcers unfocused ESWT with fractionated energy in 2 weekly steps, because in this way, there is greater regenerative activation.

6. Conclusion

From these experimental and clinical data, it is possible to conclude that ESWT would improve not only the wound healing process, but also the regeneration events. The knowledge relative to the mechanotransduction has had over the years a consolidation process, instead the modulation of gene transcription related to the regenerative processes on the treatment of chronic ulcers can be considered as a new border for other clinical studies and clinical trials.

Disclosure

The author reports no conflicts of interest in this work.

Author details

Simona Maria Carmignano[1,2*]

*Address all correspondence to: simona.carmignano@gmail.com

1 Department of Medicine, Surgery and Dentistry "Salernitan Medical School", University of Salerno, Baronissi, Italy

2 C.T.R. Rehabilitation Therapeutic Center, Basilicata, Italy

References

[1] Mustoe TA, O'Shaughnessy K, Kloeters O. Chronic wound pathogenesis and current treatment strategies: A unifying hypothesis. Plastic and Reconstructive Surgery. 2006;**117**:35-41

[2] Demidova-Rice TN, Hamblin MR, Herman IM. Acute and impaired wound healing: Pathophysiology and current methods for drug delivery, part 1: Normal and chronic wounds: Biology, causes, and approaches to care. Advances in Skin & Wound Care. 2012;**25**(7):304-314

[3] Robson MC, Barbul A. Guidelines for the best care of chronic wounds. Wound Repair and Regeneration. 2006;**14**(6):647-648

[4] Hunt TK, Hopf H, Hussain Z. Physiology of wound healing. Advances in Skin & Wound Care. 2000;**13**:6-11

[5] Schultz G, Mozingo D, Romanelli M, Claxton K. Wound healing and TIME; new concepts and scientific applications. Wound Repair and Regeneration. 2005;**13**(Suppl 4):S1-S11

[6] Falanga V. Wound bed preparation and the role of enzymes: A case for multiple actions of therapeutic agents. Wounds. 2000;**4**(Suppl 2):S47-S57

[7] Ennis WJ, Menses P. Wound healing at the local level: The stunned wound. Ostomy/Wound Management. 2000;**46**:39S-348S

[8] Dymarek R, Halski T, Ptaszkowski K, Slupska L, Rosinczuk J, Taradaj J. Extracorporeal shock wave therapy as an adjunct wound treatment: A systematic review of the literature. Ostomy/Wound Management. 2014;**60**(Suppl 7):S26-S39

[9] Mathieu D. Hyperbaric oxygen therapy in the management of non-healing wounds. In: Bakker DJ, Cramer FS, editors. Hyperbaric Surgery. Flagstaff, AZ: Best Publishing Company; 2002. pp. 317-339

[10] Al-Waili NS, Butler GJ. Effects of hyperbaric oxygen on in-flammatory response to wound and trauma: Possible mechanism of action. Scientific World Journal. 2006;**6**:425-441

[11] Morykwas MJ, Argenta LC, Shelton-Brown EI, McGuirt W. Vacuum-assisted closure: A new method for wound control and treatment: Animal studies and basic foundation. Annals of Plastic Surgery. 1997;**38**:553-562

[12] Moisidis E, Heath T, Boorer C, Ho K, Deva AK. A prospective, blinded, randomized, controlled clinical trial of topical negative pressure use in skin grafting. Plastic and Reconstructive Surgery. 2004;**114**:917-922

[13] Ubbink DT, Westerbos SJ, Evans D, Land L, Vermeulen H. Topical negative pressure for treating chronic wounds. Cochrane Database of Systematic Reviews. 2008;**3**:1-34

[14] Yu W, Naim JO, Lanzafame RJ. The effects of photo-irradiation on the secretion of TGF and PDGF from fibroblasts in vitro. Lasers in Surgery and Medicine. 1994;**6**(Suppl):8

[15] McLoda TA, Seegmiller JG, Baxter GD. Low-level laser therapy facilitates superficial wound healing in humans: A triple-blind, sham-controlled study. Journal of Athletic Training. 2004;**39**(Suppl 3):S223-S229

[16] Kloth LC. Electrical stimulation for wound healing: A review of evidence from in vitro studies, animal experiments, and clinical trials. The International Journal of Lower Extremity Wounds. 2005;**4**:23-44

[17] Notarnicola A, Moretti B. The biological effects of extracorporeal shock wave therapy (ESWT) on tendon tissue. Muscle, Ligaments and Tendons Journal. 2012;**2**(Suppl 1):S 33-S S7

[18] Wess O, Ueberle F, Dührssen RN, et al. Working group technical developments—Consensus report. In: Chaussy C, Eisenberger F, Jocham D, Wilbert D, editors. High Energy Shock Waves in Medicine. Stuttgart: Thieme; 1997. pp. 59-71

[19] Rompe JD, Kirkpatrick CJ, Küllmer K, Schwitalle M, Krischek O. Dose-related effects of shock waves on rabbit tendo Achillis. A sonographic and histological study. Journal of Bone and Joint Surgery. British Volume. 1998;**80**(suppl 3):S546-SS52

[20] Gerdesmeyer L, Henne M, Göbel M, Diehl P. Physical principles and generation of shockwaves. In: Towson, editor. Extracorporeal Shock Wave Therapy: Clinical Results, Technologies, Basics. Brooklandville, Baltimore County, Maryland, United States: Data Trace Publishing Company; 2006. pp. 11-20

[21] Shrivastava SK, Kailash. Shock wave treatment in medicine. Journal of Biosciences. 2005;**30**(Suppl 2):S269-S275

[22] Speed C. A systematic review of shockwave therapies in soft tissue conditions: Focusing on the evidence. British Journal of Sports Medicine. 2014;**48**(21):1538-1542

[23] Goertz O, Lauer H, Hirsch T, Ring A, Lehnhardt M, Langer S, et al. Extracorporeal shock waves improve angiogenesis after full thickness burn. Burns. 2012;**38**(Suppl 7):S1010-S1018

[24] Saggini R, Di Stefano A, Saggini A, Bellomo RG. Clinical application of shock wave therapy in musculoskeletal disorders: PART I. Journal of Biological Regulators and Homeostatic Agents. 2015;**29**(3):533-545

[25] Gollwitzer H, Gloeck T, Roessner M, Langer R, Horn C, Gerdesmeyer L, et al. Radial extracorporeal shock wave therapy (rESWT) induces new bone formation in vivo: Results of an animal study in rabbits. Ultrasound in Medicine & Biology. 2013;**39**(1):126-133

[26] Marks W, Jackiewicz A, Witkowski Z, Kot J, Deja W, Lasek J. Extracorporeal shock-wave therapy (ESWT) with a new-generation pneumatic device in the treatment of heel pain. A double blind randomised controlled trial. Acta Orthopaedica Belgica. 2008;**74**:98-101

[27] Thiel M. Application of shock waves in medicine. Clinical Orthopaedics and Related Research. 2001;**387**:18-21

[28] Mittermayr R, Antonic V, Hartinger J, et al. Extracorporeal shock wave therapy (ESWT) for wound healing: Technology, mechanisms, and clinical efficacy. Wound Repair and Regeneration. 2012;**20**(4):456-465

[29] Hwang Y, Barakat AI. Dynamics of mechanical signal transmission through prestressed stress fibers. PLoS One. 2012;**7**(Suppl 4):e35343

[30] Maniotis AJ, Chen CS, Ingber DE. Demonstration of mechanical connection between integrins, cytoskeletal filaments, and nucleoplasm that stabilize nuclear structure. Proceedings of the National Academy of Sciences. 1998;**94**:849-854

[31] Na S, Collin O, Chowdhury F, et al. Rapid signal transduction in living cells is a unique feature of mechanotransduction. Proceedings of the National Academy of Sciences. 2008;**105**:6626-6631

[32] d'Agostino MC, Craig K, Tibalt E, Respizzi S. Review shock wave as biological therapeutic tool: From mechanical stimulation to recovery and healing, through mechanotransduction. International Journal of Surgery. 2015;**24**:147-153

[33] Eming SA, Martin P, Tomic-Canic M. Wound repair and regeneration: Mechanisms, signaling, and translation. Science Translational Medicine. 2014;**6**(265):265sr6

[34] Tonnesen MG, Feng X, Clark RA. Angiogenesis in wound healing. The Journal of Investigative Dermatology. Symposium Proceedings. 2000;**5**(1):40-46

[35] Huang C, Holfeld J, Schaden W, Orgill D, Ogawa R. Mechanotherapy: Revisiting physical therapy and recruiting mechanobiology for a new era in medicine. Trends in Molecular Medicine. 2013;**19**(9):555-564

[36] Tara S, Miyamoto M, Takagi G, et al. Low-energy extracorporeal shock wave therapy improves microcirculation blood flow of ischemic limbs in patients with peripheral arterial disease: Pilot study. Journal of Nippon Medical School. 2014;**81**(1):19-27

[37] Tepeköylü C, Wang FS, Kozaryn R, et al. Shock wave treatment induces angiogenesis and mobilizes endogenous CD31/CD34-positive endothelial cells in a hindlimb ischemia model: Implications for angiogenesis and vasculogenesis. The Journal of Thoracic and Cardiovascular Surgery. 2013;**146**(Suppl 4):S971-S9S8

[38] Ciampa AR, de Prati AC, Amelio E, et al. Nitric oxide mediates anti-inflammatory action of extracorporeal shock waves. FEBS Letters. 2005;**579**(30):6839-6845

[39] Gotte G, Amelio E, Russo S, Marlinghaus E, Musci G, Suzuki H. Short-time non-enzymatic nitric oxide synthesis from L-arginine and hydrogen peroxide induced by shock waves treatment. FEBS Letters. 2002;**520**(Suppl 1-3):S153-S155

[40] Davis TA, Stojadinovic A, Anam K, et al. Extracorporeal shock wave therapy suppresses the early proinflammatory immune response to a severe cutaneous burn injury. International Wound Journal. 2009;**6**(1):11-21

[41] Fischer S, Mueller W, Schulte M, et al. Multiple extracorporeal shock wave therapy degrades capsular fibrosis after insertion of silicone implants. Ultrasound in Medicine & Biology. 2015;**41**(3):781-789

[42] Heine N, Prantl L, Eisenmann-Klein M. Extracorporeal shock wave treatment of capsular fibrosis after mammary augmentation—Preliminary results. Journal of Cosmetic and Laser Therapy. 2013;**15**(6):330-333

[43] Holfeld J, Tepeköylü C, Kozaryn R, et al. Shockwave therapy differentially stimulates endothelial cells: Implications on the control of inflammation via toll-like receptor 3. Inflammation. 2014;**37**(Suppl 1):S65-S70

[44] Tepeköylü C, Lobenwein D, Blunder S, et al. Alteration of inflammatory response by shock wave therapy leads to reduced calcification of decellularized aortic xenografts in mice. European Journal of Cardio-Thoracic Surgery. 2015;**47**(Suppl 3):e80-e90

[45] Mariotto S, de Prati AC, Cavalieri E, Amelio E, Marlinghaus E, Suzuki H. Extracorporeal shock wave therapy in inflammatory diseases: Molecular mechanism that triggers anti-inflammatory action. Current Medicinal Chemistry. 2009;**16**(19):2366-2372

[46] Kuo YR, Wang CT, Wang FS, Yang KD, Chiang YC, Wang CJ. Extracorporeal shock wave treatment modulates skin fibroblast recruitment and leukocyte infiltration for enhancing extended skin-flap survival. Wound Repair and Regeneration. 2009;**17**(1):80-87

[47] Shao PL, Chiu CC, Yuen CM, et al. Shock wave therapy effectively attenuates inflammation in rat carotid artery following endothelial denudation by balloon catheter. Cardiology. 2010;**115**(2):130-144

[48] Sukubo NG, Tibalt E, Respizzi S, Locati M, D'Agostino MC. Effect of shock waves on macrophages: A possible role in tissue regeneration and remodeling. International Journal of Surgery. 2015;**24**(Pt B):124-130

[49] Vulpiani MC, Vetrano M, Savoia V, Di Pangrazio E, Trischitta D, Ferretti A. Jumper's knee treatment with extracorporeal shock wave therapy: A long-term follow-up observational study. The Journal of Sports Medicine and Physical Fitness. 2007;**47**(3):323-328

[50] Zins SR, Amare MF, Tadaki DK, Elster EA, Davis TA. Comparative analysis of angiogenic gene expression in normal and impaired wound healing in diabetic mice: Effects of extracorporeal shock wave therapy. Angiogenesis. 2010;**13**(4):293-304

[51] Stojadinovic A, Elster EA, Anam K, et al. Angiogenic response to extracorporeal shock wave treatment in murine skin isografts. Angiogenesis. 2008;**11**(4):369-380

[52] DeLisser HM, Christofidou-Solomidou M, Strieter RM, et al. Involvement of endothelial PECAM-1/ CD31 in angiogenesis. The American Journal of Pathology. 1997;**151**:671-677

[53] Fujiwara K. Platelet endothelial cell adhesion molecule-1 and mechanotransduction in vascular endothelial cells. Journal of Internal Medicine. 2006;**259**:373-380

[54] Komiya Y, Habas R. Wnt signal transduction pathways. Organogenesis. 2008;**4**(Suppl 2):S68-S75

[55] Ilan N, Cheung L, Pinter E, Madri JA. Platelet-endothelial cell adhesion molecule-1 (CD31), a scaffolding molecule for selected catenin family members whose binding is mediated by different tyrosine and serine/threonine phosphorylation. The Journal of Biological Chemistry. 2000;**275**:21435-21443

[56] Wang FS, Wang CJ, Chen YJ, et al. Ras induction of superoxide activates ERK-dependent angiogenic transcription factor HIF-1alpha and VEGF-A expression in shock wave-stimulated osteoblasts. The Journal of Biological Chemistry. 2004;**279**:10331-10337

[57] Cunji G, Weiyong S, Melpo CS, et al. PECAM-1 functions as a specific and potent inhibitor of mitochondrial-dependent apoptosis. Blood. 2003;**102**:169-179

[58] Gauglitz GG, Siegfried Z, Spiegel F, et al. Functional characterization of cultured keratinocytes after acute cutaneous burn injury. PLoS One. 2012;**7**(2):e29942

[59] Berta L, Fazzari A, Ficco AM, Enrica PM, Catalano MG, Frairia R. Extracorporeal shock waves enhance normal fibroblast proliferation in vitro and activate mRNA expression for TGF-β1 and for collagen types I and III. Acta Orthopaedica. 2009;**80**(5):612-617

[60] Saggini R, Saggini A, Spagnoli AM, et al. Extracorporeal shock wave therapy: An emerging treatment modality for retracting scars of the hands. Ultrasound in Medicine & Biology. 2016;**42**(Suppl 1):S185-S195

[61] Aicher A, Heeschen C, Sasaki K, Urbich C, Zeiher AM, Dimmeler S. Low-energy shock wave for enhancing recruitment of endothelial progenitor cells: A new modality to increase efficacy of cell therapy in chronic hind limb ischemia. Circulation. 2006;**114**:2823-2830

[62] Schaden W, Thiele R, Kolpl C, et al. Shock wave therapy for acute and chronic soft tissue wounds. A feasibility study. The Journal of Surgical Research. 2007;**143**:1-12

[63] Saggini R, Figus A, Troccola A, Cocco V, Saggini A, Scuderi N. Extracorporeal shock wave therapy for management of chronic ulcers in the lower extremities. Ultrasound in Medicine & Biology. 2008;**34**(8):1261-1271

[64] Falanga V, Saap LJ, Ozonoff A. Wound bed score and its correlation with healing of chronic wounds. Dermatologic Therapy. 2006;**19**:383-390

[65] Wang CJ, Kuo YR, Wu RW, et al. Extracorporeal shockwave treatment for chronic diabetic foot ulcers. The Journal of Surgical Research. 2009;**152**(1):96-103

[66] Wang CJ, Wu RW, Yang YJ. Treatment of diabetic foot ulcers: A comparative study of extracorporeal shockwave therapy and hyperbaric oxygen therapy. Diabetes Research and Clinical Practice. 2011;**92**(Suppl 2):S187-S193

[67] Moretti B, Notarnicola A, Maggio G, et al. The management of neuropathic ulcers of the foot in diabetes by shock wave therapy. The management of neuropathic ulcers of the foot in diabetes by shock wave therapy. BMC Musculoskeletal Disorders. 2009;**10**:54-62

[68] Larking AM, Duport S, Clinton M, Hardy M, Andrews K. Randomized control of extracorporeal shock wave therapy versus placebo for chronic pressure ulceration. Clinical Rehabilitation. 2010;**24**:222-229

[69] Ottomann C, Stojadinovic A, Lavin PT, et al. Prospective randomized phase II trial of accelerated reepithelialization of superficial second-degree burn wounds using extracorporeal shock wave therapy. Annals of Surgery. 2012;**255**(Suppl 1):S23-SS9

[70] Saggini R, Fioramonti P, Bellomo RG, et al. Chronic ulcers: Treatment with unfocused extracorporeal shock waves European. Journal of Inflammation. 2013;**11**(2):99-509

[71] Omar MT, Alghadir A, Al-Wahhabi KK, Al-Askar AB. Efficacy of shock wave therapy on Ccronic diabetic foot ulcer: A single-blinded randomized controlled clinical trial. Diabetes Research and Clinical Practice. 2014;**106**(Suppl 3):S 548-SS554

[72] Nossair AA, Eid MM, Salama AB. Advanced protocol of shock wave therapy for diabetic foot ulcer. Journal of American Science. 2013;**9**(4):633-638

[73] Variji Z, Aghazadeh N, Hasanzadeh H, Flrooz A. Extraxoporeal shock wave therapy in the treatment of non-healing diabetic ulcer: A pilot study. Journal of Clinical & Experimental Dermatology Research. 2015;**6**(4):289

[74] Wang CJ, Wu CT, Yang YJ, Liu RT, Kuo YR. Long-term outcomes of extracorporeal shockwave therapy for chronic foot ulcers. The Journal of Surgical Research. 2014;**189**:e366-e372

[75] Jones KR, Fennie K, Lenihan A. Evidence-based management of chronic wounds. Advances in Skin & Wound Care. 2007;**20**(11):591-600

[76] Ryan S, Perrier L, Sibbald RG. Searching for evidence-based medicine in wound care: An introduction. Ostomy/Wound Management. 2003;**49**(11):67-75

[77] Werdin F, Tennenhaus M, Schaller HE, Rennekampff HO. Evidence-based management strategies for treatment of chronic wounds. Eplasty. 2009;**9**:e19

[78] Stanley A, Osler T. Senescence and the healing rates of venous ulcers. Journal of Vascular Surgery. 2001;**33**:1206-1211

[79] Lobmann R, Ambrosch A, Schultz G, Waldmann K, Schiweck S, Lehnert H. Expression of matrixmetalloproteinases and their inhibitors in the wounds of diabetic and non-diabetic patients. Diabetologia. 2002;**45**:1011-1016

[80] Frykberg RG, Banks J. Challenges in the treatment of chronic wounds. Advances in Wound Care. 2015;**4**(Suppl 9):S560-S582

[81] Ioannidis JP. Materializing research promises: Opportunities, priorities and conflicts in translational medicine. Journal of Translational Medicine. 2004;**2**:5-10

[82] Ingber DE. Cellular mechanotransduction: Putting all the pieces together again. The FASEB Journal. 2006;**20**(7):811-827

[83] Han SH, Lee JW, Guyton GP, Parks BG, Courneya JP, Schon LC. J. Leonard Goldner award 2008. Effect of extracorporeal shock wave therapy on cultured tenocytes. Foot & Ankle International. 2009;**30**(Suppl 2):93-98

[84] Chen YJ, Wang CJ, Yang KD, et al. Extracorporeal shock waves promote healing of collagenaseinduced Achilles tendinitis and increase TGF-beta1 and IGF-I expression. Journal of Orthopaedic Research. 2004;**22**(Suppl 4):854-861

[85] Leone L, Vetrano M, Ranieri D, Raffa S, Vulpiani MC, Ferretti A, et al. Extracorporeal shock wave treatment (ESWT) improves in vitro functional activities of ruptured human tendon-derived tenocytes. PLoS One. 2012;**7**(Suppl 11):S49-S759

[86] Wang FS, Yang KD, Chen RF, Wang CJ, Sheen-Chen SM. Extracorporeal shock wave promotes growth and differentiation of bone-marrow stromal cells towards osteoprogenitors associated with induction of TGF-beta1. The Journal of Bone and Joint Surgery. British Volume. 2002;**84**(Suppl 3):S457-S461

[87] Schaden W, Fischer A, Sailler A. Extracorporeal shock wave therapy of nonunion or delayed osseous union. Clinical Orthopaedics and Related Research. 2001;**387**:90-94

[88] Ma HZ, Zeng BF, Li XL. Upregulation of VEGF in subchondral bone of necrotic femoral heads in rabbits with use of extracorporeal shock waves. Calcified Tissue International. 2007;**81**(Suppl 2):S 124-SS131

[89] Wang CJ, Huang HY, Pai CH. Shock wave-enhanced neovascularization at the tendon-bone junction: An experiment in dogs. The Journal of Foot and Ankle Surgery. 2002;**41**(Suppl 1):S16-S22

[90] Wang FS, Wang CJ, Chen YJ, et al. Ras induction of superoxide activates ERK-dependent angiogenic transcription factor HIF-1alpha and VEGF-A expression in shock wavestimulated osteoblasts. The Journal of Biological Chemistry. 2004;**279**(Suppl 11):S10331-S10337

Section 6

Conceptual Approaches of the Physical Therapy Interventions

Chapter 12

Affect and Exercise

Sandro dos Santos Ferreira

Additional information is available at the end of the chapter

http://dx.doi.org/10.5772/intechopen.90056

Abstract

The increase in the number of studies involving affect and exercise published in the last two decades presents new directions and important advances in the field of exercise psychology, expanding the theoretical knowledge of the theme and highlighting new possibilities for practical application. This chapter aims to address the relationship between affect and exercise by defining their concepts, characteristics, and interactions with physiological and perceived exertion factors. In addition, it aims to demonstrate how different strategies in exercise prescription can influence the affective responses, provide the physiological and psychological benefits of exercise, and assist in the adherence and adoption of an active lifestyle.

Keywords: affective response, exercise, intensity, adherence, pleasure

1. Introduction

Over the past few decades, studies have found that physiological data and the appeal of health benefits are insufficient to encourage people to maintain regular physical activity. Therefore, understanding the relationship between affect and exercise is a vital step toward revealing what factors lead to maintenance of or dropout from exercise programs. This chapter presents the concept of basic affect and its distinction from moods and emotions, as well as the possibility of measuring affect in the context of exercise from a dimensional perspective. In terms of the affect-exercise relationship, it will address the importance of the intensity of the exercise prescription model (self-selected or imposed) in affective responses and the use of motivational music to stimulate pleasurable sensations or distract from the discomfort that exercise can cause.

IntechOpen

© 2019 The Author(s). Licensee IntechOpen. This chapter is distributed under the terms of the Creative Commons Attribution License (http://creativecommons.org/licenses/by/3.0), which permits unrestricted use, distribution, and reproduction in any medium, provided the original work is properly cited.

2. Affect

The analysis of affective constructs from general and abstract aspects (such as mental health, psychological well-being, and psychological health) has provided a plethora of terms, such as humor, emotion, and affect, with similar and diverse definitions, not all of which are universally accepted [1]. To understand the meaning of affect and its application in the context of exercise, it is important to define the concepts of mood and emotion. Emotions are immediate responses to specific stimuli (often directed at a specific object), typically characterized by a short duration and high intensity. In contrast, moods are characterized as diffuse and lacking a specific target, are typically associated with downward or no-action trends, and may be less intense and longer lasting than emotions [1, 2]. In this sense, moods refer to the larger and more diffuse existential issues of life, while emotions refer to an immediate response, having a specific and relatively narrow purpose in an encounter with variable environmental stimuli [1].

The term "affect" can be defined as the intrapersonal or experiential basis of all contrasting responses (positive or negative, pleasant or unpleasant), including, but not limited to, emotions and moods [2, 3]. Unlike emotions and moods, affect encompasses a more general description of the psychological response and can be considered basic and central. Therefore, the use of the word affect encompasses the notion that all emotions are affective conditions, but not all affective conditions are emotions [2, 4].

The investigation of affective phenomena can be envisioned from a categorical or dimensional perspective. In the categorical view of affect, affective states are ordered into different categories, comprising states that resemble the prototypical examples, such as anger, fear, sadness, disgust, happiness, love, and pride [4]. In the dimensional perspective, affective states are systematically interrelated, and their relationships can be modeled by a stringent set of dimensions. Although both categories have advantages and limitations, the dimensional approach provides a wider perspective, corroborating the characteristics of basic affect and providing a model or "map" of the affective space that offers a broad and balanced scope for investigation of affect in exercise [2, 4]. The dimensional model of affect allows the exercise-induced affective experience to be captured and the observation of affective changes throughout the exercise context [2, 4, 5].

2.1. Measuring affect

The measurement of affect can be performed with one- or two-dimensional models [6]. Some scales are commonly used to measure affective valence and perceived activation from both models. The Feeling Scale is used to measure affective valence (**Figure 1**). This instrument comprises an 11-point scale, ranging from +5 ("very good") to −5 ("very bad") [7]. Its purpose is to quantify the exercise-related sense of pleasure and displeasure. The Felt Arousal Scale is an instrument used to measure perceived activation [8] (**Figure 2**); the scale comprises six levels of activation, ranging from low activation (1) to high activation (6). High perceived activation can be characterized by excitement, anxiety, or anger, whereas low activation may be described as relaxation, boredom, or tranquility.

http://dx.doi.org/10.5772/intechopen.90056

+5 Very Good
+4
+3 Good
+2
+1 Fairly Good
0 Neutral
-1 Fairly Bad
-2
-3 Bad
-4
-5 Very Bad

Figure 1. Feeling scale.

1 Low arousal
2
3
4
5
6 High arousal

Figure 2. Felt arousal scale.

The circumplex model measures affect from a two-dimensional model, which involves an affective valence dimension (also called pleasure-displeasure) and a perceived activation dimension (also called arousal) [6, 9]. The use of the circumplex model in exercise is

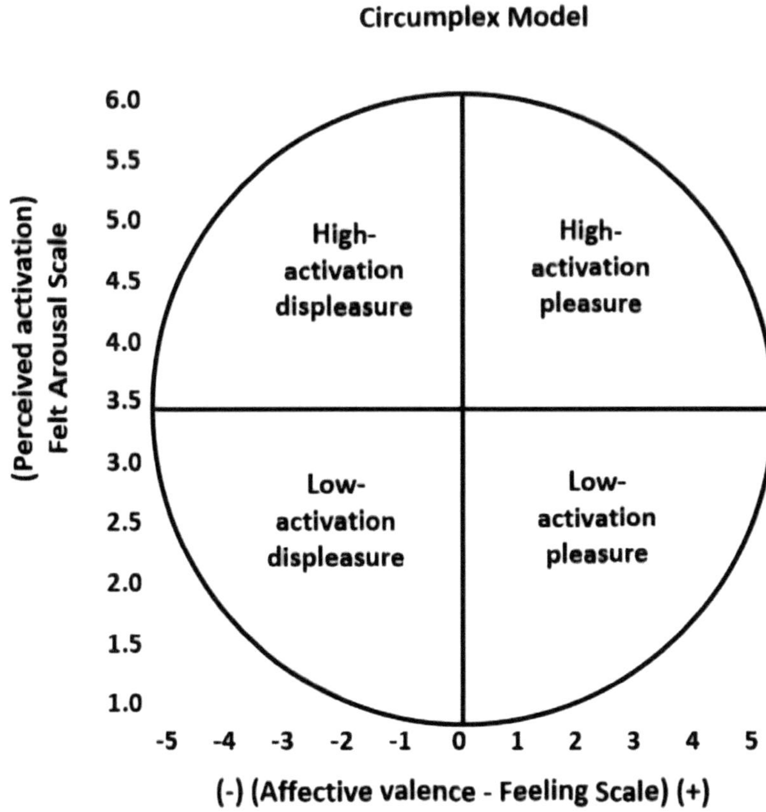

Figure 3. Circumplex model of affect (adapted [5]).

intended to avoid measuring affect with terms such as anxiety, depression, and various mood descriptions and to provide a map of affect in the broad context of exercise (before, during, and after activity) [10].

In the circumplex model (**Figure 3**), the horizontal dimension represents the affective valence (pleasure-displeasure), and the vertical dimension represents the perceived activation. Affective spaces are divided into four quadrants: quadrant 1 corresponds to a sense of high activation and displeasure (tension, nervousness, distress); quadrant 2 corresponds to a sense of high activation and pleasure (energy, excitement, vigor); quadrant 3 corresponds to a sense of low activation and displeasure (fatigue, boredom, tiredness); quadrant 4 corresponds to a sense of low activation and pleasure (tranquility, relaxation, calmness) [5, 6, 10].

Several studies using dimensional models of affect have verified the importance of measuring affective responses in exercise, as well as the factors that may influence this relationship [11–13].

3. Affective responses in exercise

The relationship between exercise and affective response is complex and multifaceted [2]. Although many studies relate exercise to affect as a single phenomenon, there is evidence that considerable complexity lies beneath this factor. This complexity is based on the nature of the affective changes and patterns in their relationship with relevant variables, such as contextual factors (exercise scenario), exercise stimulus aspects (intensity), and individual differences (physical activity level) [2, 14]. These factors may influence affective responses during exercise.

Affective valence, based on observations in neuroscience, has shown that negative affect is one of the first signs of conscious and significant changes in energy regulation and body balance [15, 16]. Neuroanatomical and neurophysiological studies suggest that interoceptive stimuli of afferent signals from baroreceptors, chemoreceptors, and mechanoreceptors located in the viscera and muscles are linked to affective responses [17]. This hypothesis suggests that changes in the transition between aerobic and anaerobic metabolism during exercise would be accompanied by unpleasant affective responses [17].

One of the main determinants of affective responses during exercise is the intensity at which the activity is performed [18]. According to the dual model theory [2], the ventilatory threshold (VT) or lactate threshold functions as a marker of exercise intensity [19–22], demonstrating that, at prescribed intensities below or around the VT, affective responses maintain a positive predominance. However, during exercise at VT, the affective valence is less pleasant and, in some cases, negative [19, 20, 22, 23]. An important aspect of intensities below or near the VT is the great variability of affective responses between individuals, in whom exercise can increase, decrease, or stabilize affective responses of pleasure. However, above VT, individual variations are smaller, and, generally, a decline in pleasure is experienced [22].

According to Dishman [24], feelings of pleasure and well-being appear to be the most compelling reasons for continued participation in an exercise program, rather than the knowledge of or belief in the health benefits of physical activity. The idea of exercise giving pleasure may indicate its usefulness to the individual, whereas discomfort indicates damage or danger [20]. The variability in affective responses may be an indication that the situation is providing substantial benefit or imminent danger. However, whenever all or most individuals respond in a similar way, with pleasure or displeasure (within a reasonable quantitative range), it can be assumed that the situation is one that has consistent (positive or negative) implications for change [20].

4. Exercise intensity and affective responses

Exercise intensity is an important factor in exercise prescription [12, 25]. Performing 30 minutes of moderate-intensity exercise, i.e., 64–76% of maximum heart rate (HR_{max}) (at least

5 days a week), or 20 minutes of vigorous intensity, i.e., 77–95% of HR_{max} (3 days a week), is the minimum recommendations proposed by the American College of Sports Medicine (ACSM) for health-related physiological benefits (ACSM, 2011). Studies published in recent decades have shown that exercise intensity is also one of the main influencers of affective exercise response [5, 26–28].

In a study by Vandoni [25], which compared the affective responses of exercise performed at moderate and vigorous intensities, the results showed that vigorous exercise promoted lower affective responses than moderate exercise. Alves [29], when observing weight training in elderly women, found higher affective pleasure responses in exercises performed with a low one-repetition maximum (1RM) percentage (35%) in relation to higher intensities (50% and 70% 1RM). Follador [30] observed that, even in moderately active adults, high-intensity protocols promoted less pleasure responses, and protocols prescribing maximal or supramaximal intensities were the most likely to stimulate the affective response of displeasure and probably have the highest negative impact on exercise program adherence.

The relevance of affective responses in the exercise program should be to prioritize the task response over the postexercise response [31]. Studies have shown that, when exercise intensity exceeds the VT, there is a decrease in affective response and this change has a greater impact on the future behavior of maintaining exercise continuity than the affective responses obtained after exercise [31, 32]. However, the difficulty and complexity of conducting medium- to long-term studies have not facilitated much investigation into adherence to exercise programs. Parfitt [28] verified the 6-month effect on physical fitness and affective responses of sedentary people after an 8-week intervention program. Three groups participated in the training: a control group, a group that exercised in PSE 13 (Borg 06-20), and group in PSE 15. Their results show that the group that performed the training at a lower intensity (PSE 13) showed more positive affective responses during the intervention, maintaining the level of physical fitness acquired during training, in relation to the control and PSE 15 groups. In the study by Perri [33], which aimed to observed the relationship between intensity, frequency, and adherence to exercise over 6 months, the results showed that exercise prescription of moderate intensity produced greater exercise adherence (66 vs. 58%) than exercise prescription of higher intensity.

4.1. Affective responses and self-selected intensity

A self-selected intensity exercise is an activity in which the participant chooses the preferred intensity [34]. For beginners, exercise at intensities above the anaerobic/VT may provide affective responses of displeasure and stimulate changes in exercise intensity toward self-selected intensities. In this sense, beginners of exercise programs seek lower perceptions of effort and greater affective pleasure responses [35].

Motivational aspects related to the practice of exercise have been investigated using behavioral theories. To better understand the factors leading to the permanence, or dropout, of beginners of exercise programs, the hedonic theory and the self-determination theory have been important in understanding self-selected exercise [36–38].

The hedonic theory of motivation suggests that when one experiences a situation that promotes pleasure, joy, or fun, one will seek to repeat that activity. However, if the situation induces displeasure, pain, or discomfort, the chance of adherence or repetition of the activity is lower [37, 39]. The self-determination theory is a general theory of human motivation that prioritizes autonomous aspects of behavior over controlled ones. Its emphasis is on providing a sense of granted autonomy and can promote a pleasant, self-gratifying feeling and greater intrinsic motivation [36, 39, 40]. The sense of autonomy and positive feelings forms the fundamental aspects of self-selected exercise.

The psychological elements of behavioral theories are linked to the physiological components of effort. Lower-intensity activities are inversely correlated with feelings of displeasure and, consequently, with adherence [34]. However, the duration of activity may also be related to displeasure, with shorter duration exercises being more conducive to adherence than very long activities [39, 41].

Self-selected intensity exercise has been proposed by several authors as a strategy to improve the participation and adherence of physical activity programs by sedentary people [3, 34]. Studies have shown that insufficiently active people are able to self-select an exercise intensity according to the ACSM parameters for maintaining and/or developing cardiorespiratory fitness, associated with lower exertion perceptions and positive affective responses [27, 28, 42]. Although some studies have addressed the fact that affective responses are more dependent on exercise intensity than on how it is prescribed (imposed or self-selected exercise) [43, 44], other studies point out that, even when the exercise session is prescribed at the same intensity as the self-selected exercise session, the affective responses may be different. Hamlyn-Williams [45] observed that aerobic exercise lowers perceptual responses and affective responses are higher during self-selected intensity than during imposed intensity. Similar results were observed in the study by Da Silva [46] on resistance training, in which three of the four exercises used in the study had lower perceptual responses, and all exercises showed higher affective responses for self-selected intensity.

In intervention studies, self-selected intensity has been shown to be an excellent strategy to provide similar or more pleasurable affective responses than imposed intensity exercises [47]. In the study by Freitas [27], which compared walking exercise programs at self-selected and imposed intensities (10% above VT) over 12 weeks of training, the results showed that self-selected exercise induced more pleasurable affective responses, where the percentage of HR and PSE responses were lower than in the imposed exercise regime. In addition, walking at a self-selected intensity was sufficient to promote improvement in maximal oxygen uptake at the end of training. Yang [48] concluded, from a 12-week study, that both self-selected and prescribed intensities improved the level of physical activity and positive affect and reduced physiological parameters (waist circumference, systolic and diastolic blood pressure) in retirees. However, the self-selected intensity was more favorable to the increase of positive affect than the prescribed intensity.

5. Influence of music on affective exercise responses

The evolution of technology in recent decades has provided facilities and amenities that were difficult or restricted to access in the past. Music has benefited in this respect, and with the creation and evolution of smartphones, headphones, MP3 players, and the Internet, access to music content of different styles and from various countries has become easier and more commonplace, and the technology has increased our capacity to transport music [3]. Nowadays, people have become more accustomed to listening to music during their various daily activities, such as walking in the park, commuting, doing homework, exercising at the gym, and leisure times [3].

In sport and exercise, music has been used for the purpose of improving performance, reducing the monotony of the activity, or as a musical background [49, 50]. Music can improve mood and emotion, reduce the perception of effort, dissociate from pain and fatigue, etc. The psychophysiological responses of music are supported by four pillars: rhythmic response, musicality, cultural impact, and association [50].

The rhythmic response represents the natural response to musical rhythm, which refers to the speed of music in beats per minute. Musicality refers to related elements such as pitch and harmony. Cultural impact is the representativeness of music to society or a cultural group. Association is the extramusical reflection that music can promote. These four factors are presented in their hierarchical order, so that there is a greater importance conferred on musical rhythm and less importance on association [49, 51]. In this sense, the use of motivational music is thought to be an important strategy in exercise for promoting acute and chronic benefits and assisting in exercise adherence [49].

Motivational music can be defined as stimulating music with a fast musical tempo and prominent beat. Studies that have investigated the acute effects of music on exercise have demonstrated the psychological and physiological influences on different populations [52, 53]. In diabetic patients, the practice of exercise with music provided greater affective responses than exercise without music [54]. In Silva's research [55], motivational music provided a greater shift of focus from feelings of discomfort and effort than when exercise was performed without music in overweight and obese women. Macone [56] found positive changes in young adults in tension, depression, mood, confusion, and fatigue and improved running performance with motivational music compared to no music. Finally, music performs different functions in the context of exercise, and its action on motivational and dissociative aspects can affect psychophysiological factors and promote a positive and enjoyable experience during physical activity.

6. Discussion

The definitions of the terms "affect," "humor," and "emotion," from a perspective that allows us to analyze their differences, are fundamental for the evolution of understanding "affect" and its application in exercise—a fact that has enabled researchers and other professionals to focus on observing "affect" from a categorical or dimensional perspective [1, 2]. In the field of exercise science, dimensional vision has allowed the appropriation and adaptation of instruments of affect measurement to be more appropriate to the context of the area, contributing to the growth of research, the comparison between studies, and the development of the field [32].

The observation of affective responses before, during, and after exercise does not replace the prescription and observation of exercise-related physiological and perceived exertion responses, but their interrelated aspects complement the importance of the psychological and physiological benefits derived from regular practice [42]. The analysis of the relationship between intensity and affective responses has challenged exercise science to investigate exercise prescription strategies that provide pleasurable sensations and achieve appropriate physiological parameters for health benefits, as well as strategies for making exercises that require a higher physiological stimulus more enjoyable [39, 55, 57].

Prescribing exercise at a self-selected intensity was one of the possibilities that emerged in order to make exercise practice more enjoyable for sedentary individuals and beginners [39]. Investigations in this area present important results, with several limitations, such as reaching physiological stimuli beyond the ventilatory threshold [2, 57]. The use of music reaches broader parameters in the context of affective responses, stimulating positive changes from its rhythmic and cultural elements, as well as dissociating feelings of discomfort arising from exercise [47, 58]Thus, the effects of music, according to its specificities, may provide benefits independent of the intensity or mode of prescription.

Using physical exercise as a nonpharmacological tool in disease prevention and treatment is a reality that tends to increase in the coming years; thus, the importance of understanding the affect-exercise relationship and its challenges will help in adhering to and, consequently, in obtaining the physiological and the psychological benefits from regular exercise.

7. Conclusions

Understanding affect from a dimensional perspective provides a broader view of the affect-exercise relationship. Although affect is understood to be a complex phenomenon, exercise intensity seems to be one of the main determinants of its quality and quantity. Selecting an appropriate exercise prescription mode and musical stimulation can also induce a more pleasurable affective experience and assist in the consistent adherence to exercise programs.

Author details

Sandro dos Santos Ferreira

Address all correspondence to: sandroferreiraef@hotmail.com

Federal Institute of Espírito Santo, ES, Brazil

References

[1] Ekkekakis P, Petruzzello SJ. Analysis of the affect measurement conundrum in exercise psychology I. Fundamental issues. Psychology of Sport and Exercise. 2000;**1**:71-88

[2] Ekkekakis P. Pleasure and displeasure from the body: Perspectives from exercise. Cognition and Emotion. 2003;**17**(2):213-239

[3] Haile L, Gallagher MJ, Robertson RJ. Perceived Exertion Laboratory Manual: From Standard Practice to Contemporary Application. New York: Springer; 2015. p. 322

[4] Ekkekakis P, Petruzzello SJ. Analysis of the affect measurement conundrum in exercise psychology: II. A conceptual and methodological critique of the exercise-induced feeling inventory. Psychology of Sport and Exercise. 2001;**2**:1-26

[5] Ekkekakis P, Parfitt G, Petruzzello SJ. The pleasure and displeasure people feel when they exercise at different intensities: decennial update and progress towards a tripartite rationale for exercise intensity prescription. Sports Medicine. 2011;**41**(8):641-671

[6] Ekkekakis P, Petruzzello SJ. Analysis of the affect measurement conundrum in exercise psychology: IV. A conceptual case for the affect circumplex. Psychology of Sport and Exercise. 2002;**3**:25-63

[7] Hardy C, Rejeski W. Not what, but how one feels: The measurement of affect during exercise. Journal of Sport & Exercise Psychology. 1989;**11**:304-317

[8] Svebak S, Murgatroyd S. Metamotivational dominance : A multimethod validation of reversal theory constructs. Journal of Personality and Social Psychology. 1985;**48**(1):107-116

[9] Russel JA. A Circumplex model of affect. Journal of Personality and Social Psychology. 1980;**39**(6):1161-1178

[10] Hall EE, Ekkekakis P, Petruzzello SJ. The affective beneficence of vigorous exercise revisited. British Journal of Health Psychology. 2002;**7**:47-66

[11] Krinski K, Machado DGS, Lirani LS, DaSilva SG, Costa EC, Hardcastle SJ, et al. Let's walk outdoors! Self-paced walking outdoors improves future intention to exercise in women with obesity. Journal of Sport & Exercise Psychology. 2017;**39**(2):145-157

[12] Lind E, Ekkekakis P, Vazou S. The affective impact of exercise intensity that slightly exceeds the preferred level: "Pain" for no additional "gain". Journal of Health Psychology. 2008;**13**(4):464-468

[13] Follador L, Alves RC, Ferreira SDS, Silva AC, Silva SG. Perceived exertion and affect from tai chi, yoga, and stretching classes for elderly women. Perceptual and Motor Skills. 2019;**126**(2):223-240

[14] Reed J, Ones DS. The effect of acute aerobic exercise on positive activated affect: A meta-analysis. Psychology of Sport and Exercise. 2006;**7**(5):477-514

[15] Damasio AR. Review toward a neurobiology of emotion and feeling: Operational concepts and hypotheses. The Neuroscientist. 1995;**1**:19-25

[16] Panksepp J. The periconscious substrates of consciousness: Affective states and the evolutionary origins of the self. Journal of Consciousness Studies. 1998;**5**(5-6):566-582

[17] Craig AD. An ascending general homeostatic afferent pathway originating in lamina I. Progress in Brain Research. 1996;**107**:225-242

[18] Rose EA, Parfitt G. Pleasant for some and unpleasant for others: A protocol analysis of the cognitive factors that influence affective responses to exercise. International Journal of Behavioral Nutrition and Physical Activity. 2010;**7**:1-15

[19] Ekkekakis P, Hall EE, Petruzzello SJ. Practical markers of the transition from aerobic to anaerobic metabolism during exercise: Rationale and a case for affect-based exercise prescription. Preventive Medicine (Baltim). 2004;**38**(2):149-59

[20] Ekkekakis P, Hall EE, Petruzzello SJ. Variation and homogeneity in affective responses to physical activity of varying intensities: An alternative perspective on dose-response based on evolutionary considerations. Journal of Sports Sciences. 2005;**23**(5):477-500

[21] Parfitt G, Rose EA, Burgess WM. The psychological and physiological responses of sedentary individuals to prescribed and preferred intensity exercise. British Journal of Health Psychology. 2006;**11**:39-53

[22] Rose EA, Parfitt G. A quantitative analysis and qualitative explanation of the individual differences in affective responses to prescribed and self-selected exercise intensities. Journal of Sport & Exercise Psychology. 2007;**29**:281-309

[23] Ekkekakis P, Petruzzello SJ. Acute aerobic exercise and affect. Current status, problems and prospects regarding dose-response. Sports Medicine. 1999;**28**(5):337-374

[24] Dishman RK, Sallis JF, Orenstein DR. The determinants of physical activity and exercise. Public Health Reports. 1985;**100**:158-171

[25] Vandoni M, Codrons E, Marin L, Correale L, Bigliassi M, Buzzachera CF. Psychophysiological responses to group exercise training sessions: Does exercise intensity matter? PLoS One. 2016;**11**(8):e0149997

[26] Alves RC, Follador L, SDS F, da Silva SG. Effect of combined training on ratings of perceived exertion and sensation of pleasure/displeasure in obese women. Revista Brasileira de Cineantropometria e Desempenho Humano. 2017;**19**(6):696-709

[27] Freitas LAG et al. The impact of a self-selected and imposed intensity on cardiorespiratory fitness and body composition in obese women. Journal of Exercise Physiology (Online). 2014;**17**(2):44-52

[28] Parfitt G, Olds T, Eston R. A hard/heavy intensity is too much: The physiological, affective, and motivational effects (immediately and 6 months post-training) of unsupervised perceptually regulated training. Journal of Exercise Science and Fitness. 2015;**13**:123-130

[29] Alves RC, SDS F, Benites ML, Krinski K, Follador L, Silva, Da SG. Exercícios com pesos sobre as respostas afetivas e perceptuais. Revista Brasileira de Medicina do Esporte. 2015;**21**(3):200-205

[30] Follador L, Alves RC, Ferreira SDS, Buzzachera CF, Andrade VFDS, EDSDA G, et al. Physiological, perceptual, and affective responses to six high-intensity interval training protocols. Perceptual and Motor Skills. 2018;**125**(2):329-350

[31] Kwan BM, Bryan A. In-task and post-task affective response to exercise: Translating exercise intentions into behaviour. British Journal of Health Psychology. 2010;**15**:115-131

[32] Rhodes RE, Kates A. Can the affective response to exercise predict future motives and physical activity behavior? A systematic review of published evidence. Annals of Behavioral Medicine. 2015;**49**(5):715-731

[33] Perri MG, Anton SD, Durning PE, Ketterson TU, Sydeman SJ, Berlant NE, et al. Adherence to exercise prescriptions: Effects of prescribing moderate versus higher levels of intensity and frequency. Health Psychology. 2002;**21**(5):452-458

[34] Ekkekakis P, Lind E, Joens-Matre RR. Can self-reported preference for exercise intensity predict physiologically defined self-selected exercise intensity? Research Quarterly for Exercise and Sport. 2006;**77**(1):81-90

[35] Cox KL, Burke V, Gorely TJ, Beilin LJ, Puddey IB. Controlled comparison of retention and adherence in home- vs center-initiated exercise interventions in women ages 40-65 years: The S.W.E.a.T. study (sedentary women exercise adherence trial). Preventive Medicine (Baltim). 2003;**36**(1):17-29

[36] Deci EL, Ryan RM. The "what" and "why" of goal pursuits: Human needs and the self-determination of behavior. Psychological Inquiry. 2000;**11**:227-268

[37] Feldman F, Kahneman D, Diener E, Schwarz N, editors. Well-Being: The Foundations of Hedonic Psychology. New York: The Russell Sage Foundation; 1999. p. 593

[38] Williams DM. Exercise, affect, and adherence: An integrated model and a case for self-paced exercise. Journal of Sport & Exercise Psychology. 2008;**30**(5):471-496

[39] Ekkekakis P. Let them roam free?: Physiological and psychological evidence for the potential of self-selected exercise intensity in public health. Sports Medicine. 2009;**39**:857-888

[40] Patrick H, Williams GC. Self-determination theory: Its application to health behavior and complementarity with motivational interviewing. International Journal of Behavioral Nutrition and Physical Activity. 2012;**9**:18

[41] Gibala MJ, et al. Macdonald MJ. Hawley JA, Physiological adaptations to low-volume, high-intensity interval training in health and disease. The Journal of Physiology. 2012; **5**(March):1077-1084

[42] ACSM. Quantity and quality of exercise for developing and maintaining cardiorespiratory, musculoskeletal, and Neuromotor fitness in apparently healthy adults: Guidance for prescribing exercise. Medicine and Science in Sports and Exercise. 2011;**43**(7):1334-59

[43] Oliveira BRR, Deslandes AC, Santos TM. Differences in exercise intensity seems to influence the affective responses in self-selected and imposed exercise: A meta-analysis. Frontiers in Psychology. 2015;**6**:1105

[44] Oliveira BRR, Deslandes AC, Nakamura FY, Viana BF, Santos TM. Self-selected or imposed exercise? A different approach for affective comparisons. Journal of Sports Science; 2015;**33**(8):777-785

[45] Hamlyn-Williams CC, Freeman P, Parfitt G. Acute affective responses to prescribed and self-selected exercise sessions in adolescent girls: An observational study. BMC Sports Science, Medicine and Rehabilitation. 2014;**6**:35

[46] da Silva SG, Garcia ED, Ferreira SS, Andrade VF, Folladar L, Alves RC, et al. Resistance exercise performed with the same load In self-selected and imposed intensities promote different affective and perceptual responses. Medicine & Science in Sports & Exercise. 2017;**49**:843

[47] Parfitt G, Hughes S. The exercise intensity-affect relationship: Evidence and implications for exercise behavior. Journal of Exercise Science and Fitness. 2009;**7**(2):34-41

[48] Yang Z, Petrini MA. Self-selected and prescribed intensity exercise to improve physical activity among inactive retirees. Western Journal of Nursing Research. 2018;**40**(9):1301 –1318

[49] Karageorghis CI, Priest DL. Music in the exercise domain: A review and synthesis (part I). International Review of Sport and Exercise Psychology. 2012;**5**(1):44-66

[50] Terry PC, Karageorghis CI. Psychophysical effects of music in sport and exercise: An update on theory, research and application. In: Psychology Bridging the Tasman: Science, Culture and Practice. Auckland, New Zealand. 26-30 Sep 2006. pp. 415-419

[51] Karageorghis CI, Terry PC, Lane AM. Development and initial validation of an instrument to assess the motivational qualities of music in exercise and sport : The Brunel M usic rating inventory. Journal of Sports Sciences. 1999;**17**:713-724

[52] Almeida FAM, Nunes RFH, SDS F, Krinski K, Elsangedy HM, Buzzachera CF, et al. Effects of musical tempo on physiological, affective, and perceptual variables and performance of self-selected walking pace. Journal of Physical Therapy Science. 2015;**27**(6):1709-1712

[53] Hutchinson JC, Karageorghis CI, Black JD. The diabetes project: Perceptual, affective and psychophysiological effects of music and music-video in a clinical exercise setting. Canadian Journal of Diabetes. 2017;**41**:90-96

[54] Jones L, Tiller NB, Karageorghis CI. Psychophysiological effects of music on acute recovery from high-intensity interval training. Physiology & Behavior. 2017;**170**:106-114

[55] Silva AC, Dos S, Ferreira S, Alves C, Follador L, Gregorio S, et al. Effect of music tempo on Attentional focus and perceived exertion during self-selected paced walking. International Journal of Exercise Science. 2016;**9**(4):536-544

[56] Macone D, Baldari C, Zelli A, Guidetti L. Music and physical activity in psychological well-being. Perceptual and Motor Skills [Internet]. 2006;**103**(1):285-295

[57] Freitas LAG, Ferreira SS, Freitas RQ, de Souza CH, de Abreu Garcia EDS, da Silva SG. Effect of a 12-week aerobic training program on perceptual and affective responses in obese women. Journal of Physical Therapy Science. 2015;**27**(7)

[58] Karageorghis CI, Priest DL. Music in the exercise domain: A review and synthesis (part II). International Review of Sport and Exercise Psychology. 2012;**5**(1):67-84

Chapter 13

A Conceptual Framework for the Inclusion of Recreational Therapy within South African Healthcare Paradigms

Terry Jeremy Ellapen, Mariette Swanepoel, Marco Barnard and Yvonne Paul

Additional information is available at the end of the chapter

http://dx.doi.org/10.5772/intechopen.91160

Abstract

Final-phase rehabilitation in South Africa is synonymous with the professions of Physiotherapy and Biokinetics; no consideration is given to the contribution of the profession of Recreational Therapy, which successfully contributes to other international healthcare paradigms. The primary aim was to determine whether collaborative relationships exist between South African recreational therapists and physiotherapists or biokineticists. A secondary aim was to review the potential inclusion of the profession of Recreational Therapy within the existing South African patient referral system of the multidisciplinary healthcare paradigm. An electronic search of the Google Scholar and Sabinet databases identified no records regarding interprofessional collaborative relationships between Recreational Therapy, Physiotherapy and Biokinetics. The authors therefore used two indirect records that prescribe interprofessional collaboration among South African healthcare practitioners during final-phase exercise rehabilitation. The quality of these individual records was appraised using the modified Downs and Black Scale in order to reduce bias. While there is a paucity of literature identifying the absence of interprofessional collaborative relationships between Recreational Therapy, Biokinetics, and Physiotherapy, the Health Professions Council of South Africa (HPCSA) guide nevertheless allows for dynamic overlap among final-phase exercise therapists, thereby providing an opportunity for the inclusion of Recreational Therapy within the existing dynamic, multidisciplinary, South African healthcare paradigm. The inclusion of the profession of Recreational Therapy, as part of a collaborative team effort, can be helpful in order to address the multifaceted challenges experienced by many South African patients.

Keywords: biokinetics, interprofessional collaboration, physiotherapy, recreational therapy

IntechOpen

© 2020 The Author(s). Licensee IntechOpen. This chapter is distributed under the terms of the Creative Commons Attribution License (http://creativecommons.org/licenses/by/3.0), which permits unrestricted use, distribution, and reproduction in any medium, provided the original work is properly cited. (cc) BY

1. Introduction

While final-phase exercise rehabilitation in South Africa is synonymous with the professions of Physiotherapy and Biokinetics [1], Recreational Therapy is another South African therapeutic profession which offers a noteworthy contribution to final-phase rehabilitation [2]. Clinical exercise rehabilitation regimes commonly adopted by Physiotherapy and Biokinetics are monotonous, resulting in poor patient rehabilitation compliance [3]. Strydom et al. [3] reported that many patients prefer fun and exciting games and playful physical activities to tedious clinically prescribed rehabilitation programmes. The inclusion of structured, fun, games and physical activities ameliorates rehabilitation compliance, thereby leading to greater rehabilitative success [3]. Playful physical activity, games, and exercises all help to develop patients' physical, cognitive, and motor skills, having a further beneficial effect on their psychosocial development [4]. Mlenzana and Frantz [5] contend that South Africa requires a multidisciplinary healthcare rehabilitation team in order to address the health and physical needs of patients who require both clinical, and non-clinical, rehabilitation.

The dynamic interaction of the profession of Recreational Therapy within the existing South African healthcare paradigm has been marginalised [6, 7]. Recreational Therapy has not been included in the South African Healthcare paradigm, and this has a detrimental effect on cross-referrals for recreational therapy [6]. Furthermore, Recreational Therapy is not acknowledged by the South African national legislative health bodies; being neither acknowledged by the Allied Health Professions Council of South Africa (AHPCSA) nor by the Health Professions Council of South Africa (HPCSA) [2]. Internationally however, the profession of Recreational Therapy has been officially recognised as a significant independent profession, contributing to the well-being of patients through their successfully rehabilitation [8]. The North Carolina Recreational Therapy Association reported that Recreational Therapy ameliorates both patients' physical conditioning (improving motor skills, joint range of motion, muscle strength, gait, and lowering blood pressure) and psychosocial development (improving mental awareness, and anxiety management skills, reducing social anxiety, depression and social isolation) [9].

In South Africa, the cross referral of patients is initiated with a visit to a general medical practitioner, who refers a patient to medical specialists or physiotherapists [6]. If surgery is warranted, the patient may undergo in-patient post-surgery physiotherapy, followed by out-patient physiotherapy, being referred to a biokineticist for final-phase functional rehabilitation [6]. The in-patient and out-patient physiotherapy is considered to form part of the acute and sub-acute (intermediate) phases of rehabilitation respectively [10].

Human health and well-being are influenced by numerous factors and the management thereof should therefore be multidisciplinary in nature [11]. Cooperative interaction within a *multidisciplinary healthcare rehabilitation team* (MDHRT) has been identified as the most effective strategy for the provision of superior healthcare [11, 12]. This ideal can only be achieved if the protagonists of the MDHRT recognise and respect each other's scope of profession (SoP), which, in turn, is reliant on their familiarity with each other's SoP [13, 14]. Pecukonis [15] and Wynn [16] underlined the need for improved multidisciplinary collaboration when they reported that the era of professional healthcare centrism and/or individualism, which restricted interprofessional healthcare partnership and effective healthcare, has passed. This is similarly emphasised by Mlenzana and Frantz [5] who contend that the need for a multidisciplinary South African healthcare exercise rehabilitation team to provide optimal patient healthcare is eminent.

The initial aim of this chapter is to determine whether a collaborative relationship among Recreational Therapy, Physiotherapy, and Biokinetics exists. A further aim was to identify the opportunities under which Recreational Therapy can make the most meaningful contribution to the South African rehabilitation healthcare paradigm.

2. Methodology

The methodology complied with the PRIMSA practises for drafting review articles, following its guidelines [17].

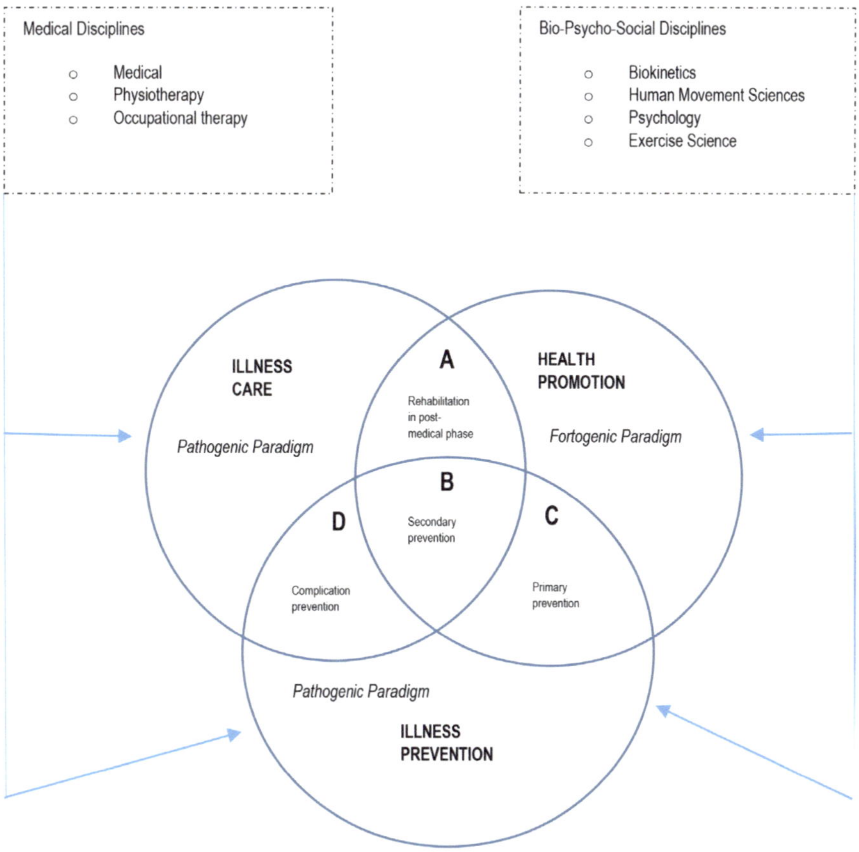

Figure 1. Articulation of the health dimensions in the health paradigms [3].

2.1 Literature surveillance

A literature exploration of professional, peer-reviewed, statutory records and grey literature was conducted using the Sabinet and Google Scholar search engines (**Figure 1**). Key search terms were: "physiotherapy," "biokinetics," "recreational therapy," and "interprofessional collaboration."

2.2 Admissibility criteria

The participants were records concerning interprofessional collaborations between the professions of Physiotherapy, Biokinetics, and Recreational Therapy. Themes of interest that emerged were proposals for interprofessional collaborations between recreational therapists and biokineticists, post final-phase physiotherapy, and the dynamics of interprofessional collaboration between recreational therapists and biokineticists within the South African rehabilitation health paradigm. The exclusion criteria employed were: collaborative relationships between biokineticists, physiotherapists, occupational therapists, physical educators, psychologists, and dieticians. Furthermore, non-English records were excluded. The screening eligibility of records was performed in the following steps: (i) title screen, (ii) abstract screen, (iii) exclusion of duplicate records, (iv) the application of the aforementioned exclusion criteria, and (v) full text screen.

3. Results

The Google Scholar and Sabinet search engines identified no records pertaining to collaborative relationships between recreational therapists, physiotherapists, and biokineticists. The literature surveillance was not limited to a specific time frame. The paucity of published research on this subject is indicative of the need for qualitative research to be undertaken in order to encourage and support interprofessional collaboration between physiotherapists, biokineticists, and recreational therapists. The researchers engaged with two indirectly related records in order to assist with the overarching discussion of the potential inclusion of Recreational Therapy within the South African final-phase rehabilitation healthcare paradigm post physiotherapy (**Table 1**). The quality of each record was appraised using the modified Downs and Black Appraisal Scale that examines both randomised controlled trials and non-randomised records [18]. The revised checklist comprised 13 questions. Each question was scored as either

Authors	Findings
Strydom et al. [3]	Provides insight into the articulation of the dimensions of health care and wellbeing that facilitate the expertise of Human Movement Science practitioners (biokineticists and recreational therapists) within the South African context.
Hall [6]	Outlines the holistic interaction of South African healthcare practitioners within a number of health dimensions and paradigms.

Table 1. Records adopted into this commentary (n = 2).

Authors	Reporting prowess (n = 5)	External validity (n = 3)	Internal validity (n = 4)	Power (n = 1)	Total (n = 13)	Grading % = x/13 × 100
Strydom et al. [3]	4	0	1	0	5	38.46
Hall [6]	4	0	0	0	4	30.76

Table 2. Appraisal of records using the modified Downs and Black appraisal scale.

1 (yes) or 0 (no). The questions selected were 1, 2, 3, 6, 10, 11, 12, 13, 14, 18, 20, 23 and 27. The assessment reviewed the evidence reporting expertise (n = 5 questions), the internal validity (n = 4 questions), the external validity (n = 3 questions) as well as the power of significance (n = 1). Thereafter the summation of the scores was expressed as a percentage, reflective of the overall quality of the paper. These percentages were categorised into weak (<50%), fair (50–69%), good (70–79%) and very good (>80%) as per the grading system proposed by Downs and Black [18] (**Table 2**). The average percentage of all the records was 34.61%.

4. Discussion

The discussion relates to the review of the SoP of Physiotherapy, Biokinetics, and Recreational Therapy, which is followed by a description of the healthcare dimensions and paradigms. The article concludes with a discussion concerning the dynamic interaction of the aforementioned healthcare professions within the South African healthcare paradigms, specifically reviewing the inclusion of Recreational Therapy in the final-phase exercise therapy.

4.1 Scope of profession of physiotherapy

The profession of Physiotherapy was established in 1924 and is a longstanding provider of rehabilitation in South Africa [19, 20]. The SoP of Physiotherapy includes the treatment of diverse pathologies that include orthopaedic, neurological, respiratory and thoracic, cardiovascular, obstetric, paediatric, and geriatric, as well as providing treatment in terms of sports medicine, intensive care, and general rehabilitation [1]. Physiotherapy's SoP does not include recreational therapy.

4.2 Scope of profession of biokinetics

The profession of Biokinetics was officially gazetted in South African Healthcare legislature in 1983 [3, 21]. Biokinetic rehabilitation improves an individual's wellbeing and quality of life through personalised evaluation and therapeutic exercise prescription within the context of chronic clinical pathologies (the illness care and illness prevention health dimensions within the pathogenic paradigm) and performance advancement, which may include apparently healthy patients who aim to enhance or preserve their health by participating in habitual exercise, but who do not have any risk of pathology (the fortogenic paradigm) [21, 22]. Biokineticists manage children, pubescent, adolescent, adult and elderly patients during final-phase rehabilitation [1, 3].

4.3 Scope of profession of therapeutic recreation

Despite the lack of official recognition, professional bodies such as the *South African National Recreation Council* (SANRC), *Recreation South Africa* and the *Leisure and Recreation Association of South Africa* (LARASA) [2] promulgate the practise of Therapeutic Recreational. *Recreation South Africa* was the initial professional body founded in 1994, whose primary objective was to perpetuate recreation and leisure fieldwork training. Subsequently, in 1998, the SANRC, whose fundamental purpose was campaigning for national recreational and leisure activity service delivery, was established [2]. Almost a decade later, in 2010, LARASA was established in order to promote Recreation as an independently recognised profession. The Leisure and Recreation Association of South Africa (LARASA) crusades against a physically inactive lifestyle by campaigning for leisure time physical activity [2]. Recreational Therapy makes use of both clinical and non-clinical components in order to facilitate the successful rehabilitation of patients (The Hull House) [8]. Recreational therapy involves a systematic process that prescribes recreation and other activity-based treatments to meet the therapeutic needs of patients with illnesses and/or disabilities, thereby facilitating their physical and psychological recovery and well-being [23]. The aim of Recreational Therapy is to improve or preserve the patient's physical, social, cognitive, emotional, and spiritual functioning so as to enhance the patient's quality of life [23]. Recreational Therapy includes therapeutic recreational activities such as arts and crafts, dance, drama, music, animal therapy, games, sports, and community outings [23]. Recreational therapists also treat the mental and emotional co-maladies of non-communicable diseases and musculoskeletal injuries by reducing depression, anxiety, and stress, while simultaneously increasing patient confidence [23].

4.3.1 Summary of the scope of profession of the aforementioned professions

Recreational therapists form part of the bio-psycho-social discipline and are amalgamated with dieticians, psychologists, and biokineticists [6] (**Figure 1**). Bio-psycho-social practitioners function within both the pathogenic and fortogenic health care paradigms [6]. Physiotherapists and occupational therapists function within the domain of the pathogenic healthcare paradigm and are considered to be primary healthcare practitioners (medical discipline) [10]. Maharaj [10] further reported that Physiotherapy is synonymous with acute and sub-acute treatment, whereas biokineticists are synonymous with final-phase or post medical rehabilitation. Recreational Therapy provides both physical and psychological rehabilitation through recreational activities and social engagement [8]. While psychological rehabilitation does not fall within the SoP of Physiotherapy and Biokinetics, it is a fundamental aspect that is needs to be addressed in order to ensure the successful re-integration of patients into work and society [1].

5. Healthcare dimensions and paradigms

Before studying the healthcare paradigms, it is crucial to appreciate the three healthcare dimensions, namely:

i. Illness care, which occurs when pathology is apparent. The principal objective is to prescribe medical treatment to remedy the pathology [3],

ii. Illness prevention, which is apparent when the patient is pathology-free but is at an inherent increased risk of a given pathology, significantly increasing the chances that he/she may develop the pathology later on in life [3]

iii. The health promotion dimension is where the patient is pathology free and/or not inherently predisposed to risks for prospective illness, but is insistent on proactively participating in physical activity (exercise and games) in order to maintain a healthy lifestyle, thus preventing or even avoiding the acquisition of chronic illness and/or inherent risk factors that may compromise their health and wellbeing [3, 24].

The aforesaid healthcare dimensions function within the two healthcare paradigms, namely the pathogenic and fortogenic paradigms. The pathogenic paradigm is comprised of the illness care and illness prevention health care dimensions, thus requiring the clinical intervention of medical disciplines (medical doctors and nurses, paediatricians, physiotherapists, and occupational therapists) [6]. In the fortogenic paradigm, the patient has neither an existing pathology nor an intrinsic susceptibility to disease, injury and/or disability, but would like to be physically active in an attempt to prevent disease, injury, or disability [3]. It is essential to consider that the health dimensions are dynamic; an overlap in healthcare dimensions and paradigms can exist thereby necessitating the clinical expertise of different healthcare practitioners. The healthcare professional should be mindful of this fact and demonstrate professional integrity, which will on occasion lead to collaborative endeavours among practitioners who, in so doing, form a MDHRT. The fundamental objective is the delivery of the best healthcare possible: conflicts arising out of the adjudication of the jurisdiction of the SoP of a given discipline are counterproductive [25, 26].

5.1 The overlay of clinical expertise in the various health care dimensions

i. The overlay between the two paradigms occurs in late stage rehabilitation in Area A (*final-phase rehabilitation or post medical phase*) (**Figure 1**). An excellent example can be given in an athlete experiencing glenohumeral (shoulder) pain and who initially presents themself to a medical doctor who will ascertain the musculoskeletal and/or ligamentous pathology and prescribe initial treatment such as PRICE (protection, rest, ice and elevation) and medication [27]. The patient is thereafter referred to a physiotherapist who performs early stage treatment entailing reduction in inflammation, and establishes normal pain-free movement. The patient would thereafter be referred to a biokineticist who would symmetrically strengthen the scapulothoracic and rotator cuff muscles, ameliorate proprioception and enhance scapulohumeral rhythm and functional movements in multidirectional planes. The glenohumeral rotator cuff muscles should be symmetrically strengthened because they orchestrate glenohumeral movement in all planes. The principal goal of the biokinetic rehabilitation is to foster normal scapulohumeral rhythm and multi-planar glenohumeral arthrokinematics under dynamic stress during vigorous physical activity [25, 27]. Biokinetic rehabilitation becomes challenging at this stage if the patient has meagre motor skills, kinanesthesia, co-ordination and proprioception. Another fundamental concern is patients' need to remain enthusiastic regarding the clinical rehabilitation in order to maintain patient compliance. Due to this fact, the biokineticist should refer such patients to a recreational therapist, who will endeavour to augment the patient's motor skills, kinanaesthesia, and proprioception as well as their body co-ordination through the prescription of individual fun functional physical activities, exercises and/or playful games. Once the patient has improved their motor skills, kinanaesthesia, proprioception and co-ordination, the patient can be referred back to the biokineticist to complete their return to sport evaluation. The biokineticist should also refer patients who are not enthusiastically engaged in sport or in a regular physical activity (exercise) to a recreational therapist so as to encourage a continuing engagement with recreational physical activity. This will encourage these patients to be physically active, abating their sedentary lifestyle. The recreational therapist can help the patient identify their recreational physical activity interests (painting, dancing, gardening, fishing, and trail walks) and subsequently encourage these activities as part of the patient's habitual lifestyle. A generally sedentary lifestyle and obesity are among two of the greatest problems that affect the health of South African children and adolescents and one of aims of the South African National Healthcare Strategy is to encourage a physical active lifestyle especially among children and adolescents. Cross-referral among South African healthcare practitioners can help achieve this goal.

ii. Area B is considered to be the *secondary prevention* of a pre-existing injury and/or pathology and the onset of co-maladies (**Figure 1**) [3]. In this scenario the patient has experienced a pathology, has undergone medical treatment and thereafter embarks on physical rehabilitation in order to prevent a reoccurrence of the pathology, the progressive deterioration of the pathology, or to prevent the development of comorbidities, while concurrently ameliorating their health status [3]. Adopting the earlier example of an athlete suffering from shoulder pain; the patient has successfully completed his/her acute and sub-acute phase physiotherapy and final-phase biokinetic rehabilitation, but would like to continue with symmetrical strengthening of the musculature of the sternoclavicular, acromioclavicular, scapulohumeral joints, seeking to improve kinaesthesia and proprioception and thereby collectively protecting the shoulder joint from a prospective relapse [27]. To this end Strydom et al. [3] reported that many patients enjoy playing structured games that have specific therapeutic benefits instead of complying with clinical final-phase exercise rehabilitation. The prescription of structured therapeutic games is known as *therapeutic recreation*, and would necessitate the referral of the patient to a recreational therapist [3]. Strydom et al. [3] recommend the prescription of fun, enjoyable games which increase patient's rehabilitation adherence, thereby increasing the success of the rehabilitative programme. Understanding the post injury stage of healing, motor and psycho-social development is imperative for the delivery of successful secondary prevention rehabilitation services to patients [27]. Therefore, the cross-referral to recreational therapists is of vital importance to this rehabilitation process. Plys [28] reported that individuals residing in assisted living communities engage in recreational activities, which enhances their quality of life. Many individuals residing in assisting living communities have suffered limb loss (paraplegics), psychological challenges and/or elderly individuals who need assistance. Supervised recreational therapy will greatly enhance their physical conditioning and thereby ameliorate their quality of life.

iii. In the second health dimension (illness prevention) the patient has no pathology but is at risk of developing non-communicable diseases due to an unhealthy lifestyle, or the patient would like to be physically active to improve their quality of life [3]. The illness prevention dimension is an extension of the illness care dimension found within the pathogenic paradigm. Patients in the illness prevention healthcare dimension require the expertise of both the medical and bio-psycho-social disciplines [3, 6]. The overlap between the illness care and illness prevention lies in Area D, which is regarded as *complication prevention* (**Figure 1**). The example of an insulin-dependent diabetic, who is overweight and adheres to medication and therapeutic exercises so as to negate auxiliary metabolic deterioration, is instructive [29]. Management of this condition requires the combined expertise of the medical discipline (paediatrician, nurse, endocrinologist and occupational therapist) and the bio-psych-social discipline (recreational therapist, dietician and psychologist) [6, 24]. The combination of the long-term duration of the *complication prevention* rehabilitation and the age of patients must be seen as factors that require the expertise of both a recreational therapist and a biokineticist [3]. The recreational therapist ensures the prescription of fun, enjoyable recreational physical activity, while concurrently maintaining a clinical therapeutic agenda [3]. This enjoyment of evidence based, age appropriate physical activity will aid in the success of the rehabilitation services subsequently provided by the recreational therapist, advancing the overall goal of habitual adherence to physical activity [24]. Patients needing clinical rehabilitation may initially be referred to a biokineticist, thereafter the biokineticist should refer them to a recreational therapist thereby helping the patient habitually continue with fun, enjoyable recreational physical activity. Patients may at times be uncooperative, and unwilling to participate in clinical rehabilitation contrary to their needs. The introduction of fun, enjoyable recreational activity may be useful in persuading uncooperative patients to engage in physical activity.

iv. In the fortogenic paradigm the person is healthy (pathology free) and is not at any intrinsic risk of injury and/or illness but enjoys being physically active [3]. These patients often consult biokineticists in order to prescribe exercise programmes, physical activity games and functional drills with the goal of enhancing their physical status and the intention of improving their health and quality of life. Practitioners should consider the age and zeal of the patient; these needs should be harnessed so as to propagate a habitual physically active lifestyle, forming positive habits that reinforce regular exercise and physical activity outside a clinical or competitive sport arena. Referral to a recreational therapist could be an outstanding choice, allowing the prescription of age appropriate therapeutic exercise and games delivered in such a way that it would make regular physical activity enjoyable, fun and habitual.

It is important to note that the stratification of final-phase exercise rehabilitation into the expertise of Biokinetics and Recreational Therapy will enhance patient experience and thereby increase physical activity well into late adulthood.

6. Conclusion

Optimal final-phase exercise rehabilitation warrants the mutual collaborative efforts of physiotherapists, occupational therapists, biokineticists, and recreational therapists, in working together towards the goal of holistic rehabilitation; cross-referrals among these exercise therapy professions is thus a necessary condition for success. This commentary touches on certain pertinent aspects of collaborative final-phase exercise rehabilitation among recreational therapists and biokineticists but is simultaneously aware that much more illustrative research and disciplinary encouragement is needed for successful cross-referrals to become a reality.

Author details

Terry Jeremy Ellapen[1*], Mariette Swanepoel[1], Marco Barnard[2] and Yvonne Paul[3]

*Address all correspondence to: tellapen1@yahoo.com

1 Department of Sport Rehabilitation and Dental Therapy, Tshwane University of Technology, Tshwane, South Africa

2 Independent Scientist

3 Physical Activity Sport and Recreation (Research Focus: PhASRec), North-West University, Potchefstroom, South Africa

References

[1] Health Professions Council of South Africa (HPCSA). No 1746 (Act 56 of 1974). Available from: http://www.hpcsa.ac.za [Retrieved: 24, 2019]

[2] Young MEM. Therapeutic recreation as a developing profession in South Africa. World Leisure Journal. 2015;**57**(1):34-45

[3] Strydom GL, Wilders CJ, Moss SJ, Bruwer E. A conceptual framework of biokinetic procedures and referral system: An integrated protocol for the various health paradigms. African Journal for Physical, Health Education, Recreation and Dance. 2009;**15**(4): 641-649

[4] Graham N, Nye C, Mandy A, Clarke C, Morris-Roberts C. The meaning of play for children and young people with physical disabilities: A systematic thematic synthesis. Child: Care, Health and Development. 2017;**44**:175-182

[5] Mlenzana N, Frantz J. Rehabilitation model to promote interprofessional practice at primary health care level in Western Cape of South Africa. African Journal for Physical Activity and Health Sciences. 2017;**1.2**(Supplementary):247-254

[6] Hall J. Scope of Professions of Physiotherapy, Podiatry and Biokinetics: Overlap identification. Physiotherapy, Podiatry and Biokinetics News. Tshwane: Health Professions Council of South Africa; 2013. p. 8

[7] Janse Van Rensburg AM. A study to identify the physiotherapy referral practices of South African practitioners in Bloemfontein for musculoskeletal patients [Published thesis]. Bloemfontein: University of Free State; 2017

[8] Robertson T, Long T. Foundations of Therapeutic Recreation. Champaign, IL: Human Kinetics; 2008. pp. 80-85

[9] NARIC (National Rehabilitation Information Center). New Resources and Hidden Gems from the NARIC Collection. 2019. Available from: https://naricspotlight.wordpress.com/2014/05/06/what-are-the-benefits-of-recreational-therapy/ [Retrieved: 23 July 2019]

[10] Maharaj S. Comments on the Overlap of Scope of Practice with Physiotherapy. Johannesburg: South African Society of Physiotherapy; 2011

[11] Macdonald MB, Bally JM, Ferguson LM, Murray BL, Fowler-Kerry SE, Anonson JMS. Knowledge of the professional role of others: A key inter-professional competency. Nurse Education in Practice. 2010;**10**:238-242

[12] Miller KL, Kontos PC. The intraprofessional and interprofessional relations of neuro-rehabilitation nurses: A negotiated order perspective. Journal of Advanced Nursing. 2013;**69**(8):1797-1807. DOI: 10.1111/jan.12041. Epub: 16 November 2012. PubMed PMID: 23157380

[13] Curran VR, Sharpe D, Forristall J, Flynn K. Attitudes of health sciences students towards inter-professional teamwork and education. Learning in Health and Social Care. 2008; **7**(3):146-156

[14] Momsen A, Rasmussen JO, Nielsen CU, Iversen MD, Lund H. Multi-disciplinary team care in rehabilitation: An overview of reviews. Journal of Rehabilitation Medicine. 2012;**44**:901-912

[15] Pecukonis E. Reducing barriers to interprofessional training: Promoting interprofessional culture competence. Journal of Interprofessional Care. 2008;**22**(4):417-428

[16] Wynn GH. Complementary and alternative medicine approaches in the treatment of PTSD. Current Psychiatry Reports. 2015;**17**(8):600. DOI: 10.1007/s11920-015-0600-2. Review. PubMed PMID: 26073362

[17] Shamseer L, Moher D, Clarke M, Ghersi D, Liberatti A, Petticrew M, et al. Preferred reporting items for systematic review and meta-analysis protocols (PRISMA-P): Elaboration and explanation. British Medical Journal. 2015;**349**:7647-7647

[18] Downs SH, Black N. The feasibility of creating a checklist for the assessment of the methodological quality both of randomized and non-randomized studies of health care interventions. Journal of Epidemiology and Community Health. 1998;**52**:377-384

[19] Bakewell S. Medical gymnastics and the Cyrian collection. Medical History. 1997;**41**: 487-495

[20] Ellapen TJ, Abrahams S, Desai FA, Mortimer J, Pillay K, Rugbeer N, et al. A profile of biokinetic services provided by the University of Kwa-Zulu Natal, 2005-2009. African Journal for Physical Health Education Recreation and Dance. 2010;**16**(4):560-569

[21] Ellapen TJ, Swanepoel M. The evolution of the profession of biokinetics. South African Journal for Research in Sport Physical Education Recreation. 2017;**39**(1):41-49

[22] Biokinetics Association of South Africa (BASA). Guidelines for Biokineticists. 2017. Available from: http://www.biokinetics.org.za [Retrieved: 24, 2019]

[23] National Council for Therapeutic Recreation Certification (NCTRC). Paths to Certification. 2018. Available from: https://nctrc.org/new-applicants/paths-to-certification/ [Retrieved: 24 July 2019]

[24] Ehrman JK, Gordon PM, Visich PS, Keteyian SJ. Clinical Exercise Physiology. 3rd ed. Champaign, IL: Human Kinetics; 2013

[25] Ellapen TJ, Swanepoel M, Hammill HV, Paul Y, Strydom GL. What Is the profession of biokinetics? In: Sport and Exercise Science. InfoTech; 2018

[26] Ellapen TJ, Paul Y, Swanepoel M, Strydom GL. Current controversy: Transgression of biokineticists onto the scope of practice of physiotherapy. African Journal for Physical Activity and Health Sciences. 2018;**24**(3):316-331

[27] Prentice WE. Rehabilitation Techniques for Sports Medicine and Athletic Training. 4th ed. New York: McGraw-Hill; 2004

[28] Plys E. Recreational activity in assisted living communities: A critical review and theoretical model. Gerontologist. 2019;**59**(3):e207-e222

[29] Durstine JL, Moore GE, Painter PL, Roberts SO. ACSM's Exercise Management for Persons with Chronic Diseases and Disabilities. 3rd ed. Champaign, IL: Human Kinetics; 2009

Chapter 14

Manual Therapy: Art or Science?

Paolo Bizzarri and Andrea Foglia

Additional information is available at the end of the chapter

http://dx.doi.org/10.5772/intechopen.90730

Abstract

Manual Therapy is one of the most widely used therapeutic solutions in the treatment of pain and musculoskeletal disorders. Its evolution began several centuries ago and culminated in the modern reference methods in the field of physiotherapy, osteopathy, and chiropractic, which mainly address the treatment of joint and myofascial tissues. The advent of evidence-based medicine and the ever-growing literature available in the field of Manual Therapy has led this therapeutic approach to be heavily criticized on the basis of studies that have shown its limitations with regard to manual and palpatory assessment techniques, the poor biomechanical validity of therapeutic methods, and the poor long-term results in the treatment of patients with musculoskeletal pain. A better understanding of the mechanisms underlying the effectiveness of Manual Therapy, as well as of the mediators of the medium- and long-term effectiveness of musculoskeletal rehabilitation processes, has made it possible to reconsider the role of Manual Therapy and the healthcare professionals specializing in manipulative therapy within the framework of the biopsychosocial model, which focuses on the patient and their functionality.

Keywords: Manual Therapy, manipulations, myofascial, biopsychosocial model, clinical reasoning, effectiveness, evidence

1. Introduction

Manual Therapy is currently one of the main therapeutic options in the field of rehabilitation and more specifically in the treatment of musculoskeletal disorders. In recent years, the advent of evidence-based medicine has led to the publication of several studies on Manual Therapy, thereby enabling a better understanding of the mechanisms underlying its effectiveness in clinical settings. However, this method originated in ancient times. Indeed, testimonies show that it was applied in very distant times and places and in very different forms, contexts, and

IntechOpen

© 2020 The Author(s). Licensee IntechOpen. This chapter is distributed under the terms of the Creative Commons Attribution License (http://creativecommons.org/licenses/by/3.0), which permits unrestricted use, distribution, and reproduction in any medium, provided the original work is properly cited.

cultures, such as by shamans in Central Asia and bone setters in Mexico, Nepal, Russia, and Norway [1]. We have direct evidence by Hippocrates (ca. 400 BC) who described the use of manipulative and physical therapy for the treatment of scoliosis and vertebral dysfunctions. Similar techniques were described by Galen, a roman surgeon (ca. 150 CE), and illustrated in his treatises [2].

In the Western world, modern Manual Therapy dates back to the seventeenth century and has undergone a progressive evolution that has led to current manual practices in physiotherapy, osteopathy, and chiropractic [1].

Most of the current clinical practice and manual techniques used by the majority of practitioners defined as "experts in manipulative treatments," are based on biomechanical assumptions at the root of the patient's symptoms, with palpatorily identifiable dysfunctions, that can be treated by means of specific techniques aimed at joint tissue [3–5], myofascial tissue [6–8], or nervous tissue [9].

All these concepts, based on anatomical theoretical models of musculoskeletal and health disorders, were born and developed as a result of the often brilliant intuitions of different authors, but they must be interpreted within the context in which they were born, the knowledge, the cultural contexts, and the technological and instrumental options available at the time [2].

Each author has, in some way, enabled the development of our approach to the patient and their management: witness symptom modification (Mulligan Concept) [4], the role of self-treatment (McKenzie Method) [3], and the need to focus clinical practice on the patient's daily demands and difficulties (Maitland Approach) [10].

However, the biomechanical effects and elements at the basis of the effectiveness of these approaches have been increasingly challenged by the advent of an evidence-based medicine culture [11]. Although expert opinion is part of the evidence pyramid that should guide clinical practice, it is only the lowest level of evidence [12].

Studies published in the last 30 years have seriously challenged both the "tissue-related" and "biomechanical" bases of these manual approaches and the validity and reliability of the techniques involving palpatory assessment as well as manual and manipulative treatment [13–15].

As healthcare professionals, we have a duty to ask ourselves questions: "Are we really able to accurately palpate a specific target tissue from an assessment point of view? [16] Are we able to identify a specific tissue as responsible for the patient's symptoms? Are we able to differentiate it from the surrounding tissues and identify any dysfunctions? [14, 17]".

From a therapeutic point of view, are we able to make structural changes to peripheral tissues, whether they consist in joint repositioning or orientation of collagen fibers in the myofascial tissue?

Above all, is the modification of peripheral tissues related, and therefore necessary, to the achievement of clinical improvements in patients experiencing musculoskeletal pain?

How important are these factors in changing the prognosis of musculoskeletal patients? How much must a manual technique and a healthcare professional be "biomechanically specialized" to achieve a positive outcome in the patient? Highlighting these elements is extremely important, as they are still the basis of the clinical practice, care, and treatment of millions of patients worldwide and thus have a major clinical impact [18]. What technique or approach can improve the symptoms of patients with musculoskeletal pain, and why?

Today, there is a wealth of literature supporting the effectiveness of Manual Therapy in improving pain and mobility in patients with musculoskeletal disorders [19–21]. However, these improvements are mainly short-term and have a reduced efficacy, particularly in subjects with chronic symptoms [21].

The limited efficacy in patients with chronic pain and the overlapping course of clinical symptoms in the long term irrespective of manual treatments [22, 23] cast doubt on the clinical assumptions that still often guide manual and manipulative clinical practice.

The lack of a shared model supported by evidence and the limited diagnostic, therapeutic, and prognostic role of approaches linked to exclusively manual and biomechanical interventions has led to the development and implementation of what has been defined as the biopsychosocial model, also in the field of rehabilitation [24].

The biopsychosocial model is currently the reference model when it comes to taking care of and managing patients with musculoskeletal disorders. It focuses on the patient as a person, particularly with regard to disability and quality of life in relation to their disorder, considering the impact that internal and external factors, including non-biomechanical ones, can have on their status and prognosis [20, 25].

Enter psychosocial factors. Elements such as fear of movement, anxiety, depression, and self-efficacy have been shown to play a central role in mediating and modulating the symptoms and prognosis of these patients [25], particularly in the transition from the acute to the chronic phase of the disorder and the resulting disability [26, 27], far more than exclusively biomechanical impairments such as range of movement (ROM) or muscle strength [28].

While a manual clinical practice based on musculoskeletal impairments and aimed at improving the patient's signs and symptoms may be useful and reasonable in the clinical management of the patient [19], it is important to consider that any therapeutic intervention is directed towards a person, with both explicit and implicit consequences on the individual's beliefs, convictions, and cognitive processes [29].

Indeed, while a manual technique can be effective in the short term, the narrative that guides it, which the practitioner presents when framing the patient and taking care of them, can have very significant consequences on the meaning that the patient gives and will give to their own disorder [30].

To date, several authors have linked pain to the body's perception of a threat/danger [31]. A manipulative technique that is effective in reducing a patient's lumbar pain may have significant long-term consequences if associated with concepts related to a "repositioning" of the intervertebral disc with respect to the nerve roots. The patient will indeed be able to convince themselves that they have a fragile back, with structures that could face possible neurological damage, thereby promoting hypervigilance, anxiety, and fear of movement [32].

In addition to short-term beneficial effects, it is therefore important to consider possible "nocebo" effects of Manual Therapy in the long term when not properly presented to the patient [32]. It is no coincidence that manual techniques have shown insignificant results in the long run, even when compared with nontreatment. However, if we want to change the patient's prognosis, we need to act on the most significant prognostic factors, which have been shown to be psychosocial [33].

All of this has an impact not only on the individual but also on the community. This is particularly the case at a time when the availability of economic resources for supporting healthcare and personal health services is constantly subject to spending review. As a matter of fact, we know that most of the resources are allocated to the treatment of chronic disorders.

The effectiveness and efficiency of health decision-making processes and the appropriateness of the therapies proposed and supported are and will increasingly be central to social choices [34]. However, these same considerations apply to every single practitioner, even in the private sector. From an ethical standpoint, what are the best therapies that can be offered to patients with musculoskeletal disorders? Which patients need complex therapies, and when can unimodal therapies achieve satisfactory clinical results? Is there an evidence-based approach to Manual Therapy that can allow for its full integration within a biopsychosocial model focused on the improvement of the patient's disability not only in the short term but also in the medium and long term? Can the patient be involved in these issues, even if mainly passive techniques are used? At the end of the day, what is Manual Therapy? What does it do, and why can it be so decisive in some cases for both the patient and the practitioner? We will try to answer all these questions in this chapter.

2. Manual Therapy: from theoretical speculations to research

Even today, most Manual Therapy approaches are based on the evaluation of biomechanical factors that may be the cause or consequence of symptoms reported by the patient, with a feeling of pain and reduction in function, either directly at the local and segmental level or indirectly in neighboring regions [35].

The basic assumption entails the possibility, on the part of the healthcare worker, to be able to identify the said dysfunctions, correlate them to the clinical picture of the patient, and correct them by the use of palpatory analyses and therapeutic techniques that can be refined over years of practice, thereby making the rehabilitation process increasingly efficient and effective. In general terms, these elements are transversally present in almost all of the most commonly suggested and used Manual Therapy methods, especially in the direct approaches to the assessment and treatment of myofascial and articular tissues [8, 36].

Being able to fully understand and judge the scientific nature and validity of the proposed notions can be complex, especially at the beginning of one's personal and professional training, especially when presented by charismatic teachers with years of experience. Moreover, at first, the disciple can often find it difficult to manually perceive the biomechanical impairments the teacher refers to.

One may intuitively think that, as with any learning process, palpation skills can be developed and learned through training, repetition, and clinical practice, as it has been observed in the improvement in in the two-point discrimination threshold [36]. But is this really the case from a clinical point of view? How much can daily clinical practice improve one's palpatory ability, with consequent clinical repercussions in the treatment of patients with musculoskeletal pain? And how much of this progressive understanding of and expertise in patient management depends on effective manual specialization?

The above example may be familiar to many of those who are reading this chapter. However, many of the theoretical assumptions upon which these models are based were wrong. Indeed, the manual assessment methods adopted in most manipulative approaches have not shown adequate levels of validity and reliability for application in the management of patients with musculoskeletal pain.

For instance, techniques for the assessment of the physiological intervertebral motion of individual vertebral levels have not shown a correlation with the actual mobility assessed by means of radiological tests [37]. As a matter of fact, vertebral levels deemed hypomobile upon manual assessment have not shown a reduction in mobility when investigated through dynamic MRI [38].

Moreover, the same possibility of investigating the passive physiological and accessory mobility of a single vertebral level by means of manual assessments has been heavily criticized. Indeed, the proposed techniques have been shown to produce movements on multiple vertebral levels [17, 39]. The same assessments, even when made by experienced clinicians, have not shown a correlation with the patient's symptoms. Indeed, the assessors were not able to tell subjects with pain from an asymptomatic control group [40].

The same palpatory identification of the target structures proved to be poorly reproducible, with little agreement also as to the identification and pinpointing of anatomically evident elements such as the posterior superior and anterior superior iliac spines [30]. It is therefore not surprising that the assessment of any hypomobility or hypermobility of the selected segments shows low agreement values among different assessors [41, 42] and that different therapists choose treat different joints [43].

This seems to be related to the technique used and the actual total mobility of the considered joints [44]. As a matter of fact, it appears to be good in the assessment of the osteokinematic mobility of large joints [45], but it is almost useless or comparable to random chance in the assessment of joints with particularly limited mobility, such as sacroiliac joints [46]. Therefore, the more emphasized the role of specialized manual skills in identifying possible dysfunctions, the more statistically insignificant the results of these tests, even when conducted by experienced clinicians [47].

Similar analyses have been performed as to the palpatory assessment of extra-articular soft tissues, thereby showing that even very experienced assessors are hardly able to identify the anatomical location of the target tissues [48], grade the muscle stiffness [49], pinpoint any tissue dysfunction, or tell a subject with pain from a healthy one. In some cases, even the creators of some of the methods proved inadequate [50].

Therefore, while different training proposals involving Manual Therapy may initially seem logical, intuitive, and fascinating, their biomechanical and tissue-related bases have often proven to be incorrect, for instance, by failing to consider the very high prevalence of bone asymmetries in 85% of the general population [51, 52].

The phenomenon defined as "pareidolia" seems to play a significant role when it comes to the lack of accuracy of these theoretical models, which were conceived in, and are therefore inevitably related to, historical periods in which the available technologies did not allow for a thorough understanding of the body and its biomechanical properties. Pareidolia [53] is the tendency to detect patterns and information known to the observer on the basis of random, vague, and undefined inputs, hence the tendency to pinpoint an alteration or a dysfunction exclusively on the basis of one's own personal experience, be it training-related or not.

However, several cognitive biases can affect the reasoning and clinical practice of a healthcare professional, particularly in Manual Therapy [54–56]: witness anchoring, confirmation, group biases, or the illusion of frequency. A group bias is the tendency to overestimate and deem more competent those who belong to one's group, such as a teacher or a colleague who uses our same assessment and treatment method, compared to other professionals. A similar mechanism is found in frequency bias, based on which we tend to detect factors and elements more easily once we have spent time studying them in depth: witness the possibility of finding an increased prevalence of positional or tissue alterations in our patients following a course focused on these aspects, regardless of their clinical significance. Anchoring bias highlights the tendency to focus on relatively unimportant aspects, thereby attaching central significance to them in the overall picture. In clinical practice, witness the tendency to focus on the restoration of ideal soft tissue consistency, thereby either underestimating or not considering the lack of improvement in the pain perceived by the patient during the rehabilitation process. On the other hand, confirmation bias refers to the tendency to irrationally focus on the first clinical hypothesis that one may have developed with regard to a specific patient and clinically research elements that confirm the said hypothesis, thereby discarding any significant aspects that would invalidate it [54–56]. All of these elements can be related to heuristics [55], that is, mental shortcuts that enable you to obtain quick answers even without considering all the factors involved. While such aspects allow for faster and more efficient reasoning, in clinical practice they can also lead to errors in the decision-making process and to a nonoptimal management of the patient and thus to an incorrect reading of clinical phenomena [57]. Such observations are obviously not only part of Manual Therapy but also of rehabilitation approaches based on therapeutic exercise [58], which, when proposed in an orthodox manner, can lead to a "guru-based" clinical practice in which the core of the rehabilitation process is no longer the patient, but the method or mental scheme of the practitioner themselves.

Therefore, an ethical model of patient treatment and care cannot be separated from a thorough understanding of the scientific literature, in which many of the aspects described above have been studied and deepened, thereby giving answers to many of the questions that may arise during daily clinical practice [34]. Only in this way is it possible to have a clinical practice that can improve the medium- and long-term prognosis of patients with musculoskeletal disorders, thereby reducing the negative influence of cognitive bias and theoretical models.

Building upon the said assumptions, it is indeed possible to strongly support the effectiveness of Manual Therapy in the improvement of various impairments that characterize the clinical pictures of patients with musculoskeletal disorders, especially with respect to pain and range of movement and with particular reference to the short and medium term, with a high level of satisfaction on the part of the patients who receive it [19, 20].

However, the mechanisms underlying its effectiveness seem different from those considered up to now. As a matter of fact, the clinical improvement observed as a result of manual techniques does not appear to be related to a realignment of the articular heads [59], a displacement of the disc tissue [60], or a structural modification of the soft tissues [61], which to date have never been demonstrated, despite years of scientific research [60]. Fortunately, these changes do not appear to be necessary in order to achieve a significant therapeutic effect, nor do they appear to be related to the clinical picture of patients with musculoskeletal pain [62].

Indeed, models based on biomedical and biomechanical assumptions have been shown to play a clinical role mostly in strictly pathoanatomical pictures and in relation to particularly significant structural alterations such as the presence of severe osteoarthritis, which are related to significant alterations in the articular surfaces where the pathognomonic data shows a marked reduction in joint ROM [63].

Nevertheless, these elements have been shown to have limited clinical or scientific value in the management of most musculoskeletal disorders. As a matter of fact, verifiable modifications observed in radiological investigations were present in a large part of the general population, without showing, in the great majority of cases, a significant correlation with the clinical picture reported by the patient [64]. This has been observed in clinical pictures related to the axial skeleton but also to the limbs: witness patellofemoral pain syndrome [65] or shoulder pain [66]. Indeed, most patients with musculoskeletal pain have multifactorial disorders. The attempt to translate the determinism typical of the biomedical model and orthopedic medicine into musculoskeletal rehabilitation is probably at the root of the limitations of many Manual Therapy methods, which show resistance to change in the face of the latest scientific findings in the field of Manual Therapy and musculoskeletal pain.

Uncertainty management in medicine is one of the most debated issues in healthcare-related clinical reasoning and can be disorienting and complex to integrate into one's vision and clinical practice [67]. However, once accepted, it enables one to confidently respond to various criticalities that may arise on a daily basis: witness patients who do not adequately respond to therapies despite the correct manipulation of specific target segments or still show symptoms despite a palpatory analysis that is normalized with respect to the initially identified dysfunctions.

The very multifactorial nature of these disorders requires multifactorial treatments also involving peripheral tissues, for example, manual techniques, which can allow for significant improvements with respect to symptoms and thus in the quality of life of the patient, regardless of the search for actual anatomical changes. Fortunately, these changes, as mentioned, do not seem to be necessary [60]. Manual Therapy can be extremely effective in reducing pain and improving ROM in these patients. Its effects seem to be mainly mediated by neurophysiological mechanisms [68].

Several studies have described the mechanical stimulus applied through Manual Therapy techniques as able to activate a cascade of peripheral, spinal, and supraspinal neurophysiological effects related to pain modulation and ROM improvement [68]. For example, as a result of joint tissue techniques, a reduction in the concentration of inflammation mediators was observed [68]. The role of spinal mechanisms was suggested by the change in temporal summation and muscle tone [69]. Finally, studies conducted using functional magnetic resonance imaging have shown the activation of areas related to mechanisms leading to a downward modulation of pain, such as the periaqueductal gray [69]. These scientifically proven observations thus seem to establish a very significant correlation between the clinical efficacy of Manual Therapy and the possibility of activating neurophysiological mechanisms linked to the modulation of pain perception. This seems to be confirmed by studies that have shown an inability to produce therapeutic effects in subjects with alterations of the said mechanisms, that is, in the presence of augmented temporal summation, which is indicative of increased dorsal horn excitability, or of a clinical state of widespread pain with a generalized reduced pressure pain threshold, which is indicative of the presence of central sensitization with regard to pain [69].

However, there are other aspects of Manual Therapy that are not closely linked to the mechanical stimulation of the technique used and can mediate its therapeutic effect. The said aspects are an integral part of the biopsychosocial model. As a matter fact, there is an affective and cognitive dimension that involves the patient in the therapeutic act linked to the therapeutic "touch" [70]. In accordance with the gate theory, in addition to a reduction of pain perception due to tactile stimulation, touch applied in an "empathic" way has proven capable of reducing pain perception in itself and acting on the concentration of biomarkers related to stress, negative emotions, and mechanisms related to the perception of threats. Furthermore, several contextual and verbal communication and relationship aspects have been shown to play a role in making a manual technique effective with regard to pain reduction. An open, positive, and empathetic style of communication adopted by a healthcare professional capable of listening to the patient and convincingly answering their questions has indeed been associated with greater short-term pain reduction and higher patient satisfaction [71]. The same can be said for the patient's possible preferences, which may be related to previous experiences or personal beliefs. All these effects are attributable to what has been defined as "placebo mechanisms," not intended as a psychological response to inert therapies, but as generalized and non-specific "psychologically and physiologically active process associated with a robust hypoalgesic response" [72, 73]. Finally, psychosocial factors such as anxiety and fear of movement or motion (kinesiophobia) and self-efficacy seem to play a very important role when it comes to the effectiveness of a given technique or approach [74].

All these observations show that, irrespective of the criticism levelled at the most commonly proposed clinical models, a scientific approach focused on the patient, based on Manual Therapy and founded on the biopsychosocial model, is possible without the need to resort to imaginative holistic or pseudoscientific theories.

The second part of this chapter will show when and how it is possible to adopt the said approach in the most common clinical pictures that can be dealt with in clinical practice.

3. Manual Therapy: from research to clinical practice

3.1. Joint manual therapy

As described, Manual Therapy techniques targeting joint or extra-articular soft tissue can be very effective in relieving pain and improving ROM in individuals with musculoskeletal disorders, both in the spine and in the limbs [21].

Joint techniques can be divided into mobilization and manipulation techniques [75]. Joint mobilization has been defined as "a Manual Therapy technique comprising a continuum of skilled passive movements involving the joint complex that are applied at varying speeds and amplitudes, which may include a small-amplitude/high velocity therapeutic movement [manipulation] with the intent to restore optimal motion and function and/or reduce pain." Joint manipulations have been defined as "passive, high velocity, low amplitude thrusts applied to a joint complex within its anatomical limit with the intent to restore optimal motion and function and/or reduce pain" [75].

In studies conducted on standardized populations of subjects with musculoskeletal pain, no manual technique could be shown to be more effective than the other. Research has shown an overlap in the therapeutic effectiveness of different techniques, be it among different types of joint mobilization techniques [76, 77] and different kinds of vertebral manipulation techniques [78] or mobilization and manipulation techniques [79]. These results have been mainly observed in non-specific spinal pain but also when comparing different techniques targeted towards peripheral joints, that is, in subjects with knee osteoarthritis [80]. Similarly, research comparing joint techniques with soft tissue techniques has shown similar clinical results [81, 82].

3.2. Myofascial Manual Therapy

Several manual techniques have been proposed for the treatment of soft tissues, from more intense manual approaches following methods that seek the elicitation of significant pain in the patient during their application [8] to painless techniques seeking the elimination of symptoms by using positionings and maneuvers primarily aimed at shortening the tissues [83].

Again, manual techniques have been shown to alleviate pain and improve ROM [84]. Likewise, no one technique can be said to be superior to another, either among different Manual Therapy techniques or between manual techniques and the use of instruments such as dry needling or instrument-assisted soft tissue manipulation (IASTM) [84, 85].

3.3. Which technique to choose? successful predictors in joint Manual Therapy

According to most Manual Therapy methods, the likelihood of therapeutic success in patients with spinal pain strictly depends on the identification of the dysfunctional vertebral level; the appropriate "corrective" technique, which is to be targeted towards the intended segment using the correct parameters of direction, is thus to be applied with the correct direction, intensity, and duration parameters with respect to the stimulus [10].

However, the need for specific therapeutic techniques is not supported by the literature. As already seen in this chapter, manual and palpatory assessment methods have been found to be ineffective and unreliable. Experienced assessors taking part in a blind study showed agreement levels equal, if not inferior, to random chance in the identification of the tissues to be treated [43]. These same models did not prove valid even with regard to the proposed therapeutic techniques. Indeed, sacroiliac [15], lumbar [15, 86], thoracic [86], and cervical [87] manipulation techniques have been shown to produce clinical and biomechanical effects on different vertebral levels, which are therefore not specific to the target segment and lead the practitioner to produce unpredictable vertebral movements [88]. This data is confirmed by clinical studies that have shown an overlap between the therapeutic effect of manipulations theoretically directed at a single vertebral level and "global" manipulation techniques involving the lumbar spine of subjects with low back pain [89].

Nevertheless, in clinical practice, very different clinical responses are commonly observed in different patients as a result of the application of the same technique. In the last 20 years, several studies have tried to identify the clinical elements present at the baseline that could indicate the best therapeutic solution for each specific patient [90]. In particular, the so-called clinical prediction rules (CPRs) [91] have been studied and developed for the issues referred to in this chapter, also with reference to manipulative treatment in patients with lumbar [92], cervical [93], and shoulder pain [94], among others. Despite promising initial studies, these rules have not proven to be good enough for application in clinical practice. In particular, evidence has shown that, upon modification of the statistical value considered as the indicator of "therapeutic success" [whether it be pain reduction or improvement of the disability, either in proportional or absolute terms], these rules also change in a very significant way [95]. In addition, subjects positively responding to CPRs with respect to lumbar manipulative treatment were found to be equally responsive to joint mobilization techniques [96] and McKenzie exercises [97]. In essence, a positive response to these rules proved able to generally predict a positive prognosis following a rehabilitation program, regardless of the proposed therapy [98].

3.4. Pain mechanisms

The presence of similar therapeutic effectiveness following treatment approaches that are sometimes in direct opposition to each other [8, 83] both in their theoretical bases and in their clinical application is a further element supporting the poor biomechanical validity of these techniques and the predominant role of neurophysiological factors in their effectiveness. Neurophysiological elements have proven to be fundamental in determining the clinical picture of the patient and mediating the effectiveness of techniques targeting peripheral tissues [68].

As a matter of fact, Manual Therapy has been shown to be more effective in the presence of mechanical pain, which is by definition elicited during the execution of specific movements and refers to clinical pictures of peripheral nociceptive pain [69]. Clinically speaking, this kind of pain is a typical feature of patients experiencing sudden problems, such as subjects with acute lumbar block following a poorly controlled movement. On the contrary, patients with constant, general pain present even at rest, which is indicative of central sensitization, have shown little response to manual treatments [69]. This aspect seems to play an important role with regard to the low effectiveness of manual techniques in subjects with chronic pain, such as patients diagnosed with fibromyalgia syndrome.

3.5. Manual techniques as modulator of peripheral afferences

When it comes to the treatment of musculoskeletal pain, Manual Therapy thus seems to be able to significantly modulate the nociceptive afferences of peripheral tissues, regardless of their structural specificity. Based on this, the literature seems to support a patient-centered clinical practice focused on the mechanisms of pain and musculoskeletal impairment that characterize it based on the reactivity of the clinical picture.

3.6. Pain as a cause of limited ROM and mobility

While no manual approach is superior to the others, the literature itself supports the use of techniques tailored to each individual patient, modulating the force applied during the technique (from low to high), the duration (from short to long), and the prepositioning of the tissues (from relaxed to pretensioned) and acting either within or away from the resistance [75].

In patients (defined by Maitland as "pain dominant") with a clinical picture characterized by severe, often nocturnal pain significantly limiting ROM, applying intense techniques will be difficult and unreasonable. It may therefore be very useful to use painless techniques, far from the tissue barrier and symptom elicitation, which have been shown to alleviate pain, but not to improve the patient's ROM [99]. Witness patients suffering from phase II frozen shoulder or symptomatic disc herniation [100, 101]. On the contrary, or progressively upon decrease in pain, patients with joint limitations and mild/moderate pain elicitable at the end of the joint range (whom Maitland defines as "stiffness dominant") will benefit from more intense, longer-lasting techniques carried out at the end of the joint range, possibly with the reproduction of a symptomatology during application, which have proven capable of improving both pain and ROM in these patients [102, 103]: phase III frozen shoulder or osteoarthritis clinical pictures can be considered as emblematic examples [100, 104].

3.7. Pain as a strength limiter

While biomechanical elements such as an increased mechanical extensibility of the joint capsule cannot be completely ruled out, improvements in functional impairments such as ROM would seem to be linked to the ability of manual techniques to modulate peripheral nociceptive afferences, thereby acting on all related clinical phenomena [105].

This would seem to be confirmed by the possibility of obtaining a short-term improvement in muscle strength following techniques specifically targeted towards soft tissues in patients with musculoskeletal pain [106, 107]. These observations have led several authors to support the usefulness of manual techniques also in the field of well-being and physical training, with the aim of achieving greater physical functionality. However, studies carried out on healthy subjects or in the absence of peripheral impairments have contradicted this hypothesis by not showing the same benefits in mobility, strength, and functionality found in patients suffering from musculoskeletal disorders [108, 109]. The link between pain and muscle strength, and the possibility that these may be modulated by manual techniques, can nonetheless be of particular clinical interest. Indeed, studies included in the literature have shown the possibility of identifying soft tissue impairments, even within non-specific frameworks, through active and resistance tests, especially when the said active and resistance tests are painful and recreate the symptoms typical of the patient [110]. For example, a dry needling treatment targeted towards multifidus muscle has been observed to be more effective if the patients reported pain while recruiting that muscle [110].

3.8. Patient-centered and impairment-based Manual Therapy

These observations hint at the clinical value of a Manual Therapy clinical practice that is evidence-based as well as focused on the patient and the impairment that can characterize both them and their daily life.

Joint and soft tissue techniques can therefore focus on and be guided by:

- Pain
  - High reactivity/low reactivity
- ROM limitation
  - Osteokinematics
- Soft tissue dysfunctions
  - Active/resistance tests

3.9. Treatment of function

The aspects described so far mainly refer to techniques directed at the anatomical regions responsible for the clinical picture of the patient. However, in accordance with a Manual Therapy model based on the improvement of the patient's function, Manual Therapy techniques can be useful in improving all the musculoskeletal impairments that can biomechanically and neurophysiologically contribute to the patient's symptoms and daily limitations [35]. For instance, sedentary patients with lower back pain may benefit from the treatment of any limitations present at hip level, which due to phenomena related to referred pain and afferent convergence may support pain perception [111–113].

These aspects can play an even more significant role in subjects with high functional requirements such as professional athletes, where the correct functionality of all the structures participating in a specific movement will be clinically central in enabling their being able to perform at high levels. A typical example is the clinical relevance of a limitation in ankle dorsiflexion in a volleyball player with patellofemoral pain syndrome [114].

3.10. Short-term benefits

The advantages and limitations of Manual Therapy should be known in order to apply it in the best possible way. We know that the clinical effects that can be obtained in the treatment of musculoskeletal disorders tend to diminish over time after the end of the treatment, thereby often overlapping with the natural history of the disorder in the long term. This aspect is often highlighted by the opponents of manual techniques, who attribute many of the benefits observed in clinical practice to the benign and self-limiting nature of musculoskeletal disorders [115].

While these observations can be statistically accurate, it is important not to underestimate the role that an immediate modification of the symptom can play in the patient's need for help [116]. Going back to professional athletes and their need for help, a rapid decrease in symptoms can enable one to resume sports activities just in time to take part in a cup final. The ability to use manual techniques in order to obtain benefits in the short term compared to mere therapeutic exercise will thus have a major impact on their daily activities and quality of life [117]. Similarly, we know that clinical pictures of symptomatic disc hernias have in most cases a positive prognosis within 3–6 months [118]. However, this data does not take into account the impact that a disorder of this type can have in the daily life of the patient in that period of time and the potential benefits of therapeutic techniques that have been shown to be able to significantly modify pain symptoms already in the first month [101]. Finally, symptom modification can play a very important educational role by enabling patients to realize that they are not the bearers of an incurable and unchangeable disorder, thereby acting on psychosocial factors that play an important prognostic role in the chronicity of the symptom [116].

3.11. Psychosocial clinical factors in Manual Therapy

As written above, the presence of biomechanical and functional impairment can be very important in guiding the choice of the therapeutic technique to be used. However, non-biomechanical elements such as psychosocial factors can also mediate the clinical results that can be obtained through Manual Therapy techniques.

In a standardized population of subjects with chronic neck pain, mobilization and joint manipulation techniques have shown to alleviate pain and improve ROM without statistically significant differences among the proposed techniques [76]. However, some elements present at the baseline, such as anxiety levels, were found to be associated with a different response to each technique [74]. As a matter of fact, patients with low anxiety levels showed more significant improvements following vertebral manipulation techniques, while more anxious subjects reported a greater reduction in pain when subjected to joint mobilization techniques. The psychosocial sphere can thus also be very important in the choice of the therapeutic method capable of producing the best clinical results, even in the short term.

3.12. The three EBP pillars

It is important to remember that evidence-based practice is based on three pillars: the preferences, needs and expectations of the patient, the expertise of the practitioner, and the available authoritative literature [11]. All these elements must be taken into account in the decision-making process. Their role is particularly significant in making clinical decisions with a risk of serious adverse events, such as choosing whether or not to perform risky heart surgery. However, they are also relevant in musculoskeletal rehabilitation and Manual Therapy.

Patient preferences have been shown to modulate the response to a specific treatment. For example, in the aforementioned study, the clinical response that could be obtained following vertebral manipulation techniques was also mediated by the opinion that the patients had of the proposed techniques [74]. Placebo mechanisms involving a descending inhibition of pain linked to expectation also seem to play a role in modulating the effectiveness of the techniques used based on the patient's preferences [119]. Useful information can thus be obtained from the patient's medical history. People who report having had negative results following soft tissue therapies and having responded very positively to manipulative techniques are likely to respond better to the latter. Clearly, the possible failure of a given therapeutic approach can be linked to purely clinical aspects, such as an incorrect classification of the patient. Subjects with pelvic pain may not respond to lumbar treatment techniques if the practitioner does not identify possible hip arthrosis as the real cause of the problem [113]. However, the information provided by the patient will play an important role by leading the practitioner to consider different evaluation and treatment hypotheses.

A second pillar of evidence-based practice involves the practitioner's expertise and clinical competence. Also in this case, the possibility of modulating clinical effectiveness may be due to exclusively clinical or non-biomechanical aspects. The literature has shown that, in applying the same technique, the physiotherapist's beliefs about the effectiveness of that specific technique were able to lead to different clinical responses in the patient [120]. This may be due once again to the expectations that, either explicitly or implicitly, the practitioner can give the patient when proposing and applying the said technique. In addition, the very mastery and confidence shown in the execution and application of the technique can convey the feeling of being in "good hands," reduce the sense of threat, and activate central pain-inhibiting mechanisms [70].

Finally, even though the overlap in the clinical effectiveness of different Manual Therapy techniques has been pointed out several times, this entails basic competence in the application of these techniques. When the practitioner is not trained to perform a given technique, or does not have adequate clinical experience, they may have trouble in identifying the correct landmarks, in particular on small joints, or determining the adequate posology, thereby producing either no results at all or even harmful consequences.

3.13. Adverse events

As a matter of fact, clinical practice in Manual Therapy is to be based on advanced knowledge enabling, first and foremost, the identification of patients who do not fall within the scope of rehabilitation and are to be referred to a physician or who may present contraindications to manual practice [121].

There is a wide debate in the literature on the dangers of manual techniques, particularly with regard to possible vascular or nerve damage as a result of cervical manipulation. These events seem to be mainly related to inadequate background checks as to the patient's medical history and ultimately to the failure to spot red flag factors [122]. In particular, ongoing cervical vascular disorders may initially arise only with symptoms related to the cervical level, thereby mimicking the presence of musculoskeletal disorders. An early identification of these clinical pictures can enable the practitioner to immediately refer the patient to a more suitable clinical management, avoiding the use of treatment techniques whose role will then have to be investigated in the medical–legal field [123]. However, it is worth remembering that there is no completely safe medical and rehabilitation procedure. Indeed, studies have described adverse events even following therapeutic massage sessions [124].

The ability to recognize the appropriateness of any technique with regard to the individual patient will lead to the choice of the most appropriate type of intervention and its modulation, particularly in populations of patients with a higher risk of adverse events, such as pediatric or geriatric patients [125], without having to apply the dictates supported by a specific Manual Therapy training method.

4. Conclusion

Manual Therapy is an extremely effective therapeutic method in the management of patients with pain and musculoskeletal disorders. Like any other therapeutic method, it has its pros but also its cons and drawbacks. Its effectiveness, as described above, is based on the ability to modify the functionality, albeit not the anatomy, of the patient's tissues by means of mainly neurophysiological mechanisms [69].

Therefore, an appropriate and effective clinical practice can only be based on the correct classification of the patient, identifying first of all those clinical pictures, including musculoskeletal ones, which, according to the scientific literature, are not suitable for Manual Therapy, thereby orienting the patient towards a medical, pharmacological [126], or surgical approach [127], or a conservative program based on therapeutic exercise [128], or simply a "wait and see" strategy. Indeed, only by acknowledging the limits of Manual Therapy is it possible to strongly affirm its great merits and potential for alleviating the patient's pain and improving their functionality in the short, medium, and long term [19, 20]. This will involve the great majority of patients with musculoskeletal pain, whose clinical picture is characterized by functional impairment, in particular reduction of ROM and peripheral hyperalgesia, with particular regard to soft tissues. In this respect, Manual Therapy is able to have a very positive effect, leading to rapid and significant improvements when properly applied in accordance with the specific clinical picture and the individual patient.

While there is no such thing as a superior Manual Therapy method, being free from the dogmas of a specific therapeutic approach allows for a truly patient-oriented clinical practice focused on the patient and their needs, choosing the most appropriate technique and modulating it from time to time on the basis of the clinical picture of that individual patient. This ability to provide a clinical framework and subsequently manage the manual approach proposed to the patient is what defines the role and real competence of healthcare professionals specializing in manual and manipulative therapy, with an approach strongly based on the biopsychosocial model.

While the current main limitation of Manual Therapy is the production of predominantly short-term responses, these observations are primarily based on studies that have investigated the effectiveness of individual techniques. However, we know that the therapeutic relationship in clinical practice is also made up of other things, such as the therapeutic alliance between practitioner and patient, understood as a person [70].

For this reason, a healthcare professional trained in Manual Therapy according to an evidence-based approach can produce results even in the long term by exploiting the immediate reduction of the symptom and the rapid improvement of the functionality as a bridge to reduce the fear of movement and the related anxiety in the patient and stimulate an active coping towards their disorder [116], thereby making them gain confidence in their ability to perform "thoughtless, fearless movement" [129] through an especially active rehabilitation process.

Only in this way can the professional improve their practice for the good of the patient, acting according to science and conscience and reaffirming the central role of their professional figure in the management of musculoskeletal disorders.

Author details

Paolo Bizzarri[1,2]* and Andrea Foglia[1,3]

*Address all correspondence to: bizzarri.paolo@gmail.com

1 Physiotherapist, Private Practitioner, Civitanova Marche (MC), Italy

2 Vrije Universiteit, Brussel, Belgium

3 University of Ferrara, Italy

References

[1] Pettman E. A history of manipulative therapy. The Journal of Manual & Manipulative Therapy. 2007;**15**(3):165-174

[2] Smith AR. Manual therapy: The historical, current, and future role in the treatment of pain. Scientific World Journal. 2007;**7**:109-120

[3] McKenzie RA, May S. The Lumbar Spine: Mechanical Diagnosis & Therapy. 2nd ed. Vol. 2. Orthopedic Physical Therapy Products: Waikanae; 2003. 700 p

[4] Mulligan BR. Manual Therapy: Nags, Snags, MWMs, etc. 6th ed. Orthopedic Physical Therapy Products: Wellington, NZ; 2010

[5] Ernst E. Chiropractic: A critical evaluation. Journal of Pain and Symptom Management. 2008;**35**(5):544-562

[6] Travell JG, Simons DG. Travell and Simon's Myofascial Pain and Dysfunction: v. 1 & v. 2: Two Volume Set: Second Edition/Volume 1 and First Edition/Volume 2: Trigger Point Manual. 2 Rev ed. Lippincott Williams and Wilkins; 1998. 1664 p

[7] Jones TA. Rolfing. Physical Medicine and Rehabilitation Clinics of North America. 2004;**15**(4):799-809 vi

[8] Stecco C, Day JA. The fascial manipulation technique and its biomechanical model: A guide to the human fascial system. International Journal of Therapeutic Massage & Bodywork. 2010;**3**(1):38-40

[9] Upledger JE. Craniosacral therapy. Physical Therapy. 1995;**75**(4):328-330

[10] Maitland GD. Manipulation—Mobilisation. Physiotherapy. 1966;**52**(11):382-385

[11] Sackett DL, Rosenberg WM, Gray JA, Haynes RB, Richardson WS. Evidence based medicine: What it is and what it isn't. BMJ. 1996;**312**(7023):71-72

[12] Murad MH, Asi N, Alsawas M, Alahdab F. New evidence pyramid. Evidence-Based Medicine. 2016;**21**(4):125-127

[13] Lucas N, Macaskill P, Irwig L, Moran R, Bogduk N. Reliability of physical examination for diagnosis of myofascial trigger points: A systematic review of the literature. The Clinical Journal of Pain. 2009;**25**(1):80-89

[14] Schomacher J, Learman K. Symptom localization tests in the cervical spine: A descriptive study using imaging verification. The Journal of Manual & Manipulative Therapy. 2010;**18**(2):97-101

[15] Beffa R, Mathews R. Does the adjustment cavitate the targeted joint? An investigation into the location of cavitation sounds. Journal of Manipulative and Physiological Therapeutics. 2004;**27**(2):e2

[16] Mieritz RM, Kawchuk GN. The accuracy of locating lumbar vertebrae when using palpation versus ultrasonography. Journal of Manipulative and Physiological Therapeutics. 2016;**39**(6):387-392

[17] Lee RYW, McGregor AH, Bull AMJ, Wragg P. Dynamic response of the cervical spine to posteroanterior mobilisation. Clinical Biomechanics (Bristol, Avon). 2005;**20**(2):228-231

[18] Beliveau PJH, Wong JJ, Sutton DA, Simon NB, Bussières AE, Mior SA, et al. The chiropractic profession: A scoping review of utilization rates, reasons for seeking care, patient profiles, and care provided. Chiropractic & Manual Therapies. 2017;**25**:35

[19] Blanpied PR, Gross AR, Elliott JM, Devaney LL, Clewley D, Walton DM, et al. Neck pain: Revision 2017. The Journal of Orthopaedic and Sports Physical Therapy. 2017;**47**(7): A1-A83

[20] Delitto A, George SZ, Van Dillen LR, Whitman JM, Sowa G, Shekelle P, et al. Low back pain. The Journal of Orthopaedic and Sports Physical Therapy. 2012;**42**(4):A1-A57

[21] Pieters L, Lewis J, Kuppens K, Jochems J, Bruijstens T, Joossens L, et al. An update of systematic reviews examining the effectiveness of conservative physiotherapy interventions for subacromial shoulder pain. The Journal of Orthopaedic and Sports Physical Therapy. 2019;**15**:1-33

[22] Rubinstein SM, Terwee CB, Assendelft WJJ, de Boer MR, van Tulder MW. Spinal manipulative therapy for acute low-back pain. Cochrane Database of Systematic Reviews. 2012;**9**:CD008880

[23] Rubinstein SM, van Middelkoop M, Assendelft WJ, de Boer MR, van Tulder MW. Spinal manipulative therapy for chronic low-back pain. Cochrane Database of Systematic Reviews. 2011;**2**:CD008112

[24] Borrell-Carrió F, Suchman AL, Epstein RM. The biopsychosocial model 25 years later: Principles, practice, and scientific inquiry. Annals of Family Medicine. 2004;**2**(6):576-582

[25] Wertli MM, Rasmussen-Barr E, Weiser S, Bachmann LM, Brunner F. The role of fear avoidance beliefs as a prognostic factor for outcome in patients with nonspecific low back pain: A systematic review. Spine Journal. 2014;**14**(5):816-836.e4

[26] Vlaeyen JW, Linton SJ. Fear-avoidance and its consequences in chronic musculoskeletal pain: A state of the art. Pain. 2000;**85**(3):317-332

[27] Lee H, Hübscher M, Moseley GL, Kamper SJ, Traeger AC, Mansell G, et al. How does pain lead to disability? A systematic review and meta-analysis of mediation studies in people with back and neck pain. Pain. 2015;**156**(6):988-997

[28] Hamberg-van Reenen HH, Ariëns GAM, Blatter BM, van Mechelen W, Bongers PM. A systematic review of the relation between physical capacity and future low back and neck/shoulder pain. Pain. 2007;**130**(1-2):93-107

[29] Bialosky JE, Bishop MD, Penza CW. Placebo mechanisms of manual therapy: A sheep in Wolf's clothing? The Journal of Orthopaedic and Sports Physical Therapy. 2017;**47**(5):301-304

[30] Palsson TS, Gibson W, Darlow B, Bunzli S, Lehman G, Rabey M, et al. Changing the narrative in diagnosis and management of pain in the sacroiliac joint area. Physical Therapy. 2019;**99**(11):1511-1519

[31] Butler D, Moseley GL. Explain Pain. Australia: NOI Group Publishing; 2003

[32] Setchell J, Costa N, Ferreira M, Makovey J, Nielsen M, Hodges PW. Individuals' explanations for their persistent or recurrent low back pain: A cross-sectional survey. BMC Musculoskeletal Disorders. 2017;**18**(1):466

[33] Burton AK, McClune TD, Clarke RD, Main CJ. Long-term follow-up of patients with low back pain attending for manipulative care: Outcomes and predictors. Manual Therapy. 2004;**9**(1):30-35

[34] Robertson-Preidler J, Biller-Andorno N, Johnson TJ. What is appropriate care? An integrative review of emerging themes in the literature. BMC Health Services Research. 2017;**17**(1):452

[35] Wainner RS, Whitman JM, Cleland JA, Flynn TW. Regional interdependence: A musculoskeletal examination model whose time has come. The Journal of Orthopaedic and Sports Physical Therapy. 2007;**37**(11):658-660

[36] Chandhok PS, Bagust J. Differences between the cutaneous two-point discrimination thresholds of chiropractic students at different stages in a 5-year course. Journal of Manipulative and Physiological Therapeutics. 2002;**25**(8):521-525

[37] Kulig K, Landel R, Powers CM. Assessment of lumbar spine kinematics using dynamic MRI: A proposed mechanism of sagittal plane motion induced by manual posterior-to-anterior mobilization. The Journal of Orthopaedic and Sports Physical Therapy. 2004;**34**(2):57-64

[38] Landel R, Kulig K, Fredericson M, Li B, Powers CM. Intertester reliability and validity of motion assessments during lumbar spine accessory motion testing. Physical Therapy. 2008;**88**(1):43-49

[39] Lee R, Evans J. An in vivo study of the intervertebral movements produced by postero-anterior mobilization, Clinical Biomechanics (Bristol, Avon). 1997;**12**(6):400-408

[40] Leboeuf-Yde C, van Dijk J, Franz C, Hustad SA, Olsen D, Pihl T, et al. Motion palpation findings and self-reported low back pain in a population-based study sample. Journal of Manipulative and Physiological Therapeutics. 2002;**25**(2):80-87

[41] Schneider M, Erhard R, Brach J, Tellin W, Imbarlina F, Delitto A. Spinal palpation for lumbar segmental mobility and pain provocation: An interexaminer reliability study. Journal of Manipulative and Physiological Therapeutics. 2008;**31**(6):465-473

[42] van Trijffel E, Anderegg Q, Bossuyt PMM, Lucas C. Inter-examiner reliability of passive assessment of intervertebral motion in the cervical and lumbar spine: A systematic review. Manual Therapy. 2005;**10**(4):256-269

[43] French SD, Green S, Forbes A. Reliability of chiropractic methods commonly used to detect manipulable lesions in patients with chronic low-back pain. Journal of Manipulative and Physiological Therapeutics. 2000;**23**(4):231-238

[44] Robinson HS, Mengshoel AM. Assessments of lumbar flexion range of motion: Intertester reliability and concurrent validity of 2 commonly used clinical tests. Spine. 2014;**39**(4):E270-E275

[45] Maricar N, Callaghan MJ, Parkes MJ, Felson DT, O'Neill TW. Interobserver and intraobserver reliability of clinical assessments in knee osteoarthritis. The Journal of Rheumatology. 2016;**43**(12):2171-2178

[46] Robinson HS, Brox JI, Robinson R, Bjelland E, Solem S, Telje T. The reliability of selected motion- and pain provocation tests for the sacroiliac joint. Manual Therapy. 2007;**12**(1):72-79

[47] Herzog W, Read LJ, Conway PJ, Shaw LD, McEwen MC. Reliability of motion palpation procedures to detect sacroiliac joint fixations. Journal of Manipulative and Physiological Therapeutics. 1989;**12**(2):86-92

[48] Lew PC, Lewis J, Story I. Inter-therapist reliability in locating latent myofascial trigger points using palpation. Manual Therapy. 1997;**2**(2):87-90

[49] Davidson MJ, Nielsen PMF, Taberner AJ, Kruger JA. Is it time to rethink using digital palpation for assessment of muscle stiffness? Neurourology and Urodynamics. 2019:1-7

[50] Wolfe F, Simons DG, Fricton J, Bennett RM, Goldenberg DL, Gerwin R, et al. The fibromyalgia and myofascial pain syndromes: A preliminary study of tender points and trigger points in persons with fibromyalgia, myofascial pain syndrome and no disease. The Journal of Rheumatology. 1992;**19**(6):944-951

[51] Badii M, Shin S, Torreggiani WC, Jankovic B, Gustafson P, Munk PL, et al. Pelvic bone asymmetry in 323 study participants receiving abdominal CT scans. Spine. 2003;**28**(12):1335-1339

[52] Neumann. Kinesiology of the Musculoskeletal System, Foundations for Rehabilitation. 3rd ed. St. Louis, Missouri: Elsevier; 2016. 784 p

[53] Foye P, Abdelshahed D, Patel S. Musculoskeletal pareidolia in medical education. The Clinical Teacher. 2014;**11**(4):251-253

[54] Saposnik G, Redelmeier D, Ruff CC, Tobler PN. Cognitive biases associated with medical decisions: A systematic review. BMC Medical Informatics and Decision Making. 2016;**16**(1):138

[55] Blumenthal-Barby JS, Krieger H. Cognitive biases and heuristics in medical decision making: A critical review using a systematic search strategy. Medical Decision Making. 2015;**35**(4):539-557

[56] O'Sullivan ED, Schofield SJ. Cognitive bias in clinical medicine. The Journal of the Royal College of Physicians of Edinburgh. 2018;**48**(3):225-232

[57] Rylander M, Guerrasio J. Heuristic errors in clinical reasoning. The Clinical Teacher. 2016;**13**(4):287-290

[58] Caldwell C, Sahrmann S, Van Dillen L. Use of a movement system impairment diagnosis for physical therapy in the management of a patient with shoulder pain. The Journal of Orthopaedic and Sports Physical Therapy. 2007;**37**(9):551-563

[59] Tullberg T, Blomberg S, Branth B, Johnsson R. Manipulation does not alter the position of the sacroiliac joint. A roentgen stereophotogrammetric analysis. Spine. 1998;**23**(10):1124-1128 discussion 1129

[60] Broetz D, Hahn U, Maschke E, Wick W, Kueker W, Weller M. Lumbar disk prolapse: Response to mechanical physiotherapy in the absence of changes in magnetic resonance imaging. Report of 11 cases. NeuroRehabilitation. 2008;**23**(3):289-294

[61] Chaudhry H, Schleip R, Ji Z, Bukiet B, Maney M, Findley T. Three-dimensional mathematical model for deformation of human fasciae in manual therapy. The Journal of the American Osteopathic Association. 2008;**108**(8):379-390

[62] Shilton M, Branney J, de Vries BP, Breen AC. Does cervical lordosis change after spinal manipulation for non-specific neck pain? A prospective cohort study. Chiropractic & Manual Therapies. 2015;**23**:33

[63] Steultjens MPM, Dekker J, van Baar ME, Oostendorp RA, Bijlsma JWJ. Range of joint motion and disability in patients with osteoarthritis of the knee or hip. Rheumatology (Oxford, England). 2000;**39**(9):955-961

[64] Nakashima H, Yukawa Y, Suda K, Yamagata M, Ueta T, Kato F. Abnormal findings on magnetic resonance images of the cervical spines in 1211 asymptomatic subjects. Spine. 2015;**40**(6):392-398

[65] van der Heijden RA, Oei EHG, Bron EE, van Tiel J, van Veldhoven PLJ, Klein S, et al. No difference on quantitative magnetic resonance imaging in patellofemoral cartilage composition between patients with patellofemoral pain and healthy controls. The American Journal of Sports Medicine. 2016;**44**(5):1172-1178

[66] Lewis JS. Subacromial impingement syndrome: A musculoskeletal condition or a clinical illusion? Research Gate. 2011;**16**(5):388-398

[67] Simpkin AL, Schwartzstein RM. Tolerating uncertainty—The next medical revolution? The New England Journal of Medicine. 2016;**375**(18):1713-1715

[68] Bialosky JE, Bishop MD, Price DD, Robinson ME, George SZ. The mechanisms of manual therapy in the treatment of musculoskeletal pain: A comprehensive model. Manual Therapy. 2009;**14**(5):531-538

[69] Bialosky JE, Beneciuk JM, Bishop MD, Coronado RA, Penza CW, Simon CB, et al. Unraveling the mechanisms of manual therapy: Modeling an approach. The Journal of Orthopaedic and Sports Physical Therapy. 2018;**48**(1):8-18

[70] Geri T, Viceconti A, Minacci M, Testa M, Rossettini G. Manual therapy: Exploiting the role of human touch. Musculoskeletal Science & Practice. 2019;**25**

[71] Testa M, Rossettini G. Enhance placebo, avoid nocebo: How contextual factors affect physiotherapy outcomes. Manual Therapy. 2016;**24**:65-74

[72] Carlino E, Benedetti F. Different contexts, different pains, different experiences. Neuroscience. 2016;**338**:19-26

[73] Bizzarri P, Buzzatti L, Cattrysse E, Scafoglieri A. Thoracic manual therapy is not more effective than placebo thoracic manual therapy in patients with shoulder dysfunctions: A systematic review with meta-analysis. Musculoskeletal Science & Practice. 2018;**33**:1-10

[74] Alonso-Perez JL, Lopez-Lopez A, La Touche R, Lerma-Lara S, Suarez E, Rojas J, et al. Hypoalgesic effects of three different manual therapy techniques on cervical spine and psychological interaction: A randomized clinical trial. Journal of Bodywork and Movement Therapies. 2017;**21**(4):798-803

[75] Mintken PE, Derosa C, Little T, Smith B. American Academy of Orthopaedic Manual Physical Therapists. A model for standardizing manipulation terminology in physical therapy practice. The Journal of Manual & Manipulative Therapy. 2008;**16**(1):50-56

[76] Izquierdo Pérez H, Alonso Perez JL, Gil Martinez A, La Touche R, Lerma-Lara S, Commeaux Gonzalez N, et al. Is one better than another?: A randomized clinical trial of manual therapy for patients with chronic neck pain. Manual Therapy. 2014;**19**(3):215-221

[77] Donaldson M, Petersen S, Cook C, Learman K. A prescriptively selected nonthrust manipulation versus a therapist-selected nonthrust manipulation for treatment of individuals with low back pain: A randomized clinical trial. The Journal of Orthopaedic and Sports Physical Therapy. 2016;**46**(4):243-250

[78] Sutlive TG, Mabry LM, Easterling EJ, Durbin JD, Hanson SL, Wainner RS, et al. Comparison of short-term response to two spinal manipulation techniques for patients with low back pain in a military beneficiary population. Military Medicine. 2009;**174**(7):750-756

[79] Cleland JA, Fritz JM, Kulig K, Davenport TE, Eberhart S, Magel J, et al. Comparison of the effectiveness of three manual physical therapy techniques in a subgroup of patients with low back pain who satisfy a clinical prediction rule: A randomized clinical trial. Spine. 2009;**34**(25):2720-2729

[80] Kaya Mutlu E, Ercin E, Razak Ozdıncler A, Ones N. A comparison of two manual physical therapy approaches and electrotherapy modalities for patients with knee osteoarthritis: A randomized three arm clinical trial. Physiotherapy Theory and Practice. 2018;**34**(8):600-612

[81] Campa-Moran I, Rey-Gudin E, Fernández-Carnero J, Paris-Alemany A, Gil-Martinez A, Lerma Lara S, et al. Comparison of dry needling versus orthopedic manual therapy in patients with myofascial chronic neck pain: A single-blind. Randomized Pilot Study. Pain Research and Treatment. 2015;**2015**:327307

[82] Griswold D, Gargano F, Learman KE. A randomized clinical trial comparing non-thrust manipulation with segmental and distal dry needling on pain, disability, and rate of recovery for patients with non-specific low back pain. The Journal of Manual & Manipulative Therapy. 2019;**27**(3):141-151

[83] Wong CK. Strain counterstrain: Current concepts and clinical evidence. Manual Therapy. 2012;**17**(1):2-8

[84] Cagnie B, Castelein B, Pollie F, Steelant L, Verhoeyen H, Cools A. Evidence for the use of ischemic compression and dry needling in the management of trigger points of the upper trapezius in patients with neck pain: A systematic review. American Journal of Physical Medicine & Rehabilitation. 2015;**94**(7):573-583

[85] De Meulemeester KE, Castelein B, Coppieters I, Barbe T, Cools A, Cagnie B. Comparing trigger point dry needling and manual pressure technique for the management of myofascial neck/shoulder pain: A randomized clinical trial. Journal of Manipulative and Physiological Therapeutics. 2017;**40**(1):11-20

[86] Ross JK, Bereznick DE, McGill SM. Determining cavitation location during lumbar and thoracic spinal manipulation: Is spinal manipulation accurate and specific? Spine. 2004;**29**(13):1452-1457

[87] Dunning J, Mourad F, Barbero M, Leoni D, Cescon C, Butts R. Bilateral and multiple cavitation sounds during upper cervical thrust manipulation. BMC Musculoskeletal Disorders. 2013;**14**:24

[88] Buzzatti L, Provyn S, Van Roy P, Cattrysse E. Atlanto-axial facet displacement during rotational high-velocity low-amplitude thrust: An in vitro 3D kinematic analysis. Manual Therapy. 2015;**20**(6):783-789

[89] McCarthy CJ, Potter L, Oldham JA. Comparing targeted thrust manipulation with general thrust manipulation in patients with low back pain. A general approach is as effective as a specific one. A randomised controlled trial. BMJ Open Sport & Exercise Medicine. 2019;**5**(1):e000514

[90] Asquini G, Bianchi AE, Heneghan NR, Rushton AB, Borromeo G, Locatelli M, et al. Predictors of pain reduction following manual therapy in patients with temporomandibular disorders: A protocol for a prospective observational study. BMJ Open. 2019;**9**(11):e032113

[91] Beattie P, Nelson R. Clinical prediction rules: What are they and what do they tell us? The Australian Journal of Physiotherapy. 2006;**52**(3):157-163

[92] Childs JD, Fritz JM, Flynn TW, Irrgang JJ, Johnson KK, Majkowski GR, et al. A clinical prediction rule to identify patients with low back pain most likely to benefit from spinal manipulation: A validation study. Annals of Internal Medicine. 2004;**141**(12):920-928

[93] Puentedura EJ, Cleland JA, Landers MR, Mintken PE, Louw A, Fernández-de-Las-Peñas C. Development of a clinical prediction rule to identify patients with neck pain likely to benefit from thrust joint manipulation to the cervical spine. The Journal of Orthopaedic and Sports Physical Therapy. 2012;**42**(7):577-592

[94] Mintken PE, Cleland JA, Carpenter KJ, Bieniek ML, Keirns M, Whitman JM. Some factors predict successful short-term outcomes in individuals with shoulder pain receiving cervicothoracic manipulation: A single-arm trial. Physical Therapy. 2010;**90**(1):26-42

[95] Schwind J, Learman K, O'Halloran B, Showalter C, Cook C. Different minimally important clinical difference (MCID) scores lead to different clinical prediction rules for the Oswestry disability index for the same sample of patients. The Journal of Manual & Manipulative Therapy. 2013;**21**(2):71-78

[96] Learman K, Showalter C, O'Halloran B, Donaldson M, Cook C. No differences in outcomes in people with low back pain who met the clinical prediction rule for lumbar spine manipulation when a pragmatic non-thrust manipulation was used as the comparator. Physiotherapy Canada. 2014;**66**(4):359-366

[97] Schenk R, Dionne C, Simon C, Johnson R. Effectiveness of mechanical diagnosis and therapy in patients with back pain who meet a clinical prediction rule for spinal manipulation. The Journal of Manual & Manipulative Therapy. 2012;**20**(1):43-49

[98] Cook CE, Learman KE, O'Halloran BJ, Showalter CR, Kabbaz VJ, Goode AP, et al. Which prognostic factors for low back pain are generic predictors of outcome across a range of recovery domains? Physical Therapy. 2013;**93**(1):32-40

[99] Klein R, Bareis A, Schneider A, Linde K. Strain-counterstrain to treat restrictions of the mobility of the cervical spine in patients with neck pain: A sham-controlled randomized trial. Complementary Therapies in Medicine. 2013;**21**(1):1-7

[100] Kelley MJ, Shaffer MA, Kuhn JE, Michener LA, Seitz AL, Uhl TL, et al. Shoulder pain and mobility deficits: Adhesive capsulitis. The Journal of Orthopaedic and Sports Physical Therapy. 2013;**43**(5):A1-A31

[101] Basson A, Olivier B, Ellis R, Coppieters M, Stewart A, Mudzi W. The effectiveness of neural mobilization for neuromusculoskeletal conditions: A systematic review and meta-analysis. The Journal of Orthopaedic and Sports Physical Therapy. 2017;**47**(9):593-615

[102] Cerezo-Téllez E, Torres-Lacomba M, Fuentes-Gallardo I, Perez-Muñoz M, Mayoral-Del-Moral O, Lluch-Girbés E, et al. Effectiveness of dry needling for chronic nonspecific neck pain: A randomized, single-blinded, clinical trial. Pain. 2016;**157**(9):1905-1917

[103] Estébanez-de-Miguel E, Fortún-Agud M, Jimenez-Del-Barrio S, Caudevilla-Polo S, Bueno-Gracia E, Tricás-Moreno JM. Comparison of high, medium and low mobilization forces for increasing range of motion in patients with hip osteoarthritis: A randomized controlled trial. Musculoskeletal Science & Practice. 2018;**36**:81-86

[104] Vermeulen HM, Rozing PM, Obermann WR, le Cessie S, Vliet Vlieland TPM. Comparison of high-grade and low-grade mobilization techniques in the management of adhesive capsulitis of the shoulder: Randomized controlled trial. Physical Therapy. 2006;**86**(3):355-368

[105] Murray GM, Peck CC. Orofacial pain and jaw muscle activity: A new model. Journal of Orofacial Pain. 2007;**21**(4):263-278. discussion 279-288

[106] Arias-Buría JL, Valero-Alcaide R, Cleland JA, Salom-Moreno J, Ortega-Santiago R, Atín-Arratibel MA, et al. Inclusion of trigger point dry needling in a multimodal physical therapy program for postoperative shoulder pain: A randomized clinical trial. Journal of Manipulative and Physiological Therapeutics. 2015;**38**(3):179-187

[107] Hall ML, Mackie AC, Ribeiro DC. Effects of dry needling trigger point therapy in the shoulder region on patients with upper extremity pain and dysfunction: A systematic review with meta-analysis. Physiotherapy. 2018;**104**(2):167-177

[108] Lake AD, Myers H, Aefsky B, Butler R. Immediate and short term effect of dry needling on triceps surae range of motion and functional movement: A randomized trial. International Journal of Sports Physical Therapy. 2018;**13**(2):185-195

[109] Corso M, Mior SA, Batley S, Tuff T, da Silva-Oolup S, Howitt S, et al. The effects of spinal manipulation on performance-related outcomes in healthy asymptomatic adult population: A systematic review of best evidence. Chiropractic & Manual Therapies. 2019;**27**:25

[110] Koppenhaver SL, Walker MJ, Smith RW, Booker JM, Walkup ID, Su J, et al. Baseline examination factors associated with clinical improvement after dry needling in individuals with low back pain. The Journal of Orthopaedic and Sports Physical Therapy. 2015;**45**(8):604-612

[111] Burns SA, Mintken PE, Austin GP, Cleland J. Short-term response of hip mobilizations and exercise in individuals with chronic low back pain: A case series. The Journal of Manual & Manipulative Therapy. 2011;**19**(2):100-107

[112] Bade M, Cobo-Estevez M, Neeley D, Pandya J, Gunderson T, Cook C. Effects of manual therapy and exercise targeting the hips in patients with low-back pain—A randomized controlled trial. Journal of Evaluation in Clinical Practice. 2017;**23**(4):734-740

[113] Poulsen E, Overgaard S, Vestergaard JT, Christensen HW, Hartvigsen J. Pain distribution in primary care patients with hip osteoarthritis. Family Practice. 2016;**33**(6):601-606

[114] Wyndow N, Collins NJ, Vicenzino B, Tucker K, Crossley KM. Foot and ankle characteristics and dynamic knee valgus in individuals with patellofemoral osteoarthritis. Journal of Foot and Ankle Research. 2018;**11**:65

[115] Hartman SE. Why do ineffective treatments seem helpful? A brief review. Chiropractic & Osteopathy. 2009;**17**:10

[116] Lehman GJ. The role and value of symptom-modification approaches in musculoskeletal practice. The Journal of Orthopaedic and Sports Physical Therapy. 2018;**48**(6):430-435

[117] Eckenrode BJ, Kietrys DM, Parrott JS. Effectiveness of manual therapy for pain and self-reported function in individuals with patellofemoral pain: Systematic review and meta-analysis. The Journal of Orthopaedic and Sports Physical Therapy. 2018;**48**(5):358-371

[118] Stochkendahl MJ, Kjaer P, Hartvigsen J, Kongsted A, Aaboe J, Andersen M, et al. National Clinical Guidelines for non-surgical treatment of patients with recent onset low back pain or lumbar radiculopathy. European Spine Journal. 2018;**27**(1):60-75

[119] Reicherts P, Gerdes ABM, Pauli P, Wieser MJ. Psychological placebo and nocebo effects on pain rely on expectation and previous experience. The Journal of Pain. 2016;**17**(2): 203-214

[120] Gracely RH, Dubner R, Deeter WR, Wolskee PJ. Clinicians' expectations influence placebo analgesia. Lancet. 1985;**1**(8419):43

[121] Cook CE, George SZ, Reiman MP. Red flag screening for low back pain: Nothing to see here, move along: A narrative review. British Journal of Sports Medicine. 2018;**52**(8):493-496

[122] Rushton A, Rivett D, Carlesso L, Flynn T, Hing W, Kerry R. International framework for examination of the cervical region for potential of cervical arterial dysfunction prior to orthopaedic manual therapy intervention. Manual Therapy. 2014;**19**(3):222-228

[123] Hutting N, Kerry R, Coppieters MW, Scholten-Peeters GGM. Considerations to improve the safety of cervical spine manual therapy. Musculoskeletal Science & Practice. 2018;**33**:41-45

[124] Yin P, Gao N, Wu J, Litscher G, Xu S. Adverse events of massage therapy in pain-related conditions: A systematic review. Evidence-based Complementary and Alternative Medicine. 2014;**2014**:480956

[125] Homola S. Pediatric chiropractic care: The subluxation question and referral risk. Bioethics. 2016;**30**(2):63-68

[126] van der Heijde D, Ramiro S, Landewé R, Baraliakos X, Van den Bosch F, Sepriano A, et al. 2016 update of the ASAS-EULAR management recommendations for axial spondyloarthritis. Annals of the Rheumatic Diseases. 2017;**76**(6):978-991

[127] Long B, Koyfman A, Gottlieb M. Evaluation and management of cauda equina syndrome in the emergency department. The American Journal of Emergency Medicine. 2019;**20**

[128] Bateman M, Smith BE, Osborne SE, Wilkes SR. Physiotherapy treatment for atraumatic recurrent shoulder instability: Early results of a specific exercise protocol using pathology-specific outcome measures. Shoulder Elbow. 2015;**7**(4):282-288

[129] Gifford LS. 'Gifford's Aches and Pains': Patients, Pain Explanations, Management Foundations and Concepts. Falmouth: CNS Press; 2006